WITHDRAWN
WRIGHT STATE UNIVERSITY LIBRARIES

MODERN MODALITIES FOR THE DIAGNOSIS OF HEMATOLOGIC NEOPLASMS: COLOR ATLAS/TEXT

MODERN MODALITIES FOR THE DIAGNOSIS OF HEMATOLOGIC NEOPLASMS: COLOR ATLAS/TEXT

Chin-Yang Li, M.D.
Professor of Laboratory Medicine and Pathology
Mayo Medical School
and
Consultant, Department of Laboratory Medicine and Pathology
Mayo Clinic
Rochester, Minnesota

Lung T. Yam, M.D.
Professor of Medicine,
University of Louisville School of Medicine
and
Chief, Division of Hematology
Veterans Affairs Medical Center
Louisville, Kentucky

Tsieh Sun, M.D.
Professor of Pathology
University of Colorado
Health Sciences Center
and
Director, Flow Cytometry Resource Center
Pathology and Laboratory Medicine Service
Veterans Affairs Medical Center
Denver, Colorado
Formerly
Professor of Clinical Pathology
Cornell University Medical College
and
Chief, Division of Clinical Pathology
North Shore University Hospital
Manhasset, New York

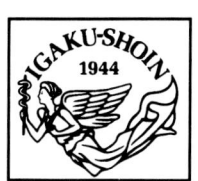

IGAKU-SHOIN   NEW YORK • TOKYO

Published and distributed by

IGAKU-SHOIN Medical Publishers, Inc.
One Madison Avenue, New York, New York 10010

IGAKU-SHOIN Ltd.,
5-24-3 Hongo, Bunkyo-ku, Tokyo 113-91.

Copyright © 1996 by IGAKU-SHOIN Medical Publishers, Inc.
All rights reserved. No part of this book may be translated or reproduced in any form by print, photo-print microfilm or any other means without written permission from the publisher.

Library of Congress Cataloging-in-Publication Data

Li, Chin-Yang. 1935-
   Modern modalities for the diagnosis of hematologic neoplasms:
color atlas/text / Chin-Yang Li, Lung T. Yam, Tsieh Sun.
     p. cm.
   Includes bibliographical references and index.
   1. Leukemia–Molecular diagnosis. I. Yam, Lung T., 1936–
II. Sun, Tsieh. III. Title
   [DNLM: 1. Leukemia–diagnosis–atlases. 2. Lymphoma–diagnosis–
atlases. 3. Histocytochemistry–atlases. 4. Immunochemistry-
atlases. WH 17 L693m 1996]
RC643.L475 1996
616.99′419075–dc20
DNLM/DLC   95-36945
for Library of Congress   CIP

ISBN: 0-89640-292-4 (New York)
ISBN: 4-260-14292-5 (Tokyo)

Printed and bound in Hong Kong
10 9 8 7 6 5 4 3 2 1

PREFACE

Before 1980, diagnosis of hematologic disorders was based mainly on morphologic assessment. Special techniques for accurate cell identification were used sparingly to aid in making diagnoses. Enzymatic and nonenzymatic cytochemical techniques were often used. Immunocytochemical techniques were still in the developmental stage and had only began to be introduced for clinical use.

In the early 1980s, we wrote to commend the virtues of these special techniques for cell identification. At that time, these techniques were performed in the traditional hematology or histology laboratories as special stains. They were intended to be simple and practical procedures that could be easily applied to commonly available clinical specimens. Much has changed since that time. We now know more about the etiology, pathophysiology, and pathogenesis of many hematologic disorders. With this new knowledge, our concepts of these diseases and their diagnoses and treatments have changed. On the other hand, refinement of immunocytochemistry has proceeded relentlessly. New better monoclonal antibodies appear frequently. In addition, there is an explosion of new knowledge, in cytogenetics, immunogenetics, cell biology, and molecular biology. Some of this new knowledge has been introduced into the fields of hematology and hematopathology for diagnostic purposes. The goal of hematologic diagnosis is no longer limited to cell identification. We now want to know the maturation, clonality, growth fraction, and DNA content of the cells. If possible, we also want to know the etiology of the disease. Obviously, this desire or requirement cannot be satisfied with the use of a few special stain in the traditional hematology or histopathology laboratories. The operation for the diagnosis of hematologic malignancies has to change. New laboratories for flow cytometry, cytogentics, and molecular biology have to be established to deal with these new and still evolving diagnostic techniques. Each of these laboratories will need to be specifically equipped and directed by staff with refined knowledge in their trade. In some medical institutions, all of these diagnostic modalities and their respective special laboratories are included within the domain of a broad-based hematopathology division. Thus, the operation for hematopathologic diagnosis has become increasingly complicated. Establishing the diagnoses for hematologic malignancies has become very expensive, if not cost-prohibitive. This is particularly true if the diagnostic tests are ordered indiscriminately and unselectively. Also, it may not be cost-effective if many tests in various developmental stages are pushed into service prematurely. In this era of increased awareness and necessity of cost containment, using the various technologies for diagnosis of hematologic malignancies selectively is not only important but critical.

Despite these new considerations and changes, the basic approach for the diagnosis of hematologic malignancies has not changed significantly. In most instances, morphologic studies are still being used to formulate a diagnostic impression. Cytochemical and immunologic studies are then used to confirm this impression. In some cases (especially in leukemias, lymphomas, and myelodysplasias), flow cytometric, cytogenetic, and molecular genetic studies are done either to provide further information or to reaffirm the diagnosis. We follow this trend in this book to provide information accordingly. We have included new information based on our experience and on recent literature. In Part One of the book, we have included nine chapters discussing the basic principles and the diagnostic use of cytochemistry, immunochemistry, flow cytometry, cytogenetics and molecular biology. Part Two provides the actual procedures to be used in the laboratory, including the technique of *in stiu* hybridization, as exemplified by the demonstration of the Epstein-Barr virus. The procedures are written in a format to accommodate the new OSHA standards formulated to reduce the risks of health care workers by exposure to bloodborne pathogens. A cautionary note has been included at the beginning of the technical section advising the use of universal precautions and personal protective equipment when working in the laboratory. Part Three gives examples of the application of these techniques through color-illustrated cases that represent most types of hematologic malignancies. The color photomicrographs and case history discussions clearly illustrate how the special techniques are applied to the diagnostic problems.

ACKNOWLEDGMENTS

It goes without saying that many friends and colleagues have contributed their help to us in such a major undertaking as the writing of this book. In particular, we wish to thank Drs. G. Dewald and J. Whang-Peng for providing detailed technical information concerning the cytogenetic studies, as well as Drs. K. C. Chow and A. J. Janckila and Mr. E. Cardwell for their many discussions and critiques of the technique of in situ hybridization. We also wish to acknowledge the contributions of Jean Henshall, Joanne Cuomo, Kathy Maher, and Debbie Rapp in the technical part (Chapter 6) of flow cytometry and Sara Brackett for her secretarial assistance.

CONTENTS

PART ONE
DIAGNOSTIC METHODS AND CLINICAL APPLICATIONS
1 Introduction   3
2 Cytochemistry   7
3 Histochemistry   20
4 Immunochemistry   27
5 Surface Markers   37
6 Flow Cytometry   48
7 Immunogenotyping and Polymerase Chain Reaction   61
8 Cytogenetics and Oncogenes   72
9 Clinical Applications   79

PART TWO
PROCEDURES
1 Buffer Solutions   103
2 Fixatives   106
3 Counterstains   109
4 Miscellaneous Solutions   110
5 Cytology and Cytochemistry   112
6 Histology and Histochemistry   128
7 Immunology and Immunofluorescence   141
8 Immunocytochemistry and Immunohistochemistry   150
9 Cytogenetics   158
10 In Situ Hybridization   163

PART THREE
CASE HISTORIES WITH COLOR ILLUSTRATIONS

1. Acute Myeloid Leukemia **169**
2. Acute Myeloblastic Leukemia (M1) **171**
3. Acute Promyelocytic Leukemia (M3) **172**
4. Acute Myelomonocytic Leukemia (M4) **173**
5. Acute Myelomonocytic Leukemia (M4 Variant) **174**
6. Acute Monoblastic Leukemia (M5a) **175**
7. Acute Erythroleukemia (M6) **176**
8. Acute Myeloid Leukemia—Basophilic Differentiation **177**
9. Acute Myeloid Leukemia—Eosinophilic Differentiation **178**
10. Acute Megakaryocytic Leukemia (M7) **179**
11. Intravascular Lymphomatosis **180**
12. Pre-T-Cell Acute Lymphoblastic Leukemia **182**
13. Common Acute Lymphoblastic Leukemia **184**
14. B-Cell Acute Lymphoblastic Leukemia (L3) **185**
15. Small Noncleaved Cell Lymphoma—Leukemic Phase (L3) **186**
16. Neuroblastoma **187**
17. Ewing's Sarcoma **188**
18. Rhabdomyosarcoma **189**
19. B-Cell Chronic Lymphocytic Leukemia **191**
20. B Small Cleaved Cell Leukemia **192**
21. Plasma Cell Leukemia **194**
22. Persistent Polyclonal B Lymphocytosis **195**
23. Helper T-Cell Chronic Lymphocytic Leukemia **197**
24. Suppressor T-Cell Chronic Lymphocytic Leukemia **199**
25. Chronic Myelocytic Leukemia **200**
26. Chronic Myelomonocytic Leukemia in Transition to M4 **201**
27. Chronic Basophilic Leukemia with Erythroblastic Transformation **203**
28. Hairy Cell Leukemia—Blood and Marrow **205**
29. Hairy Cell Leukemia—Spleen and Liver **206**
30. Systemic Mast Cell Disease—Marrow **208**

31	Mast Cell Leukemia	**210**
32	Hodgkin's Disease—Nodular Sclerosing Type	**212**
33	Malignant Lymphoma—Lymphoblastic Type	**214**
34	Burkitt's Lymphoma	**216**
35	Diffuse Large-Cell Lymphoma—Follicular Center Cell Type	**217**
36	Diffuse Large-Cell Lymphoma—B-Cell Immunoblastic Lymphoma	**218**
37	Diffuse Large-Cell Lymphoma—T-Cell Type	**219**
38	Diffuse Large-Cell Lymphoma—T-Cell Immunoblastic Lymphoma	**220**
39	Diffuse Large-Cell Lymphoma—Histiocytic Type	**221**
40	Large-Cell Lymphoma—B-Cell Type	**222**
41	Small Cleaved Follicular Center Cell Lymphoma with Bone Marrow Involvement	**224**
42	Small Lymphocytic Lymphoma with Plasmacytoid Differentiation	**225**
43	Small Lymphocytic Lymphoma—B-Cell Type with Marrow Involvement	**226**
44	Small Lymphocytic Lymphoma/Leukemia—Helper T-Cell Type with Marrow Involvement	**228**
45	Lymphoproliferative Disorder of Granular Lymphocytes	**229**
46	Peripheral T-Cell Lymphoma with Multiorgan Failure	**230**
47	Extranodal Peripheral T-Cell Lymphoma with Paraneoplastic Complications	**232**
48	Metastatic Undifferentiated Prostatic Carcinoma	**233**
49	Granulocytic Sarcoma	**234**
50	Gamma Heavy Chain Disease	**235**
51	Cutaneous T-Cell Lymphoma—Mycosis Fungoides	**236**
52	Cutaneous B-Cell Lymphoma	**237**
53	Small Lymphocytic Lymphoma of Lung	**238**
54	B-Cell Lymphoma with High Content of Epithelioid Histiocytes	**239**
55	Plasmacytoma	**240**
56	Multiple Myeloma	**241**
57	Signet-Ring-Cell Myeloma	**242**
58	Undifferentiated Myeloma	**243**

59 Primary Amyloidosis **244**

60 Primary Amyloidosis with Cardiomyopathy **245**

61 Secondary Amyloidosis **246**

62 Large-Cell Lymphoma, B-Cell Type, with Features of "Malignant Histiocytosis" **247**

63 Composite Lymphoma—B-Cell Type **249**

INDEX **251**

Part One
DIAGNOSTIC METHODS AND CLINICAL APPLICATIONS

Chapter 1
INTRODUCTION

Hematologic neoplasms comprise a great variety of tumors derived from cells of the hematopoietic system. Although these neoplasms share some common characteristics, the vast differences in their clinical features, responses to therapeutic regimens, and prognoses make it mandatory that an accurate diagnosis be established before treatment is initiated.

The traditional way of making a diagnosis was based solely on morphologic examination of the blood and tissues involved by the neoplasms. However, many hematologic neoplasms have similar morphology and require other techniques for accurate diagnosis.

Histochemical techniques developed by Raspail in 1825 have come into wide use only since the early twentieth century, mainly because of Pearse's advocacy. Even so, the merit of these techniques in the field of hematology was not fully appreciated until the refinement of cytochemistry in the 1970s.

In recent years, our knowledge of the biology and immunology of blood cells has advanced significantly, along with considerable improvement in our ability to treat patients who have hematologic neoplasms. These developments complement each other, for the diagnostic techniques based on the immunobiology of blood cells play an important role in guiding the optimal use of modern therapeutic modalities. The division of lymphocytes into T cells and B cells has proved to be useful for the immunologic classification of lymphomas and leukemias. Other developments, such as hybridoma technology for the production of monoclonal antibodies, are valuable not only for accurate diagnosis but also for their potential use in the treatment of hematologic neoplasms.

The advent of flow cytometry provides a powerful tool for multivariate analysis of blood cells. A large panel of monoclonal antibodies can be used for the study of a minute specimen in a fraction of the time required for manual techniques. The counting of cells in thousands rather than hundreds, as manual techniques do, makes the test results much more accurate and reliable, and the optical system in a flow cytometer is undoubtedly more sensitive than the human eyes in discerning immunofluorescent staining. Furthermore, the potentials of double and triple staining of the same cells, and of the combination of DNA/RNA and monoclonal antibody analyses, are unlimited.

Advanced techniques and tools reveal the phenotypes of the blood cells. The revolution of molecular biology had unveiled the other fundamental aspect: the genotype of the cells. Analyses of heavy chain, light chain, and T-cell receptor genes furnish reliable information not only on cell lineage but also on the clonality of the cell group identified. Cytogenetic studies further identify the nature of a hematologic lesion (benign, premalignant, or malignant) and, frequently, the mechanism of malignant transformation.

The diagnosis of hematologic neoplasms depends more heavily on cellular morphology than does the diagnosis of other diseases because the hematologic tumors are thought to result from developmental arrest of individual cells at various stages. During the process of cell differentiation and maturation, the chemical constituents of the cell, particularly the enzymes, may change. Through each step of differentiation, a cell may either gain or lose certain components as part of the modulation related to specific cell function. Detection of these cell-specific chemical constituents or of the differentiation antigens is extremely helpful in accurately identifying the cell types and their maturation levels and then in subclassifying the various types of hematologic neoplasms.

Many cell-specific chemical constituents, differentiation antigens, and receptors are present in or on blood cells. These include surface membrane-bound immunoglobulins on B lymphocytes, sheep erythrocyte receptors on T lymphocytes, terminal deoxynucleotidyl transferase on lymphoid progenitors, myeloperoxidase in granulocytes, and cytoplasmic immunoglobulins in plasma cells, to name just a few. A selective combination of techniques that detect these cell-specific substances is required to achieve a diagnosis satisfactory to modern demands. The techniques include cytochemistry, histochemistry, immunocytochemistry, immunohistochemistry, surface marker studies, flow cytometry, immunogenotyping, polymerase chain reaction, and cytogenetic analysis. Each technique will be discussed in the following chapters.

The clinician and pathologist must thoroughly understand the basic principles of these techniques to select and use them properly and to interpret the sometimes conflicting results caused by differences in methodology. Hence, the purpose of this text/atlas is to clearly and concisely present the theoretical background and technical details of these techniques and to discuss their specificity, sensitivity, and clinical applications.

This atlas is divided into three parts. In the first part, "Diagnostic Methods and Clinical Applications," the various types of hematologic neoplasms and current methods of classification and diagnosis are described. The applications of the diagnostic techniques and their technical and clinical limitations are discussed and presented in tables for easy reference. Detailed descriptions of the clinical and histopathologic features of the diseases are not attempted. However, the reader is encouraged to obtain this information from the textbooks, special monographs, and review articles listed at the end of this chapter and from the reference lists following the remaining chapters. These reference lists are comprehensive but not exhaustive.

The second part, "Procedures," contains detailed procedures for the diagnostic methods that we recommend. These are the techniques that the authors have adopted, modified, and used successfully in their laboratories.

The third part, "Case Histories with Color Illustrations," consists of 63 cases representing most types of hematologic neoplasms. In each case, the clinical problem is briefly stated, the laboratory data furnished by routine and special techniques are provided, and color photomicrographs of the case are presented. The diagnosis is discussed, and each case concludes with the comments on clinical or technical aspects. The number of unusual cases included is disproportionately larger than is commonly seen because we feel that it is the unusual case that requires special techniques for an accurate diagnosis. The laboratory values are given in the SI units first, followed by standard units in parentheses. The magnifications are the original ones, that is, the magnification of the objective lens times the magnification of the microscope's eyepiece lens.

GENERAL BIBLIOGRAPHY

Clinical Hematology

Beutler E, Lichtman MA, Coller BS, et al: *Williams' Hematology*, ed 5. New York, McGraw-Hill, 1995.

Block MH: *Text-Atlas of Hematology*. Philadelphia, Lea & Febiger, 1976.

Cline MJ: *The White Cell*. Cambridge, Mass, Harvard University Press, 1975.

Dameshek W, Gunz F: *Leukemia*, ed 5. Philadelphia, WB Saunders, 1990.

Hoffman R, Benz EJ Jr, Shattil SJ, et al: *Hematology: Basic Principles and Practice*. New York, Churchill Livingstone, 1991.

Hyun BH, Gulati GL, Ashton JK: *Color Atlas of Clinical Hematology*. New York, Igaku-Shoin, 1986.

Kjeldsberg C, Beutler E, Bell C, et al: *Practical Diagnosis of Hematologic Disorders*, revised. Chicago, ASCP Press, 1991.

Miale JB: *Laboratory Medicine: Hematology*, ed 6. St. Louis, CV Mosby, 1982.

Schumacher HR: *Acute Leukemia: Approach to Diagnosis*. New York, Igaku-Shoin, 1990.

Wintrobe MM: *Clinical Hematology*, ed 9. Philadelphia, Lea & Febiger, 1993.

Cytochemistry

Hayhoe FGJ, Quaglino D: *Haematological Cytochemistry*. New York, Churchill Livingstone, 1980.

Kass L: *Leukemia: Cytology and Cytochemistry*. Philadelphia, JB Lippincott, 1982.

Li CY, Yam LT: Histochemical and immunologic features of leukemic cells. *Clin Lab Annu* 1:73–104, 1982.

Li CY, Yam LT: Cytochemistry and immunochemistry in hematologic diagnoses. *Hematol Oncol Clin North Am* 8:665–681, 1994.

Scott CS: *Leukemia Cytochemistry*. Chichester, UK, Ellis Harwood, 1989.

Hematologic Cytology

Block MH: *Text-Atlas of Hematology*. Philadelphia, Lea & Febiger, 1976.

Hayhoe FGJ, Flemans RF: *A Colour Atlas of Haematological Cytology*, ed 3. St. Louis, Mosby-Year Book, 1992.

Hayhoe FGJ, Quaglino D: *Haematological Cytochemistry*. New York, Churchill Livingstone, 1980.

Hoffbrand AV, Pettit JE: *Sandoz Atlas: Clinical Hematology*. London, Gower Medical Publishing, 1988.

Kass L: *Leukemia: Cytology and Cytochemistry*. Philadelphia, JB Lippincott, 1982.

Sun NCJ: *Hematology: An Atlas and Diagnostic Guide*. Philadelphia, WB Saunders, 1983.

Undritz E: *Sandoz Atlas of Haematology*, ed 2. Basle, Switzerland, Sandoz, 1973.

Zucker-Franklin D, Greaves ME, Grossi CE, et al: *Atlas of Blood Cells: Function and Pathology*, ed. 2. Philadelphia, Lea & Febiger, 1988.

Histochemistry

Barka T, Anderson PJ: *Histochemistry, Theory, Practice and Bibliography*, ed 2. New York, Harper & Row, 1965.

Burstone MS: *Enzyme Histochemistry and Its Application in the Study of Neoplasms*. New York, Academic Press, 1963.

Li CY: Morphologic, cytochemical and immunologic diagnosis of hematologic malignancies. *Curr Hematol* 1:308–342, 1981.

Lillie RD: *Conn's Biological Stains*, ed 9. Baltimore, Williams & Wilkins, 1977.

Lillie RD, Fullmer HM: *Histopathologic Technic and Practical Histochemistry*, ed 4. New York, McGraw-Hill, 1976.

Lojda Z, Gossrau R, Schiebler TH, et al: *Enzyme Histochemistry: A Laboratory Manual*. New York, Springer-Verlag, 1979.

Luna LG (ed): *Manual of Histologic Staining Methods of the Armed Forces Institute of Pathology*, ed 3. New York, McGraw-Hill, 1968.

Pearse AGE: *Histochemistry: Theoretical and Applied*, ed 3, vol II. New York, Churchill Livingstone, 1972.

Pearse AGE: *Histochemistry: Theoretical and Applied*, ed 4, vol I. New York, Churchill Livingstone, 1980.

Histopathology

Brunning RD, McKenna RW: Tumors of the bone marrow. In Rosai J, Sobin LH: *Atlas of Tumor Pathology*, Series 3 Fascicle 9. Washington, DC, Armed Forces Institute of Pathology, 1994.

Carson F: *Histotechnology: A Self-Instructional Text*. Chicago, ASCP Press, 1990.

Fullmer HM, Lillie RD: *Histopathologic Technic and Practical Histochemistry*, ed 4. New York, McGraw-Hill, 1976.

Harris NL, Jaffe ES, Stein H, et al: A revised European-American classification of lymphoid neoplasms: A proposal from the International Lymphoma Study Group. *Blood* 84:1361–1392, 1994.

Ioachim HL: *Lymph Node Biopsy*. Philadelphia, JB Lippincott, 1982.

Jaffe ES, (ed): *Surgical Pathology of the Lymph Nodes and Related Organs*, 2nd ed., Philadelphia, W.B. Saunders, 1995.

Knowles DM: *Neoplastic Hematopathology*. Baltimore, Williams & Wilkins, 1992.

Lennert K: *Malignant Lymphoma Other Than Hodgkin's Disease*. New York, Springer-Verlag, 1978.

Luna LG (ed): *Manual of Histologic Staining Methods of the Armed Forces Institute of Pathology*, ed 3. New York, McGraw-Hill, 1968.

Mallory FB: *Pathological Technique*. 1938. Reprint; New York, Hafner Press, 1968.

Rappaport H: Tumors of the Hematopoietic System. In Subcommittee on Oncology of the Committee of Pathology of the Division of Medical Sciences of the National Academy of Sciences *Atlas of Tumor Pathology*, Section 3, Fascicle 8. Washington, DC, Armed Forces Institute of Pathology, 1966.

Sun T, Susin M (eds): *Differential Diagnosis of Lymphoid Disorders*. New York, Igaku-Shoin, 1996.

Monoclonal Antibodies

Kennett RH, McKearn TJ, Bechtol KB, et al (eds): *Monoclonal Antibodies—Hybridomas: A New Dimension in Biological Analysis*. New York, Plenum, 1980.

McMichael AJ, Fabre TJ (eds): *Monoclonal Antibodies in Clinical Medicine*. New York, Academic Press, 1982.

Reinherz EL, Haynes BF, Nadler LM, et al (eds): *Leukocyte Typing II. Volume I: Human T Lymphocytes; Volume 2: Human B Lymphocytes; Volume 3; Human Myeloid and Hematopoietic Cells*. New York, Springer-Verlag, 1986.

Immunocytochemistry and Immunohistochemistry

DeLellis RA (ed): *Advances in Immunohistochemistry*. New York, Raven Press, 1988.

Elias JM: *Principles and Techniques in Diagnostic Histopathology: Developments in Immunohistochemistry and Enzyme Histochemistry*. Park Ridge, NJ, Noyes Data Corp, 1982.

Elias JM: *Immunohistopathology: A Practical Approach to Diagnosis*. Chicago, ASCP Press, 1990.

Sternberger LA: *Immunocytochemistry*, ed 2. New York, Wiley Medical, 1979.

Taylor CR: *Immunomicroscopy: A Diagnostic Tool for the Surgical Pathologist*. Philadelphia, WB Saunders, 1986.

Tubbs RR, Gephardt GN, Petras RE: *Atlas of Immunohistology*. Chicago, ASCP Press, 1986.

Flow Cytometry

Bauer KD, Daque RE, Shankey TV (eds): *Clinical Flow Cytometry: Principles and Application*. Baltimore, Williams & Wilkins, 1993.

Coon JS, Weinstein RS (eds): *Diagnostic Flow Cytometry*. Baltimore, Williams & Wilkins, 1991.

Grogan WM, Collins JM: *Guide to Flow Cytometry Methods*. New York, Marcel Dekker, 1990.

Keren DF (ed): *Flow Cytometry and Clinical Diagnosis*, ed 2. Chicago, ASCP Press, 1993.

Laerum OD, Bjerknes R (eds): *Flow Cytometry in Hematology*. London, Academic Press, 1992.

Melamed MR, Lindmo T, Mendelsohn ML (eds): *Flow Cytometry and Sorting*, ed 2. New York, Wiley-Liss, 1990.

Riley RS, Mahin EJ, Ross W: *Clinical Application of Flow Cytometry*. New York, Igaku-Shoin, 1993.

Shapiro HM: *Practical Flow Cytometry*, ed 2. New York, Alan R Liss, 1988.

Sun T: *Color Atlas/Text of Flow Cytometric Analysis of Hematologic Neoplasms*. New York, Igaku-Shoin, 1993.

Molecular Biology

Abbas AK, Lichtman AH, Pober JS: *Cellular and Molecular Immunology*. Philadelphia, WB Saunders, 1991.

Albert B, Bray D, Lewis J, et al: *Molecular Biology of the Cell*, ed 2. New York, Garland, 1989.

Darnell J, Lodish H, Baltimore D: *Molecular Cell Biology*. New York, Scientific American Books, 1990.

Hames BD, Higgins SJ (eds): *Nucleic Acid Hybridization: A Practical Approach*. Oxford, UK, IRL Press, 1985.

Innis MA, Gelford DH, White TJ: *PCR Protocols: A Guide to Methods and Applications*. San Diego, Calif, Academic Press, 1990.

Piper MA, Unger ER: *Nucleic Acid Probes: A Primer for Pathologists*. Chicago, ASCP Press, 1989.

Watson JD, Hopkins N, Roberts K, et al: *Molecular Biology of the Gene*, ed 4. Menlo Park, Calif, Benjamin-Cummings, 1987.

Watson JD, Tooze J, Kurtz DT: *Recombinant DNA: A Short Course*. New York, WH Freeman, 1983.

Cytogenetics

Harnden DG, Klinger HP (eds): *An International System for Human Cytogenetic Nomenclature 1985; Report of the Standing Committee on Human Cytogenetic Nomenclature*. Basel, Karger, 1985.

Heim S, Mitelman F: *Cancer Cytogenetics*. New York, Alan R Liss, 1987.

Mange AP, Mange EJ: *Genetics: Human Aspects*, ed 2. Sunderland, Mass, Sinauer Associates, 1990.

Rooney DE, Czepulkowski BH: *Human Cytogenetics: A Practical Approach*. Oxford, UK, IRL Press, 1986.

Sandberg AA: *The Chromosomes in Human Cancer and Leukemia*, ed 2. New York, Elsevier, 1990.

Immunology

Abbas AK, Lichtman AH, Pober JS: *Cellular and Molecular Immunology*. Philadelphia, WB Saunders, 1994.

Alexander JW, Good RA: *Fundamentals of Clinical Immunology*. Philadelphia, WB Saunders, 1977.

Bach JF: *Immunology*, ed 2. New York, Wiley, 1982.

Bellanti JA: *Immunology III*, ed 3. Philadelphia, WB Saunders, 1985.

Klein J: *Immunology*. London, Blackwell Scientific, 1990.

Roitt I: *Essential Immunology*, ed 7. London, Blackwell Scientific, 1991.

Rose NR, Friedman H, Fahey JL: *Manual of Clinical Laboratory Immunology*, ed 3. Washington, DC, American Society for Clinical Microbiology, 1986.

Samter M (ed). *Immunological Diseases*, ed 4. Boston, Little, Brown, 1988.

Stiters DP, Stobo JD, Wells JV: *Basic and Clinical Immunology*. Norwalk, Conn, Appleton & Lange, 1987.

Chapter 2
CYTOCHEMISTRY

Cytochemistry is the microscopic study of the chemical constituents in cells. Cytologic materials used in such studies include cell suspensions, smears, and imprints. Many cytochemical studies in hematopoietic cells have been done. The aims of these studies include delineation of the chemical constituents of cells, identification of the cell types, and establishment of diagnostic criteria for hematologic diseases. Although many cytochemical reactions of hematopoietic cells have been examined, only a few have shown diagnostic potential.

PREPARATION OF SPECIMENS

Smears or imprints of blood, marrow, lymph node, and spleen are usually used, but cell suspensions are also suitable and have been used on rare occasions. These cytologic materials provide the best results when they are fresh, but most can be used after temporary storage. The maximum period of storage is determined either by the stability of the biologic substances or by the sensitivity of the cytochemical reagents. In general, the dehydrogenases and β-glucuronidase are the most unstable, and preparations containing them should be examined within 24 hr after the cytologic materials have been prepared. Nonspecific esterase, peroxidase, acid phosphatase, and tartrate-resistant acid phosphatase are fairly stable. Their activities are not appreciably decreased in air-dried smears or imprints kept at room temperature for two weeks. Chloroacetate esterase and a number of nonenzymatic stains (periodic acid–Schiff, Sudan black, toluidine blue, iron) yield stable cytochemical reaction products; therefore, these stains can be used on smears or imprints that are then stored at room temperature for many months.

For air-dried smears, storage at lower temperatures preserves enzymatic activity better. However, when unfixed air-dried smears are kept in refrigerators, moisture often condenses on the smears. The condensation then hemolyzes the erythrocytes and induces distortion of morphology of the nucleated cells. To prevent hemolysis and distortion, all cytologic material stored at 4°C to 10°C should be kept in a desiccator or wrapped in moisture-absorbing paper or cotton.

Fixatives affect the results of cytochemical studies. In general, fixatives containing heavy metals preserve the morphologic details of cells extremely well but severely inhibit the activities of most enzymes. The fixatives used in most cytochemical reactions include aqueous solutions of alcohol, acetone, or formaldehyde, or a combination of these. The composition of the fixative can be varied, depending on the cytochemical reagents used. For example, because the dehydrogenases are very labile, they should be used only in specimens fixed in cold-buffered acetone solution, which prevents significant loss of enzyme activity. The myeloperoxidases withstand most fixatives, except those that contain high concentrations of methanol. Alkaline phosphatase can be demonstrated in specimens fixed with either methanol or buffered acetone, although methanol exerts stronger inhibition of enzyme activity than does acetone.

Because cytochemical studies are most useful when several reactions occur simultaneously, we have used a general fixative containing mixtures of phosphate buffer, acetone, and formaldehyde (Part 2, Section 2-1) to preserve components in various reactions. This fixative is suitable for Sudan black, periodic acid–Schiff, chloroacetate esterase, nonspecific esterase, aminocaproate esterase, and peroxidase. It is also suitable for both acid and alkaline phosphatases, although theoretically the phosphate ion in the fixative may exert a common ion effect on these two enzymes. When it is desirable to have maximal sensitivity for the demonstration of phosphatases, fixative containing cold-buffered acetone without phosphate ions can be used (Part 2, Section 2-3).

Because the activity of many enzymes diminishes considerably in smears that have been stored after fixation (particularly if the fixatives contain alcohol or aldehyde), we prefer unfixed, air-dried smears and imprints to those preserved by the fixatives just described. Most cytochemical reactions can be satisfactorily performed on such unfixed materials, even if they have been kept at room temperature for 2 weeks or longer. When cytologic materials must be preserved for long periods of time, smears and imprints can still be kept unfixed at 4°C to 10°C. Alternatively, they can be stored in the cold after brief fixation (30 sec) in 60% buffered acetone.

Cytologic materials should be stained soon after fixation. After the reactions to the cytochemical stains are complete, the smears or imprints should be properly counterstained and mounted for microscopic observation.

PEROXIDASE REACTION

The peroxidases are enzymes capable of catalyzing the oxidation of substances by hydrogen peroxide, according to the following chemical equation, in which A stands for the oxidized substance or the indicator.

$$AH_2 + H_2O_2 \xrightarrow{\text{Peroxidase}} A + 2H_2O$$

The presence of peroxidase activity within a cell is indicated by the oxidized substance or indicator, A. In the past, benzidine and its derivatives were used as the indicator for this cytochemical reaction.[1-3] The manufacture of many benzidine compounds has ceased because of their carcinogenic potential; only 3,3-diaminobenzidine is still allowed to be used in the clinical laboratory.[1] Several substances have been introduced as indicators for the peroxidase reaction. These include 3-amino-9-ethylcarbazole[4,5]; 2,7-fluorenediamine[6,7]; α-naphtholpyronine[8]; o-toluidine[9]; and a combination of pyrocatechol and p-phenylenediamine.[10]

Since the peroxidase activity in leukocytes is derived not from a single enzyme but rather from a group of isoenzymes,[11] some of the cytochemical methods now available may demonstrate several isoenzymes; other may be specific for a single isoenzyme. For example, horseradish peroxidase can be best demonstrated at pH 5.2, whereas myeloperoxidase of human neutrophils has optimal activity at pH 7.6. By using specific monoclonal antibodies and immunochemical techniques, it is possible to demonstrate low levels of myeloperoxidase in the myeloid cells.[12]

Myeloperoxidase activity is present in neutrophils, eosinophils, and monocytes but not in lymphocytes. The enzyme in eosinophils is different from that in other cells because it remains enzymatically active in an acidic environment and in the presence of cyanide.[13-15] All myeloperoxidases are sensitive to heat and to methanol. Only erythrocytes and erythroblasts show definite staining for peroxidase after methanol treatment; however, this staining does not represent true enzyme activity but instead is due to a nonenzymatic chemical reaction between hemoglobin and the staining reagents. Nevertheless, this peculiar phenomenon has been used specifically to demonstrate hemoglobinized cells (pseudoperoxidase or Lepehne's reaction).[16,17]

Peroxidase activity is also present in human megakaryocytes, platelets,[18] and the hairy cells of hairy cell leukemia.[19] The enzyme in these cells is sensitive to a variety of fixatives, including formalin and its derivatives, and cannot be demonstrated by the conventional methods for peroxidase. This enzyme activity cannot be visualized by light microscopy, but it can be demonstrated by electron microscopy. A peroxidase reaction that demonstrates phi bodies in the leukemic cells of acute leukemia has been introduced.[20] The staining of phi bodies demonstrated by this method probably represents catalase rather than myeloperoxidase.

Myeloperoxidase activity is somewhat sensitive to storage. Enzyme activity in the neutrophils often decreases significantly when the cytologic material is kept at room temperature for more than 2 weeks or is fixed in formaldehyde. Under these circumstances, it may be necessary to use Sudan black or chloroacetate esterase instead of peroxidase.

Clinically, the peroxidase reaction has been employed either to characterize or to identify monocytes and granulocytes. It is often used in the classification of acute leukemias. In interpreting the peroxidase reaction for differential diagnosis of acute leukemias, only the enzyme activity in the blasts should be assessed. A positive reaction of the blasts in blood indicates myeloblastic or myelomonocytic leukemia. However, a positive reaction in mature granulocytes has no diagnostic value; it merely indicates that the peroxidase staining procedure is working well. Leukocytes may be deficient in or devoid of peroxidase activity. This condition may be either congenital or secondary to an association with a myeloproliferative disorder.[21-23] In some cases of poorly differentiated acute myeloid leukemia, enzyme activity is not visible by light microscopy but is demonstrable by either electron microscopy or immunochemical techniques.[12,24-26] In other cases, the leukemic cells exhibit activity of both peroxidase and terminal deoxynucleotidyl transferase (a lymphoid enzyme) and are considered to be terminal deoxynucleotidyl transferase–positive acute myeloid leukemia.[27-29]

SUDAN BLACK B STAIN

Sudan black B is a fat-soluble substance that is used for the demonstration of lipids in human cells.[30-33] The method of Sheehan and Storey[33] is most widely used for the study of blood cells. The Sudan black reaction is positive in fat cells, macrophages, and granulocytes.[33,34] Positive staining in the fat cells can be eliminated by lipid-soluble solvents, but positive staining in the granulocytes is resistant to extraction by alcohol, acetone, and other lipid-soluble solvents.[32] Therefore, the substance responsible for the positive staining of fat cells is probably lipid, but the stained component in neutrophils is uncertain and may not be lipid.

The Sudan black reaction is similar to the peroxidase reaction in the spectrum of cells that stain positively. It is as sensitive as the peroxidase reaction but is more sensitive than chloroacetate esterase in identifying myeloblasts. The Sudan black staining reaction is not significantly influenced by either heat or storage of the specimen; therefore, it can be satisfactorily applied to aged cytologic material. However, it stains both neutrophils and eosinophils strongly and thus is a less specific cell marker for neutrophilic granulocytes than is chloroacetate esterase. The Sudan black reaction is used clinically as a marker for myeloblasts and for the classification of acute leukemia. It should be cautioned that in cases of Burkitt's lymphoma and a rare case of acute lymphoblastic leukemia (ALL) in which the primitive cells have many cytoplasmic vacuoles, the lipid in these vacuoles may stain positively with Sudan black.[35–37]

CHLOROACETATE ESTERASE REACTION

Human neutrophils and mast cells have a group of enzymes capable of efficiently hydrolyzing halogenated naphthol esters in vitro. The best substrate for these enzymes appears to be naphthol AS-D chloroacetate.[38,39] These neutrophil-specific enzymes can be specifically demonstrated cytochemically under the following experimental conditions: at pH 7.4 to 7.6 for less than 30 min at room temperature.[14,40] When the incubating medium becomes acidic or when the staining time is unnecessarily prolonged, esterase activity in cells other than neutrophils may become demonstrable. These neutrophil-specific enzymes, or chloroacetate esterases, may be the enzymes chymotrypsin or elastase.[41–43] They are sensitive to chloromethyl ketone but are resistant to sodium fluoride inhibition.[40,43,44]

Several cytochemical methods are available for demonstrating chloroacetate esterase activity in the blood cells. These include the fast garnet GBC method of Moloney et al.,[39] the hexazotized pararosaniline method of Leder,[45] and the hexazotized new fuchsin method of Yam et al.[14] We prefer the new fuchsin method because of its simplicity, reproducibility, and specificity for neutrophils. Its reaction product is highly chromogenic, and is insoluble in aqueous solutions and organic solvents. When a blue reaction product is desired, fast blue BBN or fast blue BB can be used instead of new fuchsin.[14,40]

Chloroacetate esterase is most useful as a specific marker for neutrophilic granulocytes and, to a lesser extent, for mast cells.[14] It is often used to identify immature granulocytes in acute leukemia. It is very stable, and can be demonstrated in myeloid cells and even in paraffin-embedded tissues after prolonged periods of storage.[45] Cytochemical demonstration of this enzyme is particularly useful for the diagnosis of granulocytic sarcoma and extramedullary hematopoiesis.[46,47]

NONSPECIFIC ESTERASE REACTION

A group of enzymes in white blood cells are capable of hydrolyzing various aliphatic and aromatic short-chain esters. These enzymes exhibit a wide range of substrate specificity and are therefore called the *nonspecific esterases*.

Polyacrylamide gel electrophoresis studies of different types of leukocytic preparations reveal that many of the esterases are cell specific (i.e., a certain esterase is found only in a specific cell type) and that the cytochemical methods for esterase demonstrate the activity of several of the esterases.[40,43,48] By using selected substrates and specific experimental conditions, it is possible to determine which of these "nonspecific esterases" occur in a specific cell type.[40] By using the isoelectric focusing technique to examine several homogeneous populations of blood cells, it has been shown that monocytes, granulocytes, and subpopulations of lymphocytes exhibit unique patterns of esterase activity.[49–51]

The nonspecific esterase reaction is most frequently used as a specific marker for monocytes and macrophages. Several techniques are available for this purpose. When nonspecific esterases are studied in an acidic environment with α-naphthyl acetate as a substrate, they are found only in monocytes.[52] The method using naphthol AS acetate at pH 7.0 demonstrates the enzyme activity in both granulocytes and monocytes.[53,54] The nonspecific esterase activity in monocytes is inhibited by sodium fluoride, whereas that in granulocytes is resistant to fluoride.[44,54] However, differentiated histiocytes or specialized macrophages in tissues often contain strong esterase activity that is also resistant to sodium fluoride.[16,55] We believe that the method using α-naphthyl acetate or α-naphthyl butyrate with hexazotized pararosaniline in an acidic environment is better for showing monocytes because granulocytes are not demonstrable by this method.[14,40] Fluoride inhibition is used only to differentiate the blood monocytes, which are fluoride-sensitive, from the differentiated histiocytes in tissues, which are fluoride-resistant. If a more rapid and sensitive stain is desired, methods using either α-naphthyl acetate or α-naphthyl butyrate, with either fast garnet GBC, fast blue BB, or fast blue RR, are also satisfactory.[40] The activity of nonspecific esterase in human blood cells is unstable and is sensitive to heat, storage, and fixatives. Enzyme activity cannot be demonstrated in monocytes and histiocytes in paraffin-embedded tissue sections.

The nonspecific esterase reaction is useful in identifying monocytes and histiocytes, as well as in the differential diagnosis of acute leukemias and large-cell lymphomas.[55–59] It can be used with a variety of other cell marker stains to identify monocytes and other cell types simultaneously.[14,57,59,60]

ACID α-NAPHTHYL ACETATE ESTERASE REACTION

When human blood cells are studied for esterase activity by the nonspecific esterase reaction, some lymphocytes also show definite cytoplasmic enzyme activity. When stained, this lymphocytic enzyme assumes a well-demarcated, dot-like pattern in the cytoplasm of the cell. It is resistant to sodium fluoride inhibition and is best demonstrated by α-naphthyl acetate in an acidic environment with prolonged incubation.[61,63] The enzyme thus revealed is called *acid α-naphthyl acetate esterase (ANAE)*. Combined immunologic and cytochemical studies have shown that this enzyme is present almost exclusively in the helper subtype of T lymphocytes (T_h).[49,62,64–67]

The ANAE reaction is used as a marker for T-helper cells. Clinically, it is useful in identifying chronic T-lymphocytic leukemia and the T-cell lymphomas, including mycosis fungoides and Sézary syndrome.[61,62,68,69] In T-cell ALL, however, ANAE activity is variable[62] and may be weak or negative in the lymphoblasts.[61] In hairy cell leukemia, the pathognomonic hairy cells also contain abundant amounts of ANAE. The pattern of enzyme distribution in these cells is characteristic and is useful for diagnostic purposes.[70,71]

AMINOCAPROATE ESTERASE REACTION

The human mast cells contain an esterase that preferentially hydrolyzes aminocaproate esters in vitro.[72] The biochemical properties of this enzyme have not been sufficiently studied, yet it is known to be unstable and is fairly sensitive to storage and heat. When naphthol AS aminocaproate hydrobromide is used as the substrate at pH 7.0 to 7.4 for 30 min or less, aminocaproate esterase can be selectively demonstrated in the mast cells.[73,74] If the incubation time is unduly prolonged, enzyme activity may be demonstrated in the granulocytes as well. It appears that this esterase is a good marker for mast cells and is thus useful in the diagnosis of mast cell disorders.[73,75–77]

ALKALINE PHOSPHATASE REACTION

The alkaline phosphatases are enzymes capable of hydrolyzing orthomonophosphate esters in an alkaline environment. They are widely distributed in human tissues and are separable into liver, bone, intestine, placenta, and neoplastic (i.e., Regan) isoenzymes according to their tissue specificity, substrate preference, inhibitor sensitivity, and other biochemical properties.[78] In human hematopoietic tissues, alkaline phosphatase activity is present in neutrophilic granulocytes, osteoblasts, vascular endothelial cells, and sometimes lymphocytes.[79–81] Differences between the biochemical properties of alkaline phosphatases in the vascular endothelial cells and those in the mature neutrophilic granulocytes have been observed.[16] Even the enzyme within neutrophils is not homogeneous and is separable by gel electrophoresis into several molecular species.[82] Leukocyte alkaline phosphatase has been purified and characterized. This leukocytic enzyme may be different from other tissue-specific isoenzymes, although critical comparative studies on the biochemical properties of these isoenzymes are yet to be performed.

Many cytochemical methods are available for the demonstration of alkaline phosphatases. Gomori's lead nitrate method and its subsequent modifications are used mainly for ultrastructural studies.[83] Methods using naphthyl phosphate as the substrate invariably yield reaction products having relatively high solubility and imprecise localization. The method of Kaplow, which employs a substituted naphthol compound as the substrate and fast violet B salt as the coupler, produces a bright red precipitate and is satisfactory for clinical purposes.[79] Alternatively, the method of Rutenberg yields a blue reaction product and is equally satisfactory.[84]

Leukocyte alkaline phosphatase (LAP) activity in the neutrophils is increased in polycythemia vera and granulocytic leukemoid reactions, normal in secondary erythrocytosis, and decreased in most cases of chronic myelocytic leukemia (CML). Semiquantitative cytochemical assessment of LAP (i.e., the LAP score) is most useful in differentiating these disorders.[80,84]

In CML, about 90% of the cases show decreased LAP activity.[80,84] When the disease is either in its early phase or in apparent remission, the LAP score may become normal. In some atypical cases, such as CML in young children, CML in blast crisis, and CML without Ph^1 chromosome, LAP activity is often normal or increased.[80,85] In chronic neutrophilic leukemia, markedly elevated LAP activity is the rule.[86,87] Low LAP activity in granulocytes has been attributed to a number of causes, including the presence of an inhibitor in serum,[88] immaturity of the circulating neutrophils in CML,[89] and lack of production of enzyme protein in the neutrophils.[90,91] At present, the reason for low LAP activity in any given instance is uncertain. A recent study suggests that the low LAP activity in resting CML neutrophils is attributable to the absence of appropriate stimuli rather than to inability to synthesize the enzyme.[92]

Low LAP activity is not unique to CML; it may also be found in diseases such as paroxysmal nocturnal hemoglobinuria, sickle cell anemia, sideroblastic anemia, severe eosinophilia, and familial hypophosphatasemia. On rare occasions, low LAP activity may occur in healthy people. Faulty cytochemical technique may be yet another cause of the finding of low LAP activity and should be kept in mind.[80]

High LAP activity is frequently present in polycythemia vera, bacterial infections, and pregnancy, as well as in people receiving corticosteroids.[80] LAP may be a good indicator for inflammatory reactions of tissue. In Hodgkin's disease, for example, the LAP score closely parallels the progression of the disease, which is of considerable clinical value.[93]

A rare subset of human lymphocytes also possesses alkaline phosphatase activity.[81,94] These lymphocytes are found in the mantle area of lymph node follicles. In lymphocytic lymphoma of the intermediate cell type, neoplastic lymphocytes often contain alkaline phosphatase activity.[94] The clinical and biologic significance of this finding is uncertain.

Intestinal alkaline phosphatase has been used as an indicator for the immunocytochemical demonstration of tissue antigens.[95,96] This enzyme remains active at near-neutral pH (pH 7.6) and is resistant to levamisole inhibition.[97]

ACID PHOSPHATASE REACTION

The acid phosphatases are a group of enzymes capable of hydrolyzing monophosphate esters in acidic environments. In humans, these enzymes can be classified as erythrocytic and nonerythrocytic, according to their chemical properties and tissue of origin.[98] The erythrocytic isoenzymes are genetically determined and have a limited substrate specificity. The nonerythrocytic isoenzymes are not predetermined genetically. They are often tissue-specific or cell-specific and, therefore, have a restricted tissue distribution. In human blood cells, seven different nonerythrocytic isoenzymes exist: 0, 1, 2, 3, 3b, 4, and 5.[99,100] All except isoenzyme 5 are sensitive to tartrate inhibition. Isoenzymes 2 and 4 are present in neutrophils and monocytes; 3, in lymphocytes and platelets; 3b, in primitive cells and blasts; and 5, in the hairy cells of hairy cell leukemia.

Many cytochemical methods are available for the demonstration of acid phosphatase activity in blood cells. These methods vary in the substrates, couplers, and staining conditions specified. For cytologic materials, we prefer the method using naphthol AS-BI phosphate-fast garnet GBC because of its sensitivity and broad safety margins.[101] In tissue sections, this method often results in imprecise cellular enzyme localization. Therefore, the modified method[101] of Goldberg and Barka[102] using naphthol AS-BI phosphate and hexazotized pararosaniline is recommended for this purpose.

Acid phosphatase activity is increased in the neutrophils of patients with acute inflammation and CML,[103] but the magnitude of the increase is not large and is not clinically important. In the lymphocytes, enzyme activity in the T cells is much higher than that in the B cells.[58,104-107] When present in T cells, acid phosphatase activity is localized in the Golgi area and assumes a dot-like appearance. This characteristic enzymatic pattern in T cells is of considerable importance as a specific marker for these cells, particularly T lymphoblasts[108-113]; however, the erythroblasts, some myeloblasts, and an occasional null-cell lymphoblast may also show similar focal acid phosphatase activity. Therefore, when staining for acid phosphatase in T lymphoblasts, one should consider staining for other markers as well to increase the diagnostic precision for T lymphoblasts.[58]

TARTRATE-RESISTANT ACID PHOSPHATASE REACTION

The enzymatic activity of erythrocytic acid phosphatase and nonerythrocytic isoenzyme 5 is not inhibited by $l(+)$-tartrate.[98] Since the erythrocytic isoenzymes hydrolyze naphthyl phosphate compounds slowly, the tartrate-resistant enzyme activity in blood cells observed by conventional cytochemical methods is due to isoenzyme 5 exclusively.[114,115] Isoenzyme 5 is a pyrophosphatase and is present in abundance in the hairy cells of hairy cell leukemia.[116] Activated lymphocytes, particularly T cells, activated macrophages, and some specialized histiocytes (e.g., epithelioid cells, Gaucher cells) may also have considerable enzyme activity.[114] Enzyme activity in lymphocytes is often moderate and has a focal staining pattern in or around the Golgi area. Activated macrophages or specialized histiocytes may also possess strong enzyme activity; however, these cells, in addition to having distinct morphologic features, are usually fixed tissue cells with limited ability to circulate in blood. The presence in the blood of cells with strong enzyme activity is highly suggestive of hairy cell leukemia.

In blood smears, a positive reaction is denoted by the presence of more than two cells with diffuse and intense activity, i.e., more than 40 granules. The presence of cells with weak or focal enzyme activity should not be considered positive. In lymph node and spleen imprints, the diagnostic criteria require detection throughout the preparation of many cells having intense, diffuse activity. In case of doubt, histochemical studies of tissue sections are necessary to differentiate hairy cell leukemia from other disorders yielding positive tartrate-resistant acid phosphatase reactions.[114,117,118]

PERIODIC ACID–SCHIFF REACTION

The Schiff's reagent is a colorless solution obtained by the reduction of basic fuchsin by hydrogen sulfide. It is capable of reacting with R-CHO groups in tissues to form an insoluble, bright red complex (aldehyde-fuchsin-sulfurous acid compound). Therefore, glycoprotein, mucoproteins, and high molecular weight carbohydrates are positively stained by the periodic acid–Schiff (PAS) reaction. In human blood cells, the substance demonstrable by the PAS reaction is predominantly glycogen, which can be completely eliminated by pretreating tissues with diastase (α-amylase).[119] For cytologic materials, the modified technique of McManus is recommended.[120]

Many human blood cells show a positive PAS reaction in the cytoplasm. The intensity of this reaction and its staining pattern vary with the cell type. The pattern of staining can be diffuse, granular, or mixed. In normal blood cells, the staining pattern is diffuse in granulocytes and granular in lymphoid cells. In CML and polycythemia vera, PAS staining in the neutrophils is diffuse. In other hematologic malignancies, the cells involved often show intense PAS positivity in a large, granular pattern. A positive PAS reaction with the granular pattern may be present in the lymphoid cells of lymphoproliferative disorders,[121–124] in the myeloblasts of acute myeloblastic leukemia (AML)[122] and in the erythroblasts of erythroleukemia.[125] However, a positive reaction, even with the granular pattern and large areas of PAS-positive material in the cytoplasm, is not unique to neoplastic blood cells. This pattern has been seen in the lymphocytes of infectious mononucleosis,[126] in the erythroblasts of thalassemia,[127] and in chronic renal failure.[128] When these benign disorders have been treated successfully, the PAS-positive material can no longer be demonstrated. Since the PAS-positive material in human blood cells is glycogen, accumulation of this substance in blood cells is thought to be an indication of disturbed glycogen metabolism.

Significant oscillation of PAS positivity in the blood cells of hematologic neoplasms occurs. In CML, PAS reactivity in the granulocytes is less than that of the normal granulocytes. In polycythemia vera, the granulocytic glycogen is increased,[129] but the PAS positivity is difficult to quantitate cytochemically because of the diffuse staining pattern. However, the lymphoid cells and erythroblasts exhibit a granular distribution that can easily be assessed by cytochemical methods. In 80% to 90% of ALL cases, the lymphoblasts show a positive PAS reaction.[56,122] This positive reaction may be seen in the lymphoblasts of all subtypes of ALL[130,132] but is seen most often in common ALL.[133] Thus, the PAS positivity denotes a favorable clinical outcome.[133] The PAS reaction has limited value in the subclassification of the acute leukemias. Although a positive PAS reaction is often seen in ALL, it may also be seen in about 10% to 15% of the cases of AML.[56,122] Nevertheless, when the PAS reaction is used in conjunction with other cytochemical reactions, leukemic blasts that are positive for PAS and negative for Sudan black, peroxidase, or nonspecific esterase are invariably lymphoid in origin.

The PAS reaction is often positive in erythroblasts of Di Guglielmo syndrome.[125,134] The PAS-positive material is coarse and granular in the early erythroblasts but fine and diffuse in cells of later stages. For this disease, the PAS reaction is a useful diagnostic aid, particularly in those cases with intense erythroid hyperplasia and a few primitive myeloid cells. Its diagnostic value may be further enhanced if ringed sideroblasts are also present.

IRON STAIN (PERLS' REACTION)

Human tissues contain various amounts of iron. Cellular iron exists in the form of ferritin or hemosiderin and is demonstrable by cytochemical techniques.

Several cytochemical methods are available for the demonstration of iron. In the iron stain (Perls' reaction),[135] a reagent containing ferrocyanide ions reacts with ferric ions in the tissues to form ferric ferrocyanide, which appears as a green-blue precipitate at the site of the iron-containing tissues. This method is sensitive, technically simple to perform, and most widely used.

In hematopoietic tissues, cytochemically demonstrable iron exists both extracellularly and intracellularly. Extracellular iron is often seen in conditions of iron excess. Intracellular iron is present in macrophages and erythroblasts. In diseases in which total body iron is markedly increased, iron within the macrophages is also increased. In diseases of iron loading due to frequent transfusion, the iron granules within the cells are large, whereas in diseases such as familial hemochromatosis, the intracellular iron granules are small.[136–138] Intramacrophage iron is also increased in chronic diseases in which the release of iron by the macrophages is impaired. In diseases with disturbed erythropoiesis, the iron within the erythroblasts is not properly used. It accumulates within the mitochondria located around the nuclei of the cells, resulting in the appearance of ringed sideroblasts.[139,140]

Perls' reaction is most useful for evaluating iron overload due to frequent transfusion and ineffective erythropoiesis. It is particularly useful in detecting ringed sideroblastosis.

TABLE 2-1. Summary of Cytochemical Features of Blood Cells

Cytochemical Reaction	Myeloblasts	Promyelocytes	Neutrophils	Eosinophils	Basophil	Monocytes	T_h Lymphocytes	T_s Lymphocytes	T Lymphoblasts	B Lymphocytes
Peroxidase	0–3+	3+	3+	4+	0–1+	0–2+	0	0	0	0
Peroxidase with cyanide	0	0	0	3+	0	0	0	0	0	0
Pseudo-peroxidase	0	0	0	0	0	0	0	0	0	0
Sudan black B	0–3+	3+	3+	4+	0–1+	0–1+	0	0	0	0
Chloroacetate esterase	0–2+	3+	3+	0	0–1+	0–1+	0	0	0	0
α-Naphthyl acetate esterase	0–1+	0–1+	0	0	0	4+D	2+F	0–1+	0–1+F	0–1+
α-Naphthyl butyrate esterase	0	0	0	0	0	4+D	1–2+F	0–1+	0–1+	0–1+
Fluoride-resistant esterase (acetate or butyrate)	0	0	0	0	0	0	0–1+F	0–1+	0–1+F	0–1+
Aminocaproate esterase	0	0	0	0	0	0	0	0	0	0
Alkaline phosphatase	0	0	0–4+	0	0	0	0	0	0	0–1+
Acid phosphatase	0–1+	0–2+	2+	3+	1+	3–4+D	1+F	1–2+D	2–3+F	0–1+D
Tartrate-resistant acid phosphatase	0	0	0	0	0	0	0	0	0–1+F	0
PAS	0–1+	0–1+	3+	1–2+	1–2+	0–1+	0–1+	0–1+	0–1+	0–1+
Iron (Perls' reaction)	0	0	0	0	0	0	0	0	0	0
Toluidine blue O	0	0	0	0	2–3+	0	0	0	0	0

Cytochemical Reaction	B Lymphoblasts	Null Lymphoblasts	Megakaryocytes	Early Erythroblasts	Late Erythroblasts	Plasma Cells	Mast Cells	Hairy Cells	Histiocytes
Peroxidase	0	0	0	0	0	0	0	0	0
Peroxidase with cyanide	0	0	0	0	0	0	0	0	0
Pseudo-peroxidase	0	0	0	0–1+	2–3+	0	0	0	0
Sudan black B	0	0	0	0	0	0	0	0	0–1+
Chloroacetate esterase	0	0	0	0	0	0	4+	0	0–1+
α-Naphthyl acetate esterase	0	0	4+	0–2+F	0–1+F	0–2+	0	0–2+	4+
α-Naphthyl butyrate esterase	0	0	0–1+	0–1+F	0	0	0	0–1+	4+
Fluoride-resistant esterase (acetate or butyrate)	0	0	0–1+	0–1+F	0	0	0	0–1+	3–4+
Aminocaproate esterase	0	0	0	0	0	0	3+	0	0–1+
Alkaline phosphatase	0	0	0	0	0	0	0	0	0
Acid phosphatase	0–1+D	0–1+D	4+	1–2+F	1+F	3+D	3+D	4+D	4+
Tartrate-resistant acid phosphatase	0	0	0–1+	0	0	0	0–2+	4+D	3–4+D
PAS	0–1+	0–2+	4+	0	0	0–2+	2+	0–1+	0–3+
Iron (Perls' reaction)	0	0	0	0	0–2+	0	0	0	0–4+
Toluidine blue O	0	0	0	0	0	0	4+	0	0

D = diffuse staining; F = focal staining.
Note: The intensity of reaction is graded on a scale from 0 to 4+: 0 = no reaction; 4+ = strongest reaction.

The presence of many ringed sideroblasts, although not unique to neoplasia, is characteristic of myelodysplastic syndrome and Di Guglielmo syndrome, especially if the ringed sideroblasts also exhibit a positive PAS reaction.[134,141,142]

TOLUIDINE BLUE O STAIN

Toluidine blue O is a basic dye that reacts with the acid mucopolysaccharides in human blood cells to form metachromatic complexes. Since mucopolysaccharides are easily dissolved in aqueous solution, it is important to use suitable fixatives to insolubilize these substances before staining.[14]

This cytochemical reaction is a specific marker for both basophils and mast cells.[14] It is most useful in the diagnosis of acute basophilic leukemia and systemic mast cell disease.[73,143] In neoplastic disorders, however, the acid mucopolysaccharides in the neoplastic basophils and mast cells may be scarce and cannot be demonstrated. Therefore, a negative toluidine blue reaction should not be considered as an absolute criterion to exclude such neoplasms.

MISCELLANEOUS REACTIONS

Several other cytochemical reactions have also been advocated for the diagnosis of hematologic neoplasms. Arylsulfatase has been reported to selectively stain the nuclei of lymphoblasts,[144,145] but we have found this cytochemical reaction difficult to reproduce, and its clinical value has not been reaffirmed.

Oil red O is useful for staining neutral fats, especially in cases of Burkitt's lymphoma.[35,37]

Adenosine triphosphatase activity in the plasma cells is significantly lower in myeloma than in normal subjects.[146] This enzyme may be a useful marker for B lymphocytes because the adenosine triphosphatase activity is higher in B cells than in T cells,[147,148] but the clinical utility of this reaction has not been fully evaluated due to inherent technical difficulties.

Monoamine oxidase activity is not demonstrable in human blood cells, but it has been observed in neurogenic tissue and is present in neuroblastoma tumor cells.[149] Therefore, monoamine oxidase is of considerable value in the differential diagnosis between neuroblastoma and ALL (CY Li, LT Yam, unpublished data).

β-Glucuronidase is present in many types of human blood cells.[150–152] Its activity in T lymphocytes is significantly higher than that in B lymphocytes of healthy people and patients with lymphoproliferative disorders[105,153–155] β-Glucuronidase is fairly labile and difficult to demonstrate and, therefore, has not been used extensively as a marker to evaluate lymphoproliferative disorders.

Both dipeptidyl-amino-peptidase (DAPII and IV)[156,157] and N-acetyl glucosaminidase[158,159] are potentially useful markers for T lymphocytes. With the advent of flow cytometry and the immunologic markers for precise identification

TABLE 2-2. Cell Specificity and Clinical Applications of Cytochemical Reactions

Cytochemical Reactions	Cell Specificity	Clinical Applications
Peroxidase	Granulocytes, monocytes	Acute leukemia
Peroxidase with cyanide	Eosinophils	Marker for eosinophils
Pseudoperoxidase	Erythroblasts	Marker for erythroblasts
Sudan black B	Granulocytes	Acute leukemia
Chloroacetate esterase	Neutrophils	Marker for neutrophils, acute leukemia
α-Naphthyl acetate esterase	Monocytes, histiocytes, megakaryocytes, plasma cells	Monocytic leukemia, histiocytosis
α-Naphthyl butyrate esterase	Monocytes, histiocytes	Monocytic leukemia, histiocytosis
Fluoride-resistant esterase (acetate or butyrate)	Histiocytes	Marker for specialized histiocytes
Acid α-naphthyl acetate esterase	Helper T cells	T-CLL
Aminocaproate esterase	Mast cells	Mast cell disorders
Alkaline phosphatase	Neutrophils, osteoblasts, B-lymphocyte subset	CML, polycythemia vera, lymphoma
Acid phosphatase	T lymphoblasts	T-ALL, T lymphomas
Tartrate-resistant acid phosphatase	Hairy cells, histiocytes	Hairy cell leukemia
PAS	Abnormal blast cells	Acute leukemia, Di Guglielmo syndrome
Iron	Iron	Iron load, sideroblastosis
Toluidine blue O	Basophils, mast cells	Acute leukemia, mast cell disease

CML = chronic myeloid leukemia; T-ALL = T-cell acute lymphoblastic leukemia; T-CLL = T-cell chronic lymphocytic leukemia.

of subsets of T lymphocytes, these two cytochemical markers have not been used clinically as T-cell markers.

Although each cytochemical reaction is specific for one or more cell types, the selective use of certain combinations may further separate these cells into subtypes, such as suppressor T cells and helper T cells, and may identify certain diseases, such as hairy cell leukemia. Cytochemical markers for individual cell types and their clinical applications are summarized in Tables 2-1 and 2-2.

REFERENCES

1. Graham RC, Karnovski MJ: The early stages of absorption of injected horseradish peroxidase in the proximal tubules of mouse kidney: Ultrastructural cytochemistry by a new technique. *J Histochem Cytochem* 14:291–301, 1966.
2. Kaplow LS: Simplified myeloperoxidase stain using benzidine dihydrochloride. *Blood* 26:215–219, 1965.
3. Washburn AH: A combined peroxidase and Wright's stain for routine blood smears. *J Lab Clin Med* 14:246–250, 1928.
4. Graham RC, Lundholm U, Karnovsky MJ: Cytochemical demonstration of peroxidase activity with 3-amino-9-ethylcarbazole. *J Histochem Cytochem* 13:150–152, 1965.
5. Kaplow LS: Substitute for benzidine in myeloperoxidase stains. *Am J Clin Pathol* 63:451, 1975.
6. Benavides I, Catovsky D: Myeloperoxidase cytochemistry using 2,7-fluorenediamine. *J Clin Pathol* 31:114–116, 1978.
7. Inagaki A, Uno S, Yoneda M, et al: 2,7-Fluorenediamine and 2,5-fluorenediamine as peroxidase reagents for blood smears. *J Lab Clin Med* 88:334–338, 1976.
8. Lillie RD, Fullmer HM: *Histopathologic Technic and Practical Histochemistry*, ed 4. New York, McGraw-Hill, 1976, p 451.
9. Quaglino D, Flemans R: Peroxidase staining in leucocytes. *Lancet* 2:1020, 1958.
10. Hanker JS, Yates PE, Metz CB, et al: A new specific, sensitive and noncarcinogenic reagent for the demonstration of horseradish peroxidase. *Histochem J* 9:789–792, 1977.
11. Himmelhoch SR, Evans WH, Mage MG, et al: Purification of myeloperoxidases from the bone marrow of the guinea pig. *Biochemistry* 8:914–921, 1969.
12. Marishita Y, Marishima Y, Ogma M, et al: Biochemical characterization of human myeloperoxidase using three specific monoclonal antibodies. *Br J Haematol* 63:435–444, 1986.
13. Archer RK, Broome J: Studies on the peroxidase reaction of living eosinophils and other leukocytes. *Acta Haematol* 29:147–156, 1963.
14. Yam LT, Li CY, Crosby WH: Cytochemical identification of monocytes and granulocytes. *Am J Clin Pathol* 55:283–290, 1971.
15. Bolscher BGJM, Plat M, Wever R: Some properties of human eosinophil peroxidase: A comparison with other peroxidase. *Biochim Biophys Acta* 184:177–186, 1984.
16. Li CY, Yam LT, Crosby WH: Histochemical characterization of cellular and structural elements of the human spleen. *J Histochem Cytochem* 20:1049–1058, 1972.
17. Undritz E: *Sandoz Atlas of Haematology*, ed 2. Basle Switzerland, Sandoz, 1973, p 35.
18. Breton-Gorius J, Guichard J: Ultrastructural localization of peroxidase activity in human platelets and megakaryocytes. *Am J Pathol* 66:277–286, 1972.
19. Reyes F, Gourdin MF, Farcet JP, et al: Synthesis of a peroxidase activity by cells of hairy cell leukemia: A study by ultrastructural cytochemistry. *Blood* 52:537–550, 1978.
20. Hanker JS, Ambrose WW, James CJ, et al: Facilitated light microscopic cytochemical diagnosis of acute myelogenous leukemia. *Cancer Res* 39:1635–1639, 1979.
21. Breton-Gorius J, Houssay D, Dreyfus B: Partial myeloperoxidase deficiency in a case of preleukaemia, I: Studies of fine structure and peroxidase synthesis of promyelocytes. *Br J Haematol* 30:273–278, 1975.
22. Catovsky D, Galton DAG, Robinson J: Myeloperoxidase-deficient neutrophils in acute myeloid leukaemia. *Scand J Haematol* 9:142–148, 1972.
23. Salmon SE, Cline MJ, Schultz J, et al: Myeloperoxidase deficiency: Immunologic study of a genetic leukocyte defect. *N Engl J Med* 282:250–253, 1970.
24. Lee EJ, Pollak A, Leavitt RP, et al: Minimally differentiated acute nonlymphocytic leukemia. A distinct entity. *Blood* 5:1400–1406, 1987.
25. Pui CH, Behan FG, Kalwinsky DK, et al: Clinical significance of low levels of myeloperoxidase positivity in childhood acute nonlymphoblastic leukemia. *Blood* 70:51–54, 1987.
26. Matutes E, de Oliveira MP, Foroni L, et al: The role of ultrastructural cytochemistry and monoclonal antibodies in clarifying the nature of undifferentiated cells in acute leukemia. *Br J Haematol* 69:205–211, 1988.
27. Lanham GR, Bollum FJ, Williams DL, et al: Simultaneous occurrence of terminal deoxynucleotidyl transferase and myeloperoxidase in individual leukemic blasts. *Blood* 64:318–320, 1984.
28. Kaplan SS, Penchausky L, Krause JR, et al: Simultaneous evaluation of terminal deoxynucleotidyl transferase and myeloperoxidase in acute leukemias using an immunocytochemical method. *Am J Clin Pathol* 87:732–738, 1987.
29. Parreira A, de Oliveira MSP, Matutes E, et al: Terminal deoxynucleotidyl transferase positive acute myeloid leukemia: An associated with immature myeloblastic leukemia. *Br J Haematol* 69:219–224, 1988.
30. Baillif RN, Kimbrough C: Studies on leukocyte granules after staining with sudan black B and May-Grunwald-Giemsa. *J Lab Clin Med* 32:155–166, 1947.
31. Hayhoe FGJ: The cytochemical demonstration of lipids in blood and bone marrow cells. *J Pathol Bacteriol* 65:413–421, 1953.
32. Lillie RD, Burtner HJ: Stable sudanophilia of human neutrophil leukocytes in relation to peroxidase and oxidase. *J Histochem Cytochem* 1:8–26, 1953.
33. Sheehan HL, Storey GW: An improved method of staining

leukocyte granules with Sudan black B. *J Pathol Bacteriol* 59:336–337, 1947.
34. Rheingold JJ, Wislocki GB: Histochemical methods applied to hematology. *Blood* 3:641–655, 1948.
35. Berard CW, O'Conor GT, Thomas LB, et al: Histopathological definition of Burkitt's tumour. *Bull WHO* 40:601–607, 1969.
36. Tricot G, Orshoven AB-V, Van Hoof A, et al: Sudan black B positivity in acute lymphoblastic leukaemia. *Br J Haematol* 51:615–621, 1982.
37. Wright DH: Cytology and histochemistry of the Burkitt lymphoma. *Br J Cancer* 17:50–55, 1963.
38. Gomori G: Chloracyl esters as histochemical substrates. *J Histochem Cytochem* 1:469–470, 1953.
39. Moloney WC, McPherson K, Fliegelman L: Esterase activity in leukocytes demonstrated by the use of naphthol AS-D chloroacetate substrate. *J Histochem Cytochem* 8:200–207, 1960.
40. Li CY, Lam KW, Yam LT: Esterases in human leukocytes. *J Histochem Cytochem* 21:1–12, 1973.
41. Rindler R, Schmalzl F, Hörtnagl H, et al: Naphthol ASD chloroacetate esterase in granule extracts from human neutrophil leukocytes. *Blut* 23:223–227, 1971.
42. Rindler-Ludwig R, Schmalzl F, Braunsteiner H: Esterases in human neutrophil granulocytes: Evidence for their protease nature. *Br J Haematol* 27:57–64, 1974.
43. Sweetman F, Ornstein L: Electrophoresis of elastase-like esterases from human neutrophils. *J Histochem Cytochem* 22:327–339, 1974.
44. Fischer R, Schmalzl F: Über die hemmbarkeit der esterase aktivitat in blutmonocyten durch natriumfluorid. *Klin Wochenschr* 42:751, 1964.
45. Leder LD: Über die seleketive fermentcytochemische darstellung von neutrophilen myeloischen zellen und gevebsmastzellen im paraffinschmitt. *Klin Wochenschr* 42:553, 1964.
46. Neiman RS, Barcos M, Berard C, et al: Granulocytic sarcoma: A clinicopathologic study of 61 biopsied cases. *Cancer* 48:1426–1437, 1981.
47. Furebring-Fredin M, Martinsson U, Sundström C: Myelosarcoma without acute leukaemia: Immunohistochemical and clinicopathologic characterization of eight cases. *Histopathology* 16:243–250, 1990.
48. Kass L, Peters CL, Vugrin D: Electrophoretic properties of esterases in chronic granulocytic leukemia. *Am J Clin Pathol* 69:329–332, 1978.
49. Radzun HJ, Parwaresch MR, Kulenlampff C, et al: Lysosomal acid esterase: Activity and isoenzymes in separated normal human blood cells. *Blood* 55:891–897, 1980.
50. Young CW, Bittar ES: Analysis of tissue esterases from patients with Hodgkin's disease and other types of advanced cancer by isoelectric focusing in acrylamide gel. *Cancer Res* 33:2692–2700, 1973.
51. Scott CS, Morgan MAM, Limbert HJ, et al: Cytochemical, immunological, and ANAE-isoenzyme studies in acute myelomonocytic leukemia: A study of 39 cases. *Scand J Haematol* 35:284–291, 1985.
52. Braunstein H: Esterase in leukocytes. *J Histochem Cytochem* 7:202, 1959.
53. Schmalzl F, Braunsteiner H: Zytochemische Darstellung von esteraseaktivitäten in blut- und knochenmarkszellen. *Klin Wochenschr* 46:642–650, 1968.
54. Wachstein M, Wolf G: The histochemical demonstration of esterase activity in human blood and bone marrow smears. *J Histochem Cytochem* 6:457, 1958.
55. Yam LT, Tavassoli M, Jacobs P: Differential characterization of the "reticulum cells" in lymphoreticular neoplasms. *Am J Clin Pathol* 64:171–179, 1975.
56. Bennett JM, Reed CE: Acute leukemia cytochemical profile: Diagnostic and clinical implications. *Blood Cells* 1:101–108, 1975.
57. Grusovin GD, Castoldi GL: Characterization of blast cells in acute nonlymphoid leukemias by consecutive cytochemical reactions. *Acta Haematol* 55:338–345, 1976.
58. Li CY, Harrison EG Jr: Histochemical and immunohistochemical study of diffuse large cell lymphomas. *Am J Clin Pathol* 70:721–732, 1978.
59. Schmalzl F, Braunsteiner H: The application of cytochemical methods to the study of acute leukemia: A review. *Acta Haematol* 45:209–217, 1971.
60. Li CY, Phyliky RL, Yam LT: Acute myelomonocytic leukemia: An unusual variant with both granulocytic and monocytic esterases in the leukemic cells. *Mayo Clin Proc* 61:104–109, 1986.
61. Knowles DM II, Halper JP, Machin GA, et al: Acid α-naphthyl acetate esterase activity in human neoplastic lymphoid cells: Usefulness as a T-cell marker. *Am J Pathol* 96:257–278, 1979.
62. Kulenkampff J, Janossy G, Greaves MF: Acid esterase in human lymphoid cells and leukemic blasts: A marker for T lymphocytes. *Br J Haematol* 36:231–240, 1977.
63. Mueller J, Brun Del Ré G, Beurk H, et al: Nonspecific acid esterase activity: A criterion for differentiation of T and B lymphocytes in mouse lymph nodes. *Eur J Immunol* 5:270–274, 1975.
64. Armitage RJ, Linch DC, Worman CP, et al: The morphology and cytochemistry of human T-cell subpopulations defined by monoclonal antibodies and Fc receptors. *Br J Haematol* 51:605–613, 1982.
65. Grossi CE, Webb SR, Zicca A, et al: Morphological and histochemical analysis of two human T-cell subpopulations bearing receptors for IgM or IgG. *J Exp Med* 147:1405–1417, 1978.
66. Higgy KE, Burns GF, Hayhoe FGJ: Discrimination of B, T and null lymphocytes by esterase cytochemistry. *Scand J Haematol* 18:437–448, 1977.
67. Palestro G, Novero D, Godio L, et al: Acid hydrolyses in B-chronic lymphocytic leukemia (B-CLL): A comparison with normal peripheral B lymphocytes and normal B cell subset with the phenotype of B leukemic cells. *Leuk Res* 11:429–436, 1987.
68. Costello C, Catovsky D, O'Brien M, et al: Chronic T-cell leukemias, I: Morphology, cytochemistry and ultrastructure. *Leuk Res* 4:463–476, 1980.

69. Crockard AD: Cytochemistry of lymphoid cells: A review of findings in the normal and leukemic state. *Histochem J* 16:1027–1050, 1984.
70. Higgy KE, Burns GF, Hayhoe FGJ: Identification of the hairy cells of leukemic reticuloendotheliosis by an esterase method. *Br J Haematol* 38:99–106, 1978.
71. Tolksdorf G, Stein H: Acid alpha-naphthyl acetate esterase in hairy cell leukemia cells and other cells of the hematopoietic system. *Blut* 39:165–176, 1979.
72. Hopsu VK, Glenner GG: Further observations on histochemical esterase and amidase activities with similarities to trypsin. *J Histochem Cytochem* 11:520–528, 1963.
73. Webb TA, Li CY, Lam LT: Systemic mast cell disease: A clinical and hematopathologic study of 26 cases. *Cancer* 49:927–938, 1982.
74. Yam LT, Yam CF, Li CY: Eosinophilia in systemic mastocytosis. *Am J Clin Pathol* 73:48–54, 1980.
75. Travis WD, Li CY, Hoagland HC, et al: Mast cell leukemia: Report of a case and review of the literature. *Mayo Clin Proc* 61:957–966, 1986.
76. Li CY, Yam LT: Cytochemical characterization of leukemic cells with numerous cytoplasmic granules. *Mayo Clin Proc* 62:978–985, 1987.
77. Travis WD, Li CY, Bergstralh EJ, et al: Systemic mast cell disease: Analysis of 58 cases and literature review. *Medicine* 67:345–368, 1988.
78. Fishman WH: Perspective on alkaline phosphatase isoenzymes. *Am J Med* 56:617–650, 1974.
79. Kaplow LS: Cytochemistry of leukocyte alkaline phosphatase: Use of complex naphthol AS phosphates in azo dye coupling techniques. *Am J Clin Pathol* 39:439–449, 1963.
80. Kaplow LS: Leukocyte alkaline phosphatase cytochemistry: Applications and methods. *Ann NY Acad Sci* 155:911–947, 1968.
81. Kaplow LS: Alkaline phosphatase activity in peripheral blood lymphocytes. *Arch Pathol* 88:69–72, 1969.
82. Robinson JC, Pierce JE, Goldstein DP, et al: Leukocyte-alkaline-phosphatase isoenzymes. *Lancet* 2:805, 1966.
83. Gomori G: Microtechnical demonstration of phosphatase in tissue sections. *Proc Soc Exp Biol Med* 42:23–26, 1939.
84. Rutenburg AM, Rosales CL, Bennett JM: An improved histochemical method for the demonstration of leukocyte alkaline phosphatase activity: Clinical application. *J Lab Clin Med* 65:698–705, 1965.
85. Hardisty RM, Speed DE, Till M: Granulocytic leukaemia in childhood. *Br J Haematol* 10:551–566, 1964.
86. Rubin H: Chronic neutrophilic leukemia. *Ann Intern Med* 65:93–100, 1966.
87. Yam LT: Neutrophilic leukemia. *South Med J* 75:870–872, 1982.
88. Rustin GJS, Boldman JM, McCarthy D, et al: An extrinsic factor controls neutrophil alkaline phosphatase synthesis in chronic granulocytic leukemia. *Br J Haematol* 45:381–387, 1980.
89. Malaskova V, Fuksova J: Alkaline phosphatase activity in immature granulocytes. *Br J Haematol* 15:119–122, 1968.
90. Bottomly RH, Lovig CA, Holt R, et al: Comparison of alkaline phosphatase from human normal and leukemic leukocytes. *Cancer Res* 29:1866–1974, 1969.
91. Rosenblum D, Petzold SJ: Neutrophil alkaline phosphatase: Comparison of enzymes from normal subjects and patients with polycythemia vera and chronic myelogenous leukemia. *Blood* 45:335–343, 1975.
92. DeRenzo A, Micera V, Vaglio S, et al: Induction of alkaline phosphatase activity in chronic myeloid leukemia cells. In vitro studies and speculative hypothesis. *Am J Hematol* 35:278–280, 1990.
93. Bennett JM, Nathanson L, Rutenberg AM: Significance of leukocyte alkaline phosphatase in Hodgkin's disease. *Arch Intern Med* 121:338–341, 1968.
94. Nanba K, Jaffe ES, Braylan RC, et al: Alkaline phosphatase-positive malignant lymphoma: A subtype of B-cell lymphomas. *Am J Clin Pathol* 68:535–542, 1977.
95. Mason DY, Sammons R: Alkaline phosphatase and peroxidase for double immunoenzymatic labelling of cellular constituents. *J Clin Pathol* 31:454–460, 1978.
96. Yam LT, Janckila AJ, Li CY: The immunoalkaline phosphatase methods. In DeLellis RA (ed): *Advances in Immunohistochemistry*. New York, Raven Press, 1988, pp 1–29.
97. Ponder BA, Wilkinson MM: Inhibition of endogenous tissue alkaline phosphatase with the use of alkaline phosphatase conjugates in immunohistochemistry. *J Histochem Cytochem* 29:981–984, 1981.
98. Yam LT: Clinical significance of the human acid phosphatases. A review. *Am J Med* 56:604–616, 1974.
99. Li CY, Yam LT, Lam KW: Acid phosphatase isoenzyme in human leukocytes in normal and pathologic conditions. *Histochem Cytochem* 18:473–481, 1970.
100. Li CY, Yam LT, Lam KW: Studies of acid phosphatase isoenzymes in human leukocytes: Demonstration of isoenzyme cell specificity. *J Histochem Cytochem* 18:901–910, 1970.
101. Janckila AJ, Li CY, Lam KW, et al: The cytochemistry of tartrate-resistant acid phosphatase: Technical considerations. *Am J Clin Pathol* 70:45–55, 1978.
102. Goldberg AF, Barka T: Acid phosphatase activity in human blood cells. *Nature* 195:297, 1962.
103. Valentine WN, Beck WS: Biochemical studies on leucocytes. *J Lab Clin Med* 38:39–55, 1951.
104. Catovsky D, Galetto I, Okos A, et al: Cytochemical profile of B and T leukaemic lymphocytes with special reference to acute lymphoblastic leukaemia. *J Clin Pathol* 27:767–771, 1974.
105. Davey FR, Huntington SJ, Maccallum I, et al: Cytochemical reactions of normal and neoplastic lymphocytes. *J Clin Pathol* 30:653–660, 1977.
106. Huhn D, Thiel E, Rodt H: Classification of normal and malignant lymphatic cells using acid phosphatase and acid esterase. *Klin Wochenschr* 58:65–71, 1980.
107. Wehinger H, Mobius W: Cytochemical studies on T and B lymphocytes and lymphoblasts with special reference to acid phosphatase. *Acta Haematol* 56:129–136, 1976.
108. Catovsky D: T-cell origin of acid phosphatase positive lymphoblasts. *Lancet* 2:327–328, 1975.

109. Catovsky D, Greaves MF, Pain C, et al: Acid-phosphatase reaction in acute lymphoblastic leukemia. *Lancet* 1:749–751, 1978.
110. Smithson WA, Li CY, Pierre RV, et al: Acute lymphoblastic leukemia in children: Immunologic, cytochemical, morphologic, and cytogenetic studies in relation to pretreatment risk factors. *Med Pediatr Oncol* 7:83–93, 1979.
111. Stein H, Petersen N, Gaedicke G, et al: Lymphoblastic lymphoma of convoluted or acid phosphatase type: A tumor of T-precursor cells. *Int J Cancer* 17:292–295, 1976.
112. Head DR, Borowitz M, Cerezo L, et al: Acid phosphatase positivity in childhood acute lymphocytic leukemia. *Am J Clin Pathol* 86:650–653, 1986.
113. Pieters R, Veerman AJP: Prognostic significance of acid alpha naphthyl acetate esterase and acid phosphatase in childhood acute lymphoblastic leukemia. *Leuk Res* 11:995–999, 1987.
114. Mover S, Li CY, Yam LT: Semiquantitative evaluation of tartrate-resistant acid phosphatase activity of human blood cells. *J Lab Clin Med* 80:711–717, 1972.
115. Yam LT, Li CY, Lam KW: Tartrate-resistant acid phosphatase isoenzyme in the reticulum cells of leukemic reticuloendotheliosis. *N Engl J Med* 284:357–360, 1971.
116. Lam KW, Yam LT: Biochemical characterization of the tartrate-resistant acid phosphatase of human spleen with leukemic reticuloendotheliosis as a pyrophosphatase. *Clin Chem* 23:89–94, 1977.
117. Katayama I, Li CY, Yam LT: Histochemical study of acid phosphatase isoenzyme in leukemic reticuloendotheliosis. *Cancer* 29:157–164, 1972.
118. Yam LT, Janckila AJ, Li CY, et al: Cytochemistry of tartrate-resistant acid phosphatase: 15 years' experience. *Leukemia* 1:285–288, 1987.
119. Wislocki BG, Rheingold JJ, Dempsey EW: The occurrence of the periodic acid-Schiff reaction in various normal cells of blood and connective tissues. *Blood* 4:562–568, 1949.
120. McManus JFA: Histological demonstration of mucin after periodic acid (letter). *Nature* 158:202, 1946.
121. Astaldi G, Berga I: The glycogen content of the cells of lymphatic leukemia. *Acta Haematol* 17:129–135, 1957.
122. Bennett JM, Dutcher TF: The cytochemistry of acute leukemia: Observations of glycogen and neutral fat in bone marrow aspirates. *Blood* 33:341–347, 1969.
123. Mitus MJ, Bergna LJ, Mednicoff IB, et al: Cytochemical studies of glycogen content of lymphocytes in lymphocytic proliferations. *Blood* 13:748–756, 1958.
124. Quaglino D, Hayhoe FGJ: Observations of the periodic acid-Schiff reaction in lymphoproliferative diseases. *J Pathol Bacteriol* 78:521–532, 1959.
125. Quaglino D, Hayhoe FGJ: Periodic acid-Schiff positivity in erythroblasts with special reference to Di Guglielmo's disease. *Br J Haematol* 6:26–33, 1960.
126. Galbraith P, Mitus WJ, Gollerkeri, et al: The "infectious mononucleosis cell": A cytochemical study. *Blood* 22:630–638, 1963.
127. Astaldi G, Rondanelli EG, Bernardelli E, et al: An abnormal substance present in the erythroblasts of thalassaemia major: Cytochemical investigation. *Acta Haematol* 12:145–153, 1954.
128. Klein HO, Heller A: PAS-positive erythroblasts in kidney disease. *Acta Haematol* 37:225–239, 1967.
129. Valentine WN, Follette JH, Lawrence JS: The glycogen content of human leukocytes in health and in varous disease states. *J Clin Invest* 32:251–257, 1953.
130. Andreewa P, Huhn D, Thiel E, et al: Comparison of enzyme cytochemical findings and immunological marker investigations in acute lymphoblastic leukemia (ALL). *Blut* 36:299–305, 1978.
131. Feldges JA, Aur RJA, Verzosa MS, et al: Periodic acid-Schiff reaction, a useful index of duration of complete remission in acute childhood lymphocytic leukemia. *Acta Haematol* 52:8–13, 1974.
132. Humphrey GB, Nesbit ME, Brunning RD: Prognostic value of the periodic acid-Schiff reaction in acute lymphoblastic leukemia. *Am J Clin Pathol* 61:393–397, 1974.
133. Lilleyman JS, Scott CS: PAS- and acid phosphatase cytochemistry in acute lymphoblastic leukemia. In Scott SC (ed): *Leukemia Cytochemistry: Principle and Practice*. Chichester, UK, Ellis Horwood, 1989, pp 103–120.
134. Hayhoe FGJ, Quaglino D: Refractory sideroblastic anaemia and erythraemic myelosis: Possible relationship and cytochemical observations. *Br J Haematol* 6:381–387, 1960.
135. Perls M: Nachweis von eisenoxyd in gewissen pigmenten. *Virchows Arch (Pathol Anat)* 39:42–48, 1867.
136. Astaldi G, Meardi G, Lisino T: The iron content of jejunal mucosa obtained by Crosby's biopsy in hemochromatosis and hemosiderosis. *Blood* 28:70–82, 1966.
137. Cooperberg AA, Rosenberg A, Schwartz JP: Diagnostic value of bone marrow iron deposits in idiopathic hemochromatosis. *Arch Intern Med* 137:748–751, 1977.
138. Yam LT, Finkel HE, Weintraub LR, et al: Circulating iron-containing macrophages in hemochromatosis. *N Engl J Med* 279:512–514, 1968.
139. Björkman SE: Chronic refractory anemia with sideroblastic bone marrow: A study of four cases. *Blood* 11:250–259, 1956.
140. Dacie JV, Smith MD, White JC, et al: Refractory normoblastic anaemia: A clinical and haematological study of seven cases. *Br J Haematol* 5:56–81, 1959.
141. Bennett JM, Catovsky D, Daniel MT, et al: Proposals for the classification of the myelodysplastic syndromes. *Br J Haematol* 51:189–199, 1982.
142. Seo IS, Li CY, Yam LT: Myelodysplastic syndrome: Diagnostic implications of cytochemical and immunocytochemical studies. *Mayo Clin Proc* 68:47–53, 1993.
143. Wick MR, Li CY, Pierre RV: Acute nonlymphocytic leukemia with basophilic differentiation. *Blood* 60:38–45, 1982.
144. Austin JH, Bischel M: A histochemical method for sulfatase activity in hemic cells and organ imprints. *Blood* 17:216–224, 1961.
145. Ekert H, Denett X: An evaluation of nuclear aryl sulphatase activity as an aid to the cytological diagnosis of acute leukemia. *Aust Ann Med* 15:152–156, 1966.
146. Schubert VJCF, Schubert H: Die zytologische diagnose des

plasmozytoms am knochenmarkausstrich mit hilfe der adenosintriphosphatase-reaktion. *Blut* 19:78–98, 1969.
147. Harigaya K, Mikata A, Suzuki H, et al: Mg^{2+}-dependent adenosine triphosphatase as an enzyme histochemical marker for the lymphomas of B-cell origin. *Am J Pathol* 97:359–380, 1979.
148. Müller-Hermelink HR: Characterization of the B-cell and T-cell regions of human lymphatic tissue through enzyme histochemical demonstration of ATPase and 5′-nucleotidase activities. *Virchows Arch (Cell Pathol)* 16:371–378, 1974.
149. Glenner GG, Burtner HJ, Brown GW: The histochemical demonstration of monoamine oxidase activity by tetrazolium salts. *J Histochem Cytochem* 5:591–600, 1957.
150. Follette JH, Valentine WH, Lawrence JS: The beta-glucuronidase content of human leukocytes in health and in disease. *J Lab Clin Med* 40:825–840, 1952.
151. Lorbacher P, Yam LT, Mitus WJ: Cytochemical demonstration of β-glucuronidase activity in blood and bone marrow cells. *J Histochem Cytochem* 15:680–687, 1967.
152. Yam LT, Mitus WJ: The lymphocyte β-glucuronidase activity in lymphoproliferative disorders. *Blood* 31:480–489, 1968.
153. Flandrin G, Daniel MT: β:Glucuronidase activity in Sézary cells. *Scand J Haematol* 12:23–31, 1974.
154. Machin GA, Halper JP, Knowles DM II: Cytochemically demonstrable β-glucuronidase activity in normal and neoplastic human lymphoid cells. *Blood* 56:1111–1119, 1980.
155. Pangalis GA, Yataganas X, Fessas PH: β-Glucuronidase activity of lymph node imprints of malignant lymphomas and chronic lymphocytic leukemia. *J Clin Pathol* 30:812–816, 1977.
156. Chilosi M, Pizzolo G, Menestrina F, et al: Dipeptidyl-aminopeptidase (DAP IV) histochemistry in normal and pathological lymphoid tissues. *Am J Clin Pathol* 77:714–719, 1982.
157. Khalaf MR, Agel NM, Hayhoe FGJ: Histochemistry of dipeptidyl aminopeptidase (DAP II and IV) in reactive lymphoid tissues and malignant lymphoma. *J Clin Pathol* 40:480–485, 1987.
158. Orge E, Benoit Y, Roesbeke L, et al: Acetyl glucosaminidase: A new cytochemical marker of human lymphocyte subpopulations. *Histochemistry* 82:19–24, 1985.
159. Invernizzi R, Perugini O: Cytochemistry of N-acetyl-β-glucosaminidase in normal and leukemic cells. *Acta Haematol* 77:6–10, 1987.

Chapter 3
HISTOCHEMISTRY

Histochemistry, like *cytochemistry*, is defined as the science of microscopic examination and identification of the chemical constituents in tissues. These terms are often used interchangeably, but in a strict sense, histochemistry denotes chemical studies of tissue sections, whereas cytochemistry denotes studies of cytologic materials, such as cell suspensions, smears, and imprints. In this chapter, the strict definition of histochemistry is used.

Many of the enzyme reactions used in histochemistry are the same as those used in cytochemistry. Because many of these reactions were presented in detail in Chapter 2, this information will not be repeated. However, certain aspects of histochemical studies are different from cytochemical studies, such as topographic distribution of chemical reactions, method of tissue preparation, and the clinical significance of the histochemical studies (Table 3-1). These special problems will be discussed in this chapter. Studies concerning the immunochemistry of tissue antigens will be discussed in the following chapter.

PREPARATION OF TISSUES

Marrow, lymph node, spleen, and liver tissues and tumor masses in nonhematopoietic tissues are often used for histochemical studies. The results of these histochemical studies are closely related to the methods of tissue preparation.

Tissues Embedded in Paraffin

Paraffin embedding is the conventional method of preparing tissue sections for staining with hematoxylin and eosin, Giemsa, and many other nonenzymatic stains.[1,2] The embedding process involves the treatment of tissues with prolonged heating at 56°C in molten paraffin and repeated washing in organic solvents, such as xylene and alcohols. These harsh treatments inactivate most enzymes and alter the antigenic properties of many cell surface molecules. Tissues prepared by this method are, therefore, not suitable for the study of enzymes and surface antigens. However, chloroacetate esterase[3] and several cytoplasmic antigens, such as immunoglobulins[4,5] and lysozyme,[6] are not significantly affected and can be demonstrated in cells of paraffin-embedded tissues. When the tissue preparatory process is suitably modified, special studies for enzymes and tissue antigens may be made with some success.[7,8]

Fresh Frozen Tissues

Tissue sections can be prepared by cryostat sectioning of fresh specimens, with or without prior freezing in liquid nitrogen. Activity of enzymes and cell surface antigens are well preserved in tissues prepared in this manner.[9-13] The disadvantage of these methods is that cytoplasmic enzymes and antigens may leak out of the cells into surrounding areas, leading to imprecise localization. In addition, the morphology of the cells in these preparations is often less than ideal. However, both of these shortcomings can be overcome by briefly fixing the tissues with dilute formaldehyde or acetone-containing fixatives before staining.[14]

Fixed Tissues and Cryostat Sectioning

Since many enzymes and tissue antigens withstand gentle fixation, biopsy or autopsy tissues intended for histochemical studies can be prepared by fixation in cold, formaldehyde-containing compounds at neutral pH for a controlled period of time and then sectioning in a cryostat.[15-17] Cellular morphology in tissue sections prepared in this way is better than that in unfixed tissues but not as good as the cellular morphology of tissue sections prepared by embedding in paraffin or plastics. Bone marrow specimens, decalcified rapidly by strong acidic reagents, often yield poor cellular morphology and cannot be used for enzymatic histochemical studies. We prefer to decalcify these specimens more gradually (12 to 48 hr) with either

TABLE 3-1. Cell Specificity and Possible Clinical Applications of Histochemical Reactions

Histochemical Reactions	Specimen	Cell Specificity	Clinical Application
Peroxidase	F, Pl	Granulocytes	Acute leukemia
Cyanide-resistant peroxidase	F, Pl	Eosinophils	Marker for eosinophils
Sudan black B	F	Fat and cells with fat deposits	Limited
Chloroacetate esterase	F, Pl, Pa	Neutrophils, mast cells	Granulocytic sarcoma, myeloid metaplasia, mast cell disease
α-Naphthyl acetate esterase	F	Monocytes, histiocytes, megakaryocytes, plasma cells, splenic sinusoidal cells	Monocytic and histiocytic disorders
α-Naphthyl butyrate esterase	F	Monocytes, histiocytes, splenic sinusoidal cells	Monocytic and histiocytic disorders
Fluoride-resistant esterase	F	Histiocytes	Marker for specialized tissue histiocytes
Acid α-naphthyl acetate esterase	F	Helper T cells	Marker for helper T cells
Aminocaproate esterase	F, Pl	Mast cells	Mast cell disease
Naphthol AS acetate esterase	F	Splenic sinusoidal cells	Marker for splenic sinusoids
Alkaline phosphatase	F	Vascular endothelial cells, B-lymphocyte subset	Marker for blood vessels, B-cell lymphomas
Acid phosphatase	F	T lymphoblasts, transformed T cells	T-ALL, T-cell lymphomas
Tartrate-resistant acid phosphatase	F, Pl	Hairy cells, specialized histiocytes, osteoclasts	Hairy cell leukemia, early granulomas, giant cell tumors
PAS	Pl, Pa	Supporting framework	Architecture of hematopoietic tissues
β-Glucuronidase	F	Histiocytes, T lymphocytes	Limited
Reticulin stain			
Jones' silver methenamine	F, Pl, Pa	Basement membrane	Splenic sinusoidal structure
Gomori's silver impregnation	F, Pl, Pa	Reticulin fibers	Reticulin fibrosis, hairy cell leukemia, mast cell disease
Methyl green-pyronine	Pa	Primitive hematopoietic cells, plasma cells	Plasma cell disorders
Iron stain (Perls' reaction)	F, Pl, Pa	Iron, sideroblasts	Storage iron, ringed sideroblasts
Oil red O	F	Fat	Burkitt's lymphoma
Chlorazol fast pink	F, Pl, Pa	Eosinophils	Marker for eosinophils
Toluidine blue O	Pl, Pa	Basophils, mast cells	Mast cell disease

F = cryostat section of fresh frozen tissue; Pa = paraffin-embedded section; Pl = plastic-embedded section.

weak acids (i.e., formic or citric acids) or chelating agents (e.g., ethylenediaminetetraacetic acid).[18]

Tissues Embedded in Plastics

Plastics such as glycol methacrylate have been used as embedding materials for tissues and provide excellent preservation of cellular morphology.[7,19] The enzyme activities in such tissues, however, are often markedly diminished if special attention is not given to properly preparing the tissue before sectioning. To preserve the enzyme activities in such tissues, it is necessary to fix the tissues optimally and embed them at low temperatures with a reduced amount of catalyst.[7,20-24] Although some progress has been made,[25] plastic-embedded tissues are often not suitable for most of the immunohistochemical studies and are, at present, of limited clinical value for these special studies.

PEROXIDASE REACTION

Peroxidase is fairly sensitive to heat and storage, and can be best demonstrated in cryostat-cut frozen sections but not in tissues embedded in paraffin. For this reason, it is not used as often as chloroacetate esterase in tissue sections for diagnostic purposes. The peroxidase reaction, however, is more sensitive than the chloroacetate esterase reaction as a marker for primitive myeloid cells.[26] When histochemical methods for peroxidase in plastic-embedded sections have been fully developed, this enzyme marker should be used more frequently.[7,20,21] Another approach is to develop an immunohistochemical method using monoclonal anti-myeloperoxidase (MPO7) antibody, which has recently been made available and has been used in immunocytochemical identification of myeloblasts.[27,28] The methods most suitable for histochemical demonstration of the peroxidases are those of Graham and Karnovsky,[29] using 3,3-diaminobenzidine; Hanker et al.,[30] using pyrocatechol and p-phenylenediamine; and Graham et al.,[31] using aminocarbazole at pH 7.6. The peroxidase stain, when properly modified, can be used for the demonstration of hemoglobin in both erythrocytes and late stages of erythroblasts (Lepehne's or pseudoperoxidase reaction).[32,33] This stain, however, has been replaced by the more sensitive immunohistochemical technique using specific antibodies to hemoglobin.[34]

SUDAN BLACK B STAIN

Although Sudan black B has been used extensively in cytochemistry as a marker for the primitive myeloid cells and for fat-containing cells, it is technically difficult to use for such a purpose in tissue sections.

CHLOROACETATE ESTERASE REACTION

Chloroacetate esterase is very stable and is highly resistant to inactivation by storage and tissue processing.[3] Enzyme activity can be easily demonstrated in the myeloid cells in paraffin-embedded sections that have been stored for many years. However, these enzymes are readily inactivated in tissues fixed with Zenker's solution and fixatives containing mercury salts (B5 solution). The chloroacetate esterase reaction is most useful as a diagnostic aid for identifying myeloid cells in cases of myelofibrosis with myeloid metaplasia and in cases of granulocytic sarcoma.[3,35,36] However, it is not sensitive enough to stain the early myeloblasts in some cases of granulocytic sarcoma. Under such circumstances, the use of lysozyme stain may offer additional diagnostic assistance.[36] The chloroacetate esterase reaction, when applied to tissue sections, is not uniquely positive in the myeloid cells; mast cells also possess this enzyme. When tissues contain many cells positive for chloroacetate esterase, the possibility of mast cell disease also should be considered.[35,37]

NONSPECIFIC ESTERASE REACTION

Nonspecific esterase is intended for the histochemical demonstration of monocytes and true histiocytes.[9–11,14,38] Tissues suitable for this purpose include those frozen and cut by a cryostat and those embedded in plastics; tissues embedded in paraffin are not suitable for this purpose.

For staining, we prefer to use α-naphthyl butyrate and hexazotized pararosaniline.[15,20,21] When sodium fluoride is added to the incubating solution, enzyme activity in the monocytes and many tissue histiocytes is abolished. Enzyme activity is retained only in the specialized or differentiated histiocytes, such as the Gaucher's cells in Gaucher's disease, and in the epithelioid cells in the granuloma of Hodgkin's disease and in sarcoidosis.[14,15,39] Thus, the fluoride-resistant esterase may be useful in detection early or small granulomatous foci that may not be visible in specimens stained by either hematoxylin and eosin or Giemsa.[39]

ACID α-NAPHTHYL ACETATE ESTERASE REACTION

The method for demonstrating esterase in monocytes uses α-naphthyl butyrate-pararosaniline in an incubating medium with a final pH of approximately 6.1. It demonstrates enzyme activity well not only in monocytes but also in some lymphocytes[40]; these lymphocytes with esterase activity are probably helper T cells.[41]

In the ANAE reaction, α-naphthyl acetate is used instead of α-naphthyl butyrate. When α-naphthyl acetate is used as a substrate, the pH of the incubating medium is lowered to approximately 5.5 and the incubation period is prolonged; the esterase activity in monocytes is suppressed considerably, whereas that in T lymphocytes is enhanced.[42,43] Thus, ANAE demonstrates T cells only and is more specific than α-naphthyl butyrate esterase. Esterase activity in T lymphocytes can also be enhanced.[42,43] This activity can be demonstrated in an alkaline medium.[44] However, because the background staining is higher and the esterase activity in monocytes and histiocytes remains considerably stronger in the alkaline medium, this method may not be as selective for T cells as the method using the acid medium.

The histochemical method for ANAE has been used for the demonstration of topographic localization of the T lymphocytes in tissues.[45] Its clinical value, however, has not been fully realized.

AMINOCAPROATE ESTERASE REACTION

Aminocaproate esterase is a useful marker for mast cells and is clinically important for the accurate diagnosis of systemic mast cell disease. However, it is very labile and cannot be demonstrated in paraffin-embedded tissue sections.[37,46] Although enzyme activity is well preserved in frozen sections, with or without fixation, it is technically difficult to prepare sections with satisfactory cellular morphology. The availability of plastics as embedding media has facilitated the optimal staining of the mast cells for aminocaproate esterase.[20,21,47] The method using naphthol AS aminocaproate and hexazotized new fuchsin provides a very chromogenic reaction product with precise cellular localization of the enzyme. Alternatively, methods using the same substrate and either fast red ITR or fast blue BBN as a coupler are more sensitive, although the enzyme localization of these methods is less precise than that of the new fuchsin method. If the staining time for this enzyme is prolonged, weak staining activity may be seen in the immature myeloid cells in extramedullary tissues of myelofibrosis with myeloid metaplasia.

NAPHTHOL AS ACETATE ESTERASE REACTION

Cytochemical demonstration of naphthol AS acetate esterase, with or without sodium fluoride inhibition, has been used as a specific marker for granulocytes and monocytes.[48–52] The drawbacks of the method for this purpose have been discussed previously (see, in Chapter 2, "Nonspecific Esterase Reaction"). Histochemical demonstration of this enzyme under controlled experimental conditions has revealed preferential staining in the sinusoidal cells of the spleen[13,15]; however, some of the macrophages in the spleen are also positive with this stain. These macrophages may have nonspecific esterase activity that is either fluoride-sensitive or fluoride-resistant. This finding suggests that tissue macrophages are heterogeneous and that further study of these cells with several histochemical reactions for the esterases may allow separation of these cells into a number of subsets.

ALKALINE PHOSPHATASE REACTION

Histochemical demonstration of alkaline phosphatase in tissue sections is not intended to identify the neutrophils in CML and polycythemia vera but, rather, to delineate the lymphocytes in the mantle zone of lymph follicles, the osteoblasts of bone, and the vascular endothelial cells.[9–11,15,20,21,53] By decreasing the pH of the incubating solution to 8.2 or less and by using a buffer such as barbital, which exerts inhibiting effects on the neutrophilic enzyme, it is possible to increase the specificity of the alkaline phosphatase reaction for these special tissue components.[15] More recently, alkaline phosphatase has been used as an enzyme indicator for immunohistochemical identification of specific tissue antigens.[54,55] This application will be discussed in more detail in the following chapter.

ACID PHOSPHATASE REACTION

Acid phosphatase has been examined extensively from the viewpoint of cell research. The method using naphthol AS-BI phosphate and hexazotized pararosaniline is recommended for histochemical demonstration of this enzyme because it provides precise localization of the reaction product.[56,57] The acid phosphatase reaction has been used as a marker for T lymphocytes and has proved to be of considerable value for the diagnosis of T-cell lymphomas and leukemias.[14,58–60]

TARTRATE-RESISTANT ACID PHOSPHATASE REACTION

Cytochemical demonstration of tartrate-resistant acid phosphatase in leukocytes is a useful adjunct for the diagnosis of hairy cell leukemia.[61] In blood, the detection of at least two or more cells with intense activity is strongly suggestive of hairy cell leukemia.[62] In tissues other than blood, cells such as Gaucher's cells in Gaucher's disease, epithelioid cells in the granulomatous tissues, osteoclasts in bone, and some of the phagocytic histiocytes in spleen and lymph nodes also contain abundant amounts of this isoenzyme. Because the morphology and location of these tissue cells are different, these cells should not be confused with hairy cells.

The modified method of Barka and Anderson[56] is best for demonstrating tartrate-resistant acid phosphatase in tissues.[15,57] This method is less sensitive than the fast garnet GBC method,[15,57] and cells with weak enzyme activity, as demonstrated cytochemically, often fail to show unequivocal staining on tissue sections. However, histochemical study of tissue sections shows both the histologic features of the tumor and the intensity and topography of the enzyme activity in tumor cells. Therefore, for accurate diagnosis of hairy cell leukemia, histochemical study of this isoenzyme in tissue sections may be more advantageous than cytochemical study of blood cells.[15,63,64] In addition, this reaction is useful in identifying early or small granulomas that may be otherwise overlooked in sections stained with Giemsa or hematoxylin and eosin.[39,63]

PAS REACTION

The PAS reaction is employed to outline the supporting structures, reticulin fibers, and sinusoids of the spleen and marrow. It may also help to identify the granulocytes, the megakaryocytes, and, to a lesser extent, the degree of fibrosis. The PAS reaction is also useful for demonstrating the "intranuclear" inclusions or Dutcher bodies that are frequently seen in the plasmacytoid cells in macroglobulinemia.[65]

β-GLUCURONIDASE REACTION

Histochemical studies of lymph nodes and spleens have shown intense β-glucuronidase activity in areas rich in T lymphocytes.[66,67] The finding is confirmed by cytochemical findings that T lymphocytes have higher β-glucuronidase activity than do B lymphocytes; therefore, it may be a useful histochemical marker for T lymphocytes. Enzyme activity is well preserved for prolonged periods if fresh tissues are properly fixed and kept at 10°C.[15,66] Nevertheless, insufficient data exist to conclude that histochemical studies of this enzyme in tissue sections have definite clinical value.

RETICULIN STAIN

Two types of reticulin stains are recognized. The first is Jones' methenamine–silver stain for basement membrane and reticulin, which is most useful for outlining the sinusoidal structures of the spleen.[13,15,68] It is not intended for use in marrow specimens for the assessment of myelofibrosis.

The other type of reticulin stain, such as Gomori's silver impregnation,[2] is intended for the evaluation of fibrosis. This technique is helpful in confirming myelofibrosis in agnogenic myeloid metaplasia and CML, and in demonstrating the fine intercellular reticulin networks characteristic of hairy cell leukemia and mast cell disease. These methods, however, are less useful than the methenamine-silver stain in outlining sinusoidal structures of the spleen.

METHYL GREEN-PYRONINE REACTION

The methyl green–pyronine histochemical reaction is intended for demonstrating cellular RNA content and for identifying many of the primitive hematopoietic cells rich in this chemical component. This reaction is simple in principle, but it is difficult to achieve optimal staining results due to the difficulty in obtaining satisfactory reagents for clinical use. Methyl green is the nuclear stain; pyronine is the RNA stain. However, impurities in these reagents often overshadow the greenish nuclear stain with a purple hue and greatly reduce both the nucleolar and the cytoplasmic pyroninophilia. RNA content also can be assessed by the intensity of cytoplasmic basophilia caused by the Giemsa stain. When it becomes difficult to obtain optimal results by the methyl green–pyronine reaction, the Giemsa stain can be used instead.

MISCELLANEOUS REACTIONS

The Perls' reaction is useful for evaluating the tissue iron store. It is also used for demonstrating ringed sideroblasts. Oil red O is useful for staining the fatty droplets in tumor cells.[69] To achieve technical success, however, care must be taken not to dissolve the lipid material in tissues by the organic solvents during tissue processing. Chlorazol fast pink is useful in selectively demonstrating the eosinophils.[70] Toluidine blue O may be used to demonstrate metachromasia and is useful for the detection of mast cells, basophils, and, to a lesser extent, plasma cells.[71] However, the neoplastic mast cells may have few cytoplasmic granules, and they may not demonstrate metachromasia by either the toluidine blue stain or the Giemsa stain.[35,37] In rare instances, stain for mucin of cells of adenocarcinoma may be useful to differentiate the adenocarcinomas from the lymphomas.[72]

The enzyme dipeptidyl (amino) peptidase IV (DAP IV, or glycylproline naphthyl–amidase) was noted to have definite enzyme activity in the lymphocytes but no activity in the monocytes or neutrophils.[73] The lymphocytes with strong enzyme activity are T cells.[74] This finding was extended by Feller et al.,[75] who showed that the DAP IV–positive lymphocytes are either Tμ-positive (T-helper) or Tμγ-negative cells. Thus, DAP IV may be used as a marker for T lymphocytes, but it is more accurate to use a surface marker, such as CD4.

Adenosine triphosphatase was studied by Harigaya et al.[76] and found to be a fairly specific marker for B lymphocytes, plasma cells, and the supporting reticulum cells in human peripheral lymphoid tissues. This enzyme is also found in the plasma membrane of many B-lymphoma cells and may be useful as a marker for differentiating the various types of lymphomas.

In conclusion, histochemical reactions are useful for cell identification in tissues. The advantage of using histochemical stains is that several stains can be applied simultaneously to the same tissue section to identify several types of cells and the interactions among them.

REFERENCES

1. Lillie RD, Fullmer HM: *Histopathologic Technic and Practical Histochemistry*, ed 4. New York, McGraw-Hill, 1976.
2. Luna LG (ed): *Manual of Histologic Staining Methods of the AFIP*, ed 3. New York, McGraw-Hill, 1968.
3. Leder LD: Über die Seleketive ferment cytochemische darstellung von neutrophilen myeloischen zellen und gevebsmastzellen in paraffinschmitt. *Klin Wochenschr* 42:553, 1964.
4. Pangalis GA, Nathwani BN, Rappaport H: Detection of cytoplasmic immunoglobulin in well-differentiated lymphoproliferative diseases by the immunoperoxidase method. *Cancer* 45:1334–1339, 1980.
5. Pinkus GS, Said JW: Specific identification of intracellular

immunoglobulin in paraffin sections of multiple myeloma and macroglobulinemia using an immunoperoxidase technique. *Am J Pathol* 87:45–57, 1977.
6. Mason DY, Taylor CR: The distribution of muramidase (lysozyme) in human tissues. *J Clin Pathol* 28:124–132, 1975.
7. Ashford AE, Allaway WG, McCully ME: Low temperature embedding in glycol methacrylate for enzyme histochemistry in plant and animal tissues. *J Histochem Cytochem* 20:986–990, 1972.
8. Dorsett BH, Ioachim H: A method for the use of immunofluorescence on paraffin-embedded tissue. *Am J Clin Pathol* 69:66–72, 1978.
9. Braunstein H, Freiman DG, Gall EA: A histochemical study of the enzymatic activity of lymph nodes, I: The normal and hyperplastic lymph nodes. *Cancer* 11:829–837, 1958.
10. Braunstein H, Freiman DG, Thomas WJ Jr, et al: A histochemical study of the enzymatic activity of lymph nodes, II: Further investigations of normal and hyperplastic lymph nodes. *Cancer* 15:130–138, 1962.
11. Braunstein H, Freiman DG, Thomas WJ Jr, et al: A histochemical study of the enzymatic activity of lymph nodes, III: Granulomatous and primary neoplastic conditions of lymphoid tissue. *Cancer* 15:139–152, 1962.
12. Curran RC, Gregory J: Demonstration of immunoglobulin in cryostat and paraffin sections of human tonsil by immunofluorescence and immunoperoxidase techniques: Effects of processing on immunohistochemical performance of tissues and on the use of proteolytic enzymes to unmask antigens in sections. *J Clin Pathol* 31:974–983, 1978.
13. Stutte HJ: Nature of human spleen red pulp cells with special reference to sinus lining cells. *Z Zell Forsch* 91:300–314, 1968.
14. Li CY, Harrison EG Jr: Histochemical and immunohistochemical study of diffuse large-cell lymphoma. *Am J Clin Pathol* 70:721–732, 1978.
15. Li CY, Yam LT, Crosby WH: Histochemical characterization of cellular and structural elements of the human spleen. *J Histochem Cytochem* 20:1049–1058, 1972.
16. Monis B, Wasserkrug H, Seligman AM: Comparison of fixatives and substrates for aminopeptidase. *J Histochem Cytochem* 13:503–509, 1965.
17. Yam LT, Li CY, Wolfe HJ, et al: Histochemical study of acute leukemia. *Arch Pathol* 97:129–135, 1974.
18. Mori M, Ito M, Fukui S; Decalcification for histochemical demonstration of hydrolytic and oxidative enzymes. *Histochemie* 5:185–195, 1965.
19. TeVelde J, Burkhardt R, Kleiverda K, et al: Methyl-methacrylate as an embedding medium in histopathology. *Histopathology* 1:319, 1977.
20. Beckstead JH, Bainton DF: Enzyme histochemistry on bone marrow biopsies: Reactions useful in the differential diagnosis of leukemia and lymphoma applied to 2-micron plastic sections. *Blood* 55:386–394, 1980.
21. Beckstead JH, Halverson PS, Ries CA, et al: Enzyme histochemistry and immunohistochemistry on biopsy specimens of pathologic human bone marrow. *Blood* 57:1088–1098, 1981.
22. Chilosi M, Pizzolo G, Menestrina F, et al: Enzyme histochemistry on normal and pathologic paraffin-embedded lymphoid tissues. *Am J Clin Pathol* 76:729–736, 1981.
23. Mitrenga D, Arnold W, Mayersbach HV: Freeze-drying and embedding in glycol methacrylate (GMA): The results of morphological, histochemical and immunohistochemical investigation. *Histochemistry* 39:313–326, 1974.
24. Vykoupil K-F, Thide J, Georgii A: Histochemical and immunohistochemical techniques on acrylate-embedded bone biopsies. *Blut* 32:215–218, 1976.
25. Casey TT, Cousar JB, Collin RD: A simplified plastic embedding and immunohistologic technique for immunophenotypic analysis of human hematopoietic and lymphoid tissues. *Am J Pathol* 131:183–189, 1988.
26. Scott SC: Cytochemistry of acute myeloid leukemia with particular reference to myeloperoxidase. In Scott CS (ed): *Leukemia Cytochemistry: Principles and Practice.* Chichester, UK, Ellis Horwood, 1989, pp 91–102.
27. Storr J, Dolan G, Constan-Smith C, et al: Value of monoclonal anti-myeloperoxidase (MPO7) for diagnosing acute leukemia. *J Clin Pathol* 43:847–849, 1990.
28. Burchori V, Shetty V, Yoshida N, et al: The role of an anti-myeloperoxidase antibody in the diagnosis and classification of acute leukemia: A comparison with light and electron microscopy cytochemistry. *Br J Haematol* 80:62–68, 1992.
29. Graham RC, Karnovsky MJ: The early stages of absorption of injected horseradish peroxidase in the proximal tubules of mouse kidney: Ultrastructural cytochemistry by a new technique. *J Histochem Cytochem* 14:291–301, 1966.
30. Hanker JS, Yates PE, Metz CB, et al: A new specific sensitive and noncarcinogenic reagent for the demonstration of horseradish peroxidase. *Histochem J* 9:789–792, 1977.
31. Graham RC, Lundholm U, Karnovsky MJ: Cytochemical demonstration of peroxidase activity with 3-amino-9-ethylcarbazole. *J Histochem Cytochem* 13:150–152, 1965.
32. Picworth FA: A new method of study of the brain capillaries and its application to the regional localization of mental disorder. *J Anat* 69:62–71, 1934.
33. Undritz E: *Sandoz Atlas of Haematology*, ed 2. Basle, Switzerland, Sandoz, 1973, p 35.
34. Neiman RS: Erythroblastic transformation in myeloproliferative disorders: Confirmation by an immunohistologic technique. *Cancer* 46:1636–1640, 1980.
35. Lennert K, Parwaresch MR: Mast cells and mast cell neoplasia: A review. *Histopathology* 3:349–365, 1979.
36. Neiman RS, Barcos M, Berard CW, et al: Granulocytic sarcoma: A clinicopathologic study of 61 biopsied cases. *Cancer* 48:1426–1437, 1981.
37. Webb TA, Li CY, Yam LT: Systemic mast cell disease: A clinical and hematopathologic study of 26 cases. *Cancer* 49:927–938, 1982.
38. Dorfman RF: Enzyme histochemistry of the cells in Hodgkin's disease and allied disorders. *Nature* 190:925–926, 1961.
39. Yam LT, Li CY: Histogenesis of splenic lesions in Hodgkin's disease. *Am J Clin Pathol* 66:976–985, 1976.
40. Li CY, Lam KW, Yam LT: Esterases in human leukocytes. *J Histochem Cytochem* 21:1–12, 1973.
41. Grossi CE, Webb SR, Zicca A, et al: Morphological and histochemical analysis of two human T-cell subpopulations

bearing receptors for IgM or IgG. *J Exp Med* 147:1405–1417, 1978.
42. Knowles DM II, Halper JP, Machin GA, et al: Acid α-naphthyl acetate esterase activity in human neoplastic lymphoid cells: Usefulness as a T-cell marker. *Am J Pathol* 96:257–278, 1979.
43. Mueller J, Brun Del Ré G, Buerk H, et al: Nonspecific esterase activity: A criterion for differentiation of T and B lymphocytes in mouse lymph nodes. *Eur J Immunol* 5:270–274, 1975.
44. Higgy KE, Burns GF, Hayhoe FGJ: Discrimination of B, T, and null lymphocytes by esterase cytochemistry. *Scand J Haematol* 18:437–448, 1977.
45. Knowles DM II, Holck S: Tissue localization of T lymphocytes by the histochemical demonstration of acid α-naphthyl acetate esterase. *Lab Invest* 39:70–76, 1978.
46. Yam LT, Yam CF, Li CY: Eosinophilia in systemic mastocytosis. *Am J Clin Pathol* 73:48–54, 1982.
47. Li CY, Travis WD, Van Hale PC, et al: Useful cytochemical stains for the diagnosis of systemic mast cell disease (SMCD). *J Histochem Cytochem* 34:1355, 1986.
48. Bennett JM, Reed CE: Acute leukemia cytochemical profile: Diagnostic and clinical implications. *Blood Cells* 1:202–208, 1975.
49. Fischer R, Schmalzl F: Über die hemmbarkeit der esteraseaktivitat in blutmonocyten durch natriumfluorid. *Klin Wochenschr* 42:751, 1964.
50. Rozensznjn L, Leibovich M, Shoham D, et al: The esterase activity in megaloblasts, leukemic and normal haematopoietic cells. *Br J Haematol* 14:650–610, 1968.
51. Schmalzl F, Braunsteiner H: The application of cytochemical methods to the study of acute leukemia: A review. *Acta Haematol* 45:209–217, 1971.
52. Wachstein M, Wolf G: The histochemical demonstration of esterase activity in human blood and bone marrow smears. *J Histochem Cytochem* 6:457, 1958.
53. Nanba K, Jaffe ES, Braylan RC, et al: Alkaline phosphatase-positive malignant lymphoma: A subtype of B-cell lymphoma. *Am J Clin Pathol* 68:535–542, 1977.
54. Mason DY, Sammons R: Alkaline phosphatase and peroxidase for double immunoenzymatic labelling of cellular constituents. *J Clin Pathol* 31:454–460, 1978.
55. Yam LT, Janckila AI, Li CY: The immunoalkaline phosphatase methods. In De Lellis RA (ed): *Advances in Immunohistochemistry.* New York, Raven Press, 1988, pp 1–29.
56. Barka T, Anderson PJ: Histochemical methods for acid phosphatase using hexazonium pararosanilin as coupler. *J Histochem Cytochem* 10:741–753, 1962.
57. Janckila AJ, Li CY, Lam KW, et al: The cytochemistry of tartrate-resistant acid phosphatase: Technical considerations. *Am J Clin Pathol* 70:45–55, 1978.
58. Catovsky D, Greaves MF, Pain C, et al: Acid phosphatase reaction in acute lymphoblastic leukemia. *Lancet* 1:749–751, 1978.
59. Stein H, Petersen N, Gaedicke G, et al: Lymphoblastic lymphoma of convoluted or acid phosphatase type. A tumor of T precursor cells. *Int J Cancer* 17:292–295, 1976.
60. Krishnan J, Li CY, Su WPD: Cutaneous lymphomas: Correlation of histochemical and immunohistochemical characteristics and clinicopathologic features. *Am J Clin Pathol* 79:157–165, 1983.
61. Li CY, Yam LT, Lam KW: Studies of acid phosphatase isoenzymes in human leukocytes: Demonstration of isoenzyme cell specificity. *J Histochem Cytochem* 18:901–910, 1970.
62. Mover S, Li CY, Yam LT: Semiquantitative evaluation of tartrate-resistant acid phosphatase activity in human blood cells. *J Lab Clin Med* 80:711–717, 1972.
63. Katayama I, Li CY, Yam LT: Histochemical study of acid phosphatase isoenzyme in leukemic reticuloendotheliosis. *Cancer* 29:157–164, 1972.
64. Yam LT, Janckila AJ, Chan CH, et al: Hepatic involvement in hairy cell leukemia. *Cancer* 51:1497–1504, 1983.
65. Dutcher TF, Fahey JL: The histopathology of the macroglobulinemia of Waldenström. *J Natl Cancer Inst* 22:887–917, 1959.
66. Hayashi M: Distribution of β-glucuronidase activity in rat tissues employing the naphthol AS-BI glucuronide hexazonium pararosanilin method. *J Histochem Cytochem* 12:659–669, 1964.
67. Tamaoki N, Essner E: Distribution of acid phosphatase, β-glucuronidase and N-acetyl-β-glucosaminidase activities in lymphocytes of lymphatic tissues of man and rodents. *J Histochem Cytochem* 17:238–243, 1969.
68. Jones DB: nephrotic glomerulonephritis. *Am J Pathol* 33:313–330, 1957.
69. Wright DH: Cytology and histochemistry of the Burkitt lymphoma. *Br J Cancer* 17:50–55, 1963.
70. Maeda R, Kanazawa K, Nakano E, et al: Studies on the specificity of the chorazol fast pink staining method. *Acta Histochem Cytochem* 3:65–73, 1970.
71. Kramer H, Windrum GM: the metachromatic staining reaction. *J Histochem Cytochem* 3:227–237, 1955.
72. Mallory FB: *Pathological Technique.* New York, Hafner Press, 1961.
73. Lojda Z: Studies on glycyl-proline naphthylamidase, I: Lymphocytes. *Histochemistry* 54:299–309, 1977.
74. Chilosi M, Pizzolo G, Menestrina F, et al: Dipeptidyl (amino) peptidase IV (DAP-IV) histochemistry on normal and pathologic lymphoid tissues. *Am J Clin Pathol* 77:714–719, 1982.
75. Feller AC, Heijnen CJ, Ballieux RE, et al: Enzyme histochemical staining of Tμ lymphocytes for glycyl-proline-4-methoxy-beta-naphthylamide-peptidase (DAP-IV). *Br J Haematol* 51:227–234, 1982.
76. Harigaya K, Mikata A, Suzuki H, et al: Mg^{2+}-dependent adenosine triphosphatase as an enzyme histochemical marker for the lymphomas of B-cell origin. *Am J Pathol* 97:359–380, 1979.

Chapter 4
IMMUNOCHEMISTRY

Immunochemical studies have been used frequently for both cytologic and histologic materials. Fresh tissues provide the most consistent results, although those fixed with formaldehyde or other agents and embedded in paraffin or plastics may sometimes be suitable as well. Both immunocytochemistry and immunohistochemistry use visible indicators to identify cell or tissue antigens through the bindings of a specific antibody to a particular antigen. With light microscopy, fluorochrome and enzymatic indicators are most commonly used. The fluorescent indicators are visualized by fluorescence microscopy and the enzyme indicators by cytochemical stains.[1,2] Linkage between the antigen and the indicator–antibody conjugate may be direct, indirect, or in a series of steps ("sandwich"), as illustrated in Figure 4-1. In addition, a method with several steps exploiting the specificity of antibody reactions and the sensitivity of avidin–biotin binding has been introduced to increase the sensitivity of immunochemical detection of specific antigens.[3-5] Subsequently, a similar method using streptavidin instead of avidin has been introduced to further improve the specificity by decreasing the intensity of the background staining.[6]

PREPARATION OF TISSUES

Tissues that may be used for immunochemistry include fresh cell suspensions, unfixed frozen tissue sections, and tissues embedded in paraffin or plastics.[7-13] Fresh cell suspensions and unfixed frozen sections are most suitable for demonstration of the cell surface antigens.[9,13,14] Although antigens are best preserved in fresh unfixed tissues, the cell morphology of these preparations is poor.[7] Tissues embedded in plastics provide excellent preservation of cell morphology, although often at the expense of inactivation of antigenic sites.[11,12] The surface antigens are the most labile, and their antigenicity usually becomes significantly reduced after fixation and is abolished in paraffin- or plastic-embedded tissues. Other antigens, such as the cytoplasmic immunoglobulins and factor VIII antigen, withstand fixations and tissue embedding well, although some of their antigenic sites may be masked by these processes and may need reactivation by a trypsin or pepsin digestion or microwave antigen retrieval process.[15-22] Antigens such as lysozyme are very stable and maintain their antigenicity through fixation, embedding, and treatment of tissues with strong acidic solutions. The clinical applicability of the various types of specimens and the immunochemical studies most often used for the diagnosis of the hematologic neoplasms are listed in Table 4-1 and discussed in the next sections. The surface markers will be discussed in Chapter 5.

IMMUNOFLUORESCENCE TECHNIQUES

In the direct technique, the antigen is identified by a fluorochrome-labeled specific antibody (Figure 4-1A). This method is simple but relatively insensitive. It is most suitable for the study of tissues with a high concentration of the antigen of interest. In the indirect methods, an unlabeled specific primary antibody is allowed to react with the tissue antigen. The excess antibody is then washed off. A fluorochrome-conjugated second antibody (anti-immunoglobulin) capable of binding to the primary antibody is then applied (Figure 4-1B). The sensitivity of this method is greater than that of the direct method, and it can be further enhanced when it is incorporated with the avidin–biotin complex system (Figure 4-1D).[23]

The immunofluorescence technique is simple in principle and is easy to perform. Since fresh, unfixed tissues are frequently used in this technique, antigens sensitive to fixation can be studied.[10,24-26] The drawback of this technique is that the morphology of the unfixed cells is not as good as in paraffin- or plastic-embedded tissue sections; therefore, it may be difficult to identify the cells accurately in tissues. In addition, since the immunofluorescent stain may fade with storage, results must be recorded and photo-

ENZYME IMMUNOCHEMISTRY

Enzyme immunochemistry involves the demonstration of substances on the surface, in the cytoplasm, or in the nucleus of cells. The staining technique most commonly used is the immunoperoxidase method, in which the plant enzyme horseradish peroxidase is used as the indicator.[28-31] Other staining techniques now available include those using either intestinal alkaline phosphatase[32,33] or glucose oxidase[34,35] as the enzyme indicator.

Immunoperoxidase Technique

Several immunoperoxidase techniques are available, but the most widely used has been the peroxidase-antiperoxidase technique (PAP) of Sternberger et al.,[29,31,36] which is based on the principle of amplifying the specific staining through a series of immunologic reactions ending in the linkage of soluble peroxidase–antiperoxidase complexes to the tissue antigen of interest (Figure 4-1C). This technique is both specific and sensitive and has certain advantages over the other techniques.[36]

After the "sandwich" has been properly made, the peroxidase activity can be demonstrated cytochemically by using 3,3-diaminobenzidine as the indicator at pH 7.6. The reaction product of 3,3-diaminobenzidine is brownish; the background staining is relatively intense, especially when the tissue is inadequately fixed; and the endogenous peroxidase activity is considerable. With suitable modifications, this technique can be further improved. Thus, the peroxidase staining can be made more sensitive if imidazole is used to replace Tris as the incubating buffer at pH 7.6.[37,38] The reaction product can be made more chromogenic by copper salt treatment[39] and by the use of 3-amino-9-ethylcarbazole as the indicator.[40,41]

The background staining may be minimized in a number of ways: (1) by ensuring proper fixation of the tissue to prevent leakage of antigen into surrounding tissues; (2) by saturating the nonspecific binding sites for immunoglobulin in the tissues before specific antibodies are applied[42,43]; (3) by lowering the pH of the incubating medium to below 7.6 to minimize the spontaneous degradation of hydrogen peroxide[44]; and (4) by adding detergent (Brij or Tween 20) in the rinsing solution to reduce the hydrophobic interactions between tissue and protein reagents.[45] The endogenous peroxidase activity can be inhibited by pretreatment of tissues with either methanol–hydrogen peroxide[46] or periodate[47] and by using tissues embedded in paraffin or fixed with hydrochloric acid and ethanol. Recently, a more gentle and effective method using azide and hydrogen peroxide has been developed for inhibition of endogenous peroxidase activity.[48] This method will make possible better

A. Direct Method

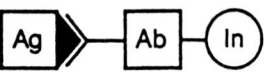

B. Indirect Method

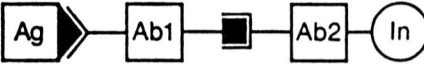

C. Enzyme-Antienzyme Complex

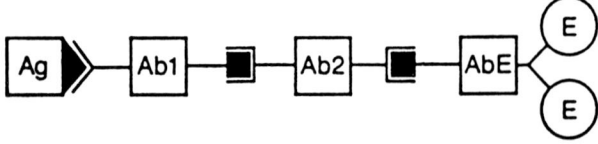

D. Avidin-Biotin-Enzyme Complex

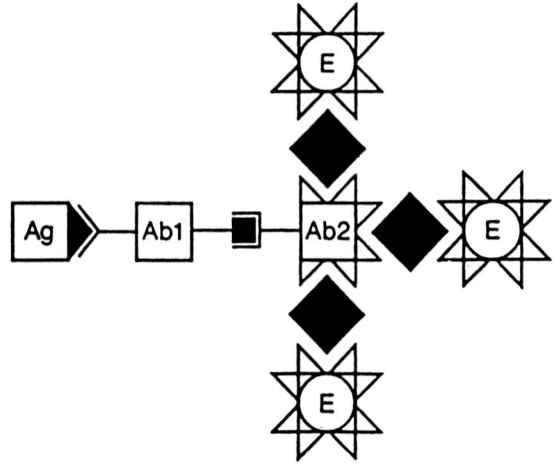

FIGURE 4-1. Four major immunohistochemical methods for detection of tissue antigens. Ab = antibody; Ab1 = primary antibody; Ab2 = secondary antibody; AbE = antienzyme antibody; Ag = antigen; E = enzyme; In = indicators (either fluorochrome or enzyme); ♦ = avidin; ◊ = biotin.

graphs must be taken to have a permanent record of the results. Although the use of fixed tissues may alleviate some of these technical limitations, fixation decreases staining sensitivity.[16,20,26,27]

TABLE 4-1. Cell Specificity and Clinical Applications of Immunochemical Reactions Excluding the Surface Markers

Immunochemical Reactions	Type of Specimen	Cell Specificity	Clinical Application
Cytoplasmic immunoglobulin	Pa, Pl, CS	B lymphocytes, plasma cells	Lymphomas, myelomas
Myeloperoxidase (MPO7)	Pa, F, I, S	Granulocytes	Granulocytic sarcoma, myeloid metaplasia
Lysozyme	Pa, Pl, CS	Granulocytes Monocytes, histiocytes	Granulocytic sarcoma, myeloid metaplasia Monocytic and histiocytic disorders
CD68 (PG-M$_1$, KP1)	Pa, Pl, F, I, S	Monocytes, histiocytes	Monocytic and histiocytic disorders
Terminal deoxynucleotidyl transferase (TdT)	F, S, I, CS	Lymphoblasts	CML in blastic crisis, ALL, lymphoblastic lymphoma
Factor VIII antigen	F, Pa	Megakaryocytes	Megakaryocytic leukemia, acute myelofibrosis, myeloid metaplasia
		Vascular endothelium	Vascular neoplasms
Hemoglobin	Pa	Erythroblasts	Myeloid metaplasia, erythroleukemia
Tryptase (AA1)	Pa, F, S	Mast cells	Mast cell disease

ALL = acute lymphoblastic leukemia; CML = chronic myelogenous leukemia; CS = cell suspension, F = cryostat section of fresh frozen tissue; I = imprint; Pa = paraffin sections; Pl = plastic section; S = smear.

application of immunoperoxidase techniques for immunocytochemical evaluation of cells in blood and bone marrow.

Since the optimum pH for horseradish peroxidase lies between 4 and 6, which is considerably lower than that of myeloperoxidase, staining for peroxidase activity in tissues in this pH range not only increases the specificity for exogenous horseradish peroxidase but also minimizes nonspecific background staining.[49] We prefer the technique using 3-amino-9-ethylcarbazole at pH 5.2 over other techniques for the immunoperoxidase reaction.[41,50]

It is technically feasible to apply the immunoperoxidase method to cell suspensions, fresh tissue sections, and tissues embedded in either paraffin or plastics; however, the immunofluorescence technique is most often used for the study of cell suspensions and frozen sections. In fresh, unfixed tissues, the immunoperoxidase technique is commonly used in those with minimal endogenous peroxidase activity and in those in which the tissue antigens of interest are resistant to procedures for inhibiting endogenous peroxidase activity.

Immunoalkaline Phosphatase Technique

In the immunoalkaline phosphatase (IAP) technique, calf intestinal alkaline phosphatase is used to replace horseradish peroxidase as the enzymic indicator for the demonstration of specific tissue agents.[32,33] The IAP technique is performed according to the principle of the indirect method or enzyme–antienzyme complex, as illustrated in Figures 4-1B and 4-1C. In the indirect method, the tissue antigen is allowed to react with a specific primary antibody. An alkaline phosphatase–conjugated anti-immunoglobulin then reacts with the primary antibody. Cytochemical disclosure of alkaline phosphatase then indicates the presence of antigen.

The IAP technique may not be as sensitive as the PAP technique, yet it is simple and specific, with certain advantages over the PAP technique. The reaction product for IAP is highly chromogenic, and the background staining is negligible. Cytochemical demonstration of calf intestinal alkaline phosphatase activity is carried out at pH 7.6 to 8.2 in the presence of specific inhibitors such as levamisole.[51] Under such control conditions, activity of the endogenous alkaline phosphatase in human tissues is either completely abolished or kept at a minimum, while that of the exogenous intestinal enzyme is not significantly diminished. Tissue antigens, including those on the surface of human blood cells, are not affected and can be demonstrated with their corresponding monoclonal antibodies by the IAP technique.

The Avidin–Biotin Complex System

Both avidin and biotin are naturally occurring substances with a strong affinity for each other. The affinity of this pair can be used to develop sensitive immunochemical methods.[3,5,52] One of the methods is depicted in Figure 4-1D. In the avidin–biotin complex (ABC) system, tissue sections are incubated with a primary antibody to the tissue antigen of interest. A biotinylated secondary antibody is then added, followed by the addition of avidin. The final step is to add a biotin–enzyme indicator complex. The tissue antigen is demonstrated by cytochemical staining of the enzyme indicator in the complex. The enzyme indicator most commonly used is horseradish peroxidase. Other enzymes such as alkaline phosphatase or glucose oxidase have also been used.

The ABC system is more sensitive than the conventional immunohistochemical methods in detecting tissue antigens when the antigen concentration or the antibody concentration is low.[53] The inherent problem with this technique is the presence in tissues of biotin that will bind with the avidin and link to the biotinyl enzyme indicator, resulting in false-positive staining. This nonspecific staining reaction can be blocked by pretreating the tissue with avidin and biotin before applying the biotinylated secondary antibody to tissue sections.[54]

Of the enzyme immunochemical techniques available, we use PAP and peroxidase-labeled streptavidin biotin techniques mainly for the demonstration of intracellular antigens in tissues embedded in either paraffin or plastics. The IAP technique is reserved for the labile surface antigens in cell suspensions, smears, or frozen sections cut in a cryostat. However, with the development of an effective method for inhibiting endogenous peroxidase,[48] the immunoperoxidase method can also be used on smears or frozen sections.

CYTOPLASMIC IMMUNOGLOBULIN DETECTION

The immunoglobulins (Ig) are synthesized by the B lymphocytes. During the maturation process, cytoplasmic immunoglobulin (CIg) first appears in pre-B cells, disappears in mature B cells, and reappears when B cells develop into plasma cells. Subsequent to the pre-B cell stage, the surface immunoglobulin appears on immature and mature B cells but eventually disappears when B cells develop into plasma cells. Each B cell is preprogrammed to produce a single class and type of immunoglobulin of a given antigenic specificity. Hence, in healthy people and in patients with reactive lymphoid hyperplasia, the B cells are of diverse types, each producing or displaying its own immunoglobulin specificity. In neoplastic proliferations of the B lymphocytes, with a few exceptions, only a single type or clone of B cells proliferates. The immunoglobulin produced by this new clone is predominantly of the same type and specificity (monoclonal). Thus, recognition of the immunoglobulin classes and types contained within the lymphoid cells is useful in determining the nature of lymphoid proliferations. The immunoglobulin molecules are composed of both heavy chains ($\gamma, \alpha, \mu, \delta, \epsilon$) and light chains ($\kappa$ and λ). It is possible to examine either the heavy chains or the light chains to determine monoclonal proliferation of the lymphoid cells. From a practical point of view, however, it is easier to examine the two light chains than the five heavy chains.

CIg can be demonstrated by either immunofluorescence techniques or enzymatic immunochemistry on fixed cytologic material and fixed or unfixed tissue sections.[13] The immunofluorescence technique is used most often for cytologic preparations. The cells in these preparations are properly fixed, so that the cell membrane is permeable enough to allow the staining reagents to react with the CIg. The immunoperoxidase technique of Sternberger et al.[31] is most often used to demonstrate CIg in tissues embedded in either paraffin or methacrylate. The antigenicity of the immunoglobulins, however, is diminished or partially masked during tissue processing. It is often necessary to unmask the antigenic sites for optimal staining by pretreating the tissues with proteolytic enzymes such as trypsin or pepsin.[15,16,18-20] Prolonged tissue fixation with formaldehyde or digestion with trypsin will invariably lead to decreased staining of the immunoglobulins. Poorly processed or fixed tissues may also allow leakage of CIg into intercellular spaces, causing intense background staining in such specimens. It is often necessary to include as controls additional sections for staining of serum albumin (the major plasma protein). When positive, these controls identify areas where plasma proteins (including immunoglobulin) may be present.[55,56]

Because of the frequent occurrence of cells with endogenous peroxidase activity in tissues used for demonstration of CIg, it is necessary to eliminate this type of enzyme activity with hydrogen peroxide and methanol or periodic acid.[46,47] The inclusion of this step, although effective in eliminating the endogenous myeloperoxidase activity in tissues, cannot totally eliminate the chemical reaction between hemoglobin and the reagents for the peroxidase stain. This chemical reaction (pseudoperoxidase or Lepehne's reaction)[57,58] is undesirable and becomes a problem when the immunoperoxidase technique is employed to examine tissues with either many erythrocytes or multiple hemorrhagic areas. In small tissue specimens with many erythrocytes, such as those from marrow biopsy specimens, the edges of the specimen are often hemorrhagic and often cause heavy background staining. This may cause considerable difficulty in interpreting the results.

Proper interpretation of the immunoperoxidase reaction for CIg requires a thorough understanding of both the staining techniques and the significance of cytologic changes in tissues. B cells with plasmacytoid features and large, activated lymphocytes frequently show intense staining for CIg, whereas the small, inactive lymphocytes seldom do so.[9,59-65] When the light chains of CIg are examined, positive staining in the lymphoid cells for a single chain (κ or λ) should be considered evidence of monoclonal proliferation. The number of positively stained cells in tissue sections varies considerably from case to case. The minimal number of cells needed for meaningful interpretation, however, has not been defined. The staining pattern of cells in areas with inflammatory changes should not be taken into consideration because it frequently will show polyclonal staining patterns.

Studies for CIg are most useful in differentiating neoplastic B-cell proliferations from reactive lymphoid hyperplasia. A monoclonal staining pattern strongly favors neoplasia of the B cells, although a negative staining reaction does not exclude such a possibility.[60,61] CIg can also be seen in macrophages as a result of phagocytosis. This is the major controversial point in the dispute about the origin of Reed-Sternberg cells, which contain CIg.[66–72] The J chain is considered a good marker to distinguish Ig-synthesizing cells from Ig-phagocytizing cells.[73,74] The J chain is a polypeptide that links the monomers in IgM and secretory IgA and has been detected in circulating immunoblasts, plasma cells, myeloma cells, and follicular center cells of human tonsils. It is present in tumors with a monoclonal light chain pattern but not in Reed-Sternberg cells or other lymphoma cells with a polyclonal pattern. It is assumed that the J chain is produced by the Ig-synthesizing cells and that its presence rules out phagocytosis or passive absorption of immunoglobulins.

LYSOZYME DETECTION

Lysozyme (muramidase) is a low molecular weight basic protein that is found in the cytoplasm of the granulocytes and monocytes.[75] It is not detectable in lymphocytes, plasma cells, erythroblasts, or megakaryocytes. It can be demonstrated by cytochemical, immunofluorescence, or immunocytochemical techniques.[69,76–80] The immunoperoxidase method appears to be the most practical for detecting this enzyme. Lysozyme is fairly stable and retains its antigenic properties after fixation with formaldehyde derivatives and Zenker's solution. It is not adversely affected by the processing of tissues, including paraffin or methacrylate embedding and decalcification in strongly acidic solutions. For these reasons, immunohistochemical study of lysozyme may be most desirable when it is necessary to identify the granulocytes and monocytes in decalcified, paraffin-embedded marrow biopsy specimens. Immunohistochemical study of lysozyme is particularly useful for the diagnosis of granulocytic sarcoma, malignant histiocytosis, and true histiocytic lymphoma[79,81,82] Lysozyme is a marker for both granulocytes and monocytes. Additional markers are needed to differentiate further between these two types of cells in tissue sections. Furthermore, nonhematopoietic cells, such as proximal renal tubular cells, serous salivary acinar cells, Paneth's cells, and the lactating epithelial cells of the breast, also contain lysozyme.[78] Interpretation of positive staining of lysozyme in tissue sections should be made with caution.

CD68 ANTIGEN (KP1) DETECTIONS

CD68 antigen, recognized by monoclonal antibody KP1, was initially isolated from a lysosomal fraction of the human macrophage and has a molecular weight of about 110 kd. Immunohistochemically, the monoclonal antibody KP1 recognizes a fixation-resistant epitope in a wide variety of tissue macrophages including Kupffer cells; osteoclasts, monocytes, and monocyte precursors; and macrophages in lung, germinal centers, spleen, bone marrow, and lamina propria. Lymphocytes, megakaryocytes, and cells of erythroid lineage are not labeled by KP1 in smears or sections of bone marrow. KP1 stains granulocytes strongly in bone marrow and blood smears, but the staining is very weak or negative in routinely processed tissue sections.[83] Recently, a new monoclonal antibody (PG-M1), directed against a fixative-resistant epitope on the macrophage-restricted form of the CD68 molecule, was produced.[84] PG-M1 showed a more restricted reactivity with elements of the monocyte-macrophage lineage without cross-reactivity with granulocytes. Immunohistochemical study of the antigens of CD68 (PG-M1) using routinely processed tissue is particularly useful for diagnosis of the disorders of the monocyte-macrophage system such as malignant histiocytosis, true histiocytic lymphoma, and monocytic and myelomonocytic leukemia.[84–87]

MYELOPEROXIDASE DETECTION

Myeloperoxidase (MPO) is a lysosomal enzyme found in the primary granules of cells of the myeloid series and is a specific enzyme marker for granulocytes and monocytes. Besides the use of conventional cytochemical methods to demonstrate the enzyme activity (Chapters 2 and 3), the MPO antigen can now be detected by immunochemical techniques using monoclonal anti-myeloperoxidase antibody (MPO7). This immunocytochemical method has been effectively used in the diagnosis of acute myeloid leukemia.[88,89]

Terminal Deoxynucleotidyl Transferase Detection

Terminal deoxynucleotidyl transferase (TdT) is an intranuclear enzyme that catalyzes the addition of deoxynucleotides to the 3'-hydroxy end of oligonucleotides or polydeoxynucleotides without the need for a template.[90] In human tissues, TdT activity can be detected in thymocytes, primitive lymphocytes, and a small number of cells in the marrow.[90] TdT activity is negligible in B lymphoblasts and mature B lymphocytes. In hematopoietic malignancies, strong TdT activity is seen in the lymphoblasts of approximately 90% of ALL and lymphoblastic lymphoma cases. It is present in the lymphoblasts of uALL, cALL, T-ALL, and occasionally pre-B-ALL, but not B-ALL.[52,91–93] This enzyme, however, is not a unique marker for either T lymphoblasts or T lymphocytes. The leukemic blasts of

CML in blastic crisis,[94–96] as well as a rare case of proven AML, have also been shown to be positive for TdT.[94,97,98]

TdT appears useful in the prognosis of CML with blastic crisis because those cases with TdT activity in many of the blasts seem to respond favorably to chemotherapy and have a better prognosis than those cases that have no TdT activity in the blasts.[94–96] TdT is also useful in detecting small foci of tumor cells. It can be used to search for lymphoma or leukemic cells in bone marrow during remission and in body fluids.

TdT can be assessed by radioimmunoassay, by biochemical assay, and by techniques of immunofluorescence and immunoperoxidase.[92,94,99–101] Under most circumstances, immunofluorescence staining is the method of choice, as it can be used to detect small numbers of tumor cells on smears from different sources.[92,99] The technique is relatively simple, and smears kept at room temperature for as long as 2 weeks can still be stained. Immunoperoxidase staining has certain advantages over immunofluorescence staining but is also more time-consuming. Both the biochemical method and radioimmunoassay require fresh specimens and are more complicated than the immunofluorescence technique.

FACTOR VIII ANTIGEN DETECTION

Factor VIII antigen is a component of the coagulation factor VIII. Factor VIII antigen is produced by both the vascular endothelial cells and the megakaryocytes.[102,103] Its presence in these cells can be demonstrated by immunochemical techniques.[17,103–105] The clinical significance of factor VIII antigen as a cell marker has not been adequately explored, although factor VIII antigen can be used as a specific marker for both the vascular endothelial cells and the megakaryocytes, and it has been used for the diagnosis of megakaryocytic leukemia.[104]

Demonstration of factor VIII antigen has also been successful for identification of other vascular neoplasms such as Kaposi's sarcoma[106,107] and vinyl chloride–related hepatic angiosarcoma,[108] as well as other vascular lesions.[109,110]

MISCELLANEOUS MARKERS

Hemoglobin has also been successfully demonstrated by the immunoperoxidase method.[111] It appears as a useful marker for the erythroblasts. Heparin in tissue mast cells has been successfully demonstrated in tissues embedded in paraffin or plastics.[112] Recently, a mouse monoclonal antibody (AA1), specific for human mast cell tryptase, became available. It can be used on routinely processed, formalin-fixed, paraffin-embedded tissue sections for identification of mast cells and the diagnosis of mast cell diseases.[113,114] Lactoferrin,[79] α-antichymotrypsin,[69] and 5′-nucleotidase[115,116] have also been examined, but their clinical diagnostic value for hematologic neoplasms has not been established. Many other tissue antigens are now demonstrable by the immunoperoxidase method and can be applied to the identification of tumors. These include several hormones for endocrine tumors,[117,118] prostatic acid phosphatase and prostatic-specific antigen for prostatic carcinoma,[50,119] keratin for squamous cell carcinoma,[120] epithelial membrane antigen (EMA) for small-cell carcinoma,[121] chromogranin and synaptophysin for neuroblastoma,[121–123] muscle actin and desmin for rhabdomyosarcoma,[124,125] placental alkaline phosphatase for germ cell tumors,[126] melanoma-specific antigen recognized by monoclonal antibody HMB-45 for melanoma,[127–129] and the secretory component of IgA for adenocarcinomas.[130] These markers are useful for distinguishing undifferentiated tumors from the lymphomas. The proper selection of an appropriate marker and the interpretation of results will depend on the clinical features of the patient and the discretion of the pathologist.

EPITOPE ENHANCEMENT

Successful immunohistochemical staining depends on the sensitivity of the methods, the specificity of the antibodies, and the optimal preparation of tissue for study. Although the specificity and sensitivity of immunohistochemical stains can be improved by good staining technique and better antibodies, a limiting factor continues to be attenuation of antigen by fixation. In paraffin-embedded tissues fixed with formaldehyde or other aldehydes, reactive epitopes of tissue antigens may be masked by cross-linking, thus go undetected by traditional immunohistochemical staining. Many methods have been tried to retain or restore the antigenic activity in paraffin-embedded tissues. These include: use of coagulant fixatives, reduction of fixation time in formaldehyde, addition of heavy metal salts such as zinc to formaldehyde, proteolytic digestion, or microwave irradiation of tissues sections.[131] Proteolytic digestion and, more recently, microwave irradiation of tissue sections have been found to be the most effective methods for unmasking reactive epitopes.[132,133] Solutions such as urea, heavy metals, citrate or Tris at various pH often help to increase the effectiveness of microwave irradiation for epitope enhancement.[133,134,135] In most instances of antigenic attenuation by formaldehyde fixation, the restoration (or enhancement) of antigenic activity can be achieved by either proteolytic digestion or microwave irradiation of tissue sections in buffered solutions of 10 to 100mM citrate at pH 6 or 500mM Tris, pH 8.0. However, the optimal conditions for epitope enhancement for each specific antibody may not be the same and should be determined individually.[135,136]

REFERENCES

1. Taylor CR: Immunoperoxidase techniques: Practical and theoretical aspects. *Arch Pathol Lab Med* 102:112–121, 1978.
2. Warnke R, Pederson M, Williams C, et al: A study of lymphoproliferative diseases comparing immunofluorescence with immunohistochemistry. *Am J Clin Pathol* 70:867–875, 1978.
3. Guesdon J-L, Ternynck T, Avramens S: The use of avidin–biotin interaction in immunoenzymatic techniques. *J Histochem Cytochem* 27:1131–1139, 1979.
4. Hsu S-M, Raine L, Fanger H: Use of avidin–biotin-peroxidase complex (ABC) in immunoperoxidase techniques: A comparison between ABC and unlabeled antibody (PAP) procedures. *J Histochem Cytochem* 29:577–580, 1981.
5. Warnke R, Ley R: Detection of T- and B-cell antigens with hybridoma monoclonal antibodies: A biotin–avidin horseradish peroxidase method. *J Histochem Cytochem* 28:771–776, 1980.
6. Shi ZR, Itzkowitz SH, Kim YS: A comparison of three immunoperoxidase techniques for antigen detection in colorectal carcinoma tissues. *J Histochem Cytochem* 36:317–322, 1988.
7. Borowitz MJ, Croker BP, Burchette J: Immunocytochemical detection of lymphocyte surface antigens in fixed tissue sections. *J Histochem Cytochem* 30:171–174, 1982.
8. Falini B, Solas ID, Halverson C, et al: Double labeled-antigen method for demonstration of intracellular antigens in paraffin-embedded tissues. *J Histochem Cytochem* 30:21–26, 1982.
9. Filippa DA, Lieberman PH, Erlandson RA, et al: A study of malignant lymphomas using light and ultramicroscopic, cytochemical, and immunologic technics: Correlation with clinical features. *Am J Med* 64:259–268, 1978.
10. Jaffe ES, Shevach EM, Frank MM, et al: Nodular lymphoma: Evidence of origin from follicular B lymphocytes. *N Engl J Med* 290:813–819, 1974.
11. Mitrenga D, Arnold W, Mayersbach HV: Freeze-drying and embedding in glycol methacrylate (GMA): The results of morphological, histochemical, and immunohistological investigations. *Histochemistry* 39:313–326, 1974.
12. Vykoupil K-F, Thide J, Georgii A: Histochemical and immunohistochemical techniques on acrylate-embedded bone biopsies. *Blut* 32:215–218, 1976.
13. Warnke R, Levy R: Immunopathology of follicular lymphomas: A model of B-lymphocyte homing. *N Engl J Med* 298:481–486, 1978.
14. Laruent G, Gourdin MF, Reyes F: Detection of surface immunoglobulins of human lymphoid cells: A comparative study of live and fixed cells using a direct immunoperoxidase procedure. *J Clin Pathol* 35:139–143, 1982.
15. Hautzer NW, Wittkuhn JF, McCoughey WTE: Trypsin digestion in immunoperoxidase staining. *J Histochem Cytochem* 28:52–53, 1980.
16. Mason DY, Biberfeld P: Technical aspects of lymphoma immunohistology. *J Histochem Cytochem* 28:731–745, 1980.
17. McComb RP, Jones TR, Pizzo SV, et al: Specificity and sensitivity of immunohistochemical detection of factor VIII/von Willebrand factor antigen in formalin-fixed paraffin-embedded tissue. *J Histochem Cytochem* 30:371–377, 1982.
18. Reading M: A digestion technique for the reduction of background staining in the immunoperoxidase method. *J Clin Pathol* 30:88–90, 1977.
19. Takamiya H, Batsford S, Vogt A: An approach to postembedding staining of protein (immunoglobulin) antigen embedded in plastic: Prerequisites and limitations. *J Histochem Cytochem* 28:1041–1049, 1980.
20. Taylor CR: Immunohistologic studies of lymphoma: Past, present, and future. *J Histochem Cytochem* 28:777–787, 1980.
21. Shi SR, Key ME, Kalra KL: Antigen retrieval in formalin-fixed, paraffin-embedded tissues: An enhancement method for immunohistochemical staining based on microwave oven heating of tissue sections. *J Histochem Cytochem* 39:741–748, 1991.
22. Cuevas EC, Bateman AC, Wilkins BS, et al: Microwave antigen retrieval in immunocytochemistry: A study of 80 antibodies. *J Clin Pathol* 47:448–452, 1994.
23. Heggeness MH, Ash J: Use of the avidin–biotin complex for the localization of actin and myosin with fluorescence microscopy. *J Cell Biol* 73:783–788, 1977.
24. Levy R, Warnke R, Dorfuran RF, et al: The monoclonality of human B-cell lymphomas. *J Exp Med* 145:1014–1028, 1977.
25. Tubbs RR, Sheibani K, Sebek BA: Immunohistochemistry versus immunofluorescence for non-Hodgkin's lymphomas. *Am J Clin Pathol* 73:144–145, 1980.
26. Warnke R: Alteration of immunoglobulin-bearing lymphoma cells by fixation. *J Histochem Cytochem* 27:1195–1196, 1979.
27. Dorsett BH, Joachim HL: A method for the use of immunofluorescence on paraffin-embedded tissues. *Am J Clin Pathol* 69:66–72, 1978.
28. Avrameas S: Coupling of enzymes to proteins with glutaraldehyde: Use of the conjugates for the detection of antigens and antibodies. *Immunochemistry* 6:43–52, 1969.
29. Heyderman E: Immunoperoxidase technique in histopathology: Applications, methods and controls. *J Clin Pathol* 32:971–978, 1979.
30. Nakane PK, Pierce GB: Enzyme-labeled antibodies: Preparation and application for the localization of antigens. *J Histochem Cytochem* 14:929–931, 1967.
31. Sternberger LA, Hardy PH, Cuculis JJ, et al: The unlabeled antibody enzyme method of immunohistochemistry. *J Histochem Cytochem* 18:315–333, 1970.
32. Mason DY, Sammons R: Alkaline phosphatase and peroxidase for double immunoenzymatic labelling of cellular constituents. *J Clin Pathol* 31:454–460, 1978.
33. Yam LT, Janckila AJ, Li CY: The immunoalkaline phosphatase methods. In De Lellis RA (ed): *Advances in Immunohistochemistry*. New York, Raven Press, 1988, pp 1–29.
34. Clark CA, Downs EC, Primus FJ: An unlabeled antibody method using glucose oxidase–antiglucose oxidase complexes (GAG): A sensitive alternative to immunoperoxidase for the detection of tissue antigens. *J Histochem Cytochem* 30:27–34, 1982.
35. Suffin SC, Much KB, Young JC, et al: Improvement of the

glucose oxidase immunoenzyme technic: Use of a tetrazolium whose formazan is stable without heavy metal chelation. *Am J Clin Pathol* 7:492–496, 1979.
36. Ordronneau P, Lindström PB-M, Petrusz P: Four unlabeled antibody bridge techniques: A comparison. *J Histochem Cytochem* 29:1397–1404, 1981.
37. Strauss W: Peroxidase procedures: Technical problems encountered during their application. *J Histochem Cytochem* 27:1349–1351, 1979.
38. Strauss W: Imidazole increases the sensitivity of the cytochemical reaction for peroxidase with diaminobenzidine at a neutral pH. *J Histochem Cytochem* 30:491–493, 1982.
39. Hanker JS, Ambrose WW, James CJ, et al: Facilitated light microscopic cytochemical diagnosis of acute myelogenous leukemia. *Cancer Res* 39:1635–1639, 1979.
40. Graham RC, Lundholm U, Karnovsky MJ: Cytochemical demonstration of peroxidase activity with 3-amino-9-ethylcarbazole. *J Histochem Cytochem* 13:150–152, 1965.
41. Yam LT, Janckila AJ, Lam WKW, et al: Immunohistochemistry of prostatic acid phosphatase. *Prostate* 2:97–107, 1981.
42. Burns J: Background staining and sensitivity of the unlabelled antibody enzyme (PAP) method: Comparison with the peroxidase-labelled antibody sandwich method using formalin-fixed paraffin-embedded material. *Histochemistry* 43:291–294, 1975.
43. Zehr DR: Use of hydrogen peroxide–egg albumin to eliminate nonspecific staining in immunoperoxidase techniques. *J Histochem Cytochem* 26:415–416, 1978.
44. Maehly AC, Chance B: The assay of catalases and peroxidases. In Glick D (ed): *Methods of Biochemical Analysis*, vol 1. New York, Interscience Publishers, 1954, pp 357–424.
45. Wasdahl DA, Li CY, Morris MA: Paraffin section immunoperoxidase (IP) lymph node staining methodology for use with the Fisher Automated Stainer (FAS). *J Histochem Cytochem* 37:939, 1989.
46. Streefkerk JG: Inhibition of erythrocyte pseudoperoxidase activity by treatment with hydrogen peroxide following methanol. *J Histochem Cytochem* 20:829–831, 1972.
47. Isaacson P, Judd MA: Immunohistochemistry of carcinoembryonic antigen: Characterization of cross-reactions with other glycoproteins. *Gut* 18:779–785, 1977.
48. Li CY, Ziesmer SC, Lazcano-Villareal O: Use of azide and hydrogen peroxide as an inhibitor for endogenous peroxidase in the immunoperoxidase method. *J Histochem Cytochem* 35:1457–1460, 1987.
49. Weir EE, Pretlow TG, Pitts A, et al: A more sensitive and specific histochemical peroxidase stain for the localization of cellular antigen by the enzyme–antibody conjugate method. *J Histochem Cytochem* 22:1135–1140, 1974.
50. Li CY, Lam WKW, Yam LT: Immunohistochemical diagnosis of prostatic cancer with metastasis. *Cancer* 46:706–712, 1980.
51. Ponder BA, Wilkinson MM: Inhibition of endogenous tissue alkaline phosphatase with the use of alkaline phosphatase conjugates in immunohistochemistry. *J Histochem Cytochem* 29:981–984, 1981.
52. Habeshaw JA, Catley PF, Stansfield AG, et al: Terminal deoxynucleotidyl transferase activity in lymphoma. *Br J Cancer* 39:566–569, 1979.
53. Sternberger LA, Sternberger NH: The unlabeled antibody method: Comparison of peroxidase–antiperoxidase with avidin–biotin complex by a new method of quantification. *J Histochem Cytochem* 34:599–605, 1986.
54. Wood GS, Warnke R: Suppression of endogenous avidin-binding activity in tissues and its relevance to biotin–avidin detection systems. *J Histochem Cytochem* 29:1196–1204, 1981.
55. Banks PM: Diagnostic applications of an immunoperoxidase method in hematopathology. *J Histochem Cytochem* 27:1192–1194, 1979.
56. Hitzman JL, Li CY, Kyle RA: Immunoperoxidase staining of bone marrow sections. *Cancer* 48:2438–2446, 1981.
57. Picworth FA: A new method of study of the brain capillaries and its application to the regional localization of mental disorder. *J Anat* 69:62–71, 1934.
58. Undritz E: *Sandoz Atlas of Haematology*, ed 2. Basle, Switzerland, Sandoz, 1973, p 35.
59. Humphrey DM, Cortez EA, Spira DA: Immunohistologic studies of cytoplasmic immunoglobulin in rheumatic diseases including two patients with monoclonal patterns and subsequent lymphoma. *Cancer* 49:2049–2069, 1982.
60. Pangalis GA, Nathwani BN, Rappaport H: Detection of cytoplasmic immunoglobulin in well-differentiated lymphoproliferative diseases by the immunoperoxidase method. *Cancer* 45:1334–1339, 1980.
61. Pangalis GA, Nathwani BN, Rappaport H: An immunocytochemical study of non-Hodgkin's lymphomas. *Cancer* 48:915–922, 1981.
62. Pinkus GS, Said JW: Specific identification of intracellular immunoglobulin in paraffin sections of multiple myeloma and macroglobulinemia using an immunoperoxidase technique. *Am J Pathol* 87:45–57, 1977.
63. Taylor CR, Burns J: The demonstration of plasma cells and other immunoglobulin-containing cells in formalin-fixed, paraffin-embedded tissues using peroxidase-labelled antibody. *J Clin Pathol* 27:14–20, 1974.
64. Taylor CR: Immunohistologic studies of lymphomas: New methodology yields new information and poses new problems. *J Histochem Cytochem* 27:1189–1191, 1979.
65. Van Heerde P, Feltkamp CA, Feltkamp-Vroom TM, et al: Non-Hodgkin's lymphoma: Immunohistochemical and electron microscopical findings in relation to light microscopy: A study of 74 cases. *Cancer* 46:2210–2220, 1980.
66. Garvin AJ, Spicer SS, Parmley RT, et al: Immunohistochemical demonstration of IgG in Reed-Sternberg and other cells in Hodgkin's disease. *J Exp Med* 139:1077–1083, 1974.
67. Hayhoe FGJ, Burns GF, Cawley JC, et al: Cytochemical, ultrastructural and immunological studies of circulating Reed-Sternberg cells. *Br J Haematol* 38:485–490, 1978.
68. Kaplan HS, Gartner S: "Sternberg-Reed" giant cells of Hodgkin's disease: Cultivation in vitro, heterotransplantation, and characterization as neoplastic macrophages. *Int J Cancer* 19:511–525, 1977.
69. Papadimitriou CS, Stein H, Lennert K: The complexity

of immunohistochemical staining pattern of Hodgkin and Sternberg-Reed cells: Demonstration of immunoglobulin, albumin, alpha-1-antichymotrypsin and lysozyme. *Int J Cancer* 21:531–541, 1978.
70. Payne SV, Wright DH, Jones K, et al: Macrophage origin of Reed-Sternberg cells: An immunohistochemical study. *J Clin Pathol* 35:159–166, 1982.
71. Poppema S: The diversity of the immunohistological staining pattern of Sternberg-Reed cells. *J Histochem Cytochem* 28:788–791, 1980.
72. Taylor CR: The nature of Reed-Sternberg cells and other malignant "reticulum" cells. *Lancet* 2:802–806, 1974.
73. Isaacson P: Immunochemical demonstration of J chain: A marker of B-cell malignancy. *J Clin Pathol* 32:802–807, 1979.
74. Isaacson P, Wright DH: Anomalous staining patterns in immunohistologic studies of malignant lymphoma. *J Histochem Cytochem* 27:1197–1199, 1979.
75. Osserman EF, Lawlor DP: Serum and urinary lysozyme (muramidase) in monocytic and monomyelocytic leukemia. *J Exp Med* 124:921–951, 1966.
76. Asamer H, Schmalzl F, Braunsteiner H: Der immunzytologische lysozymnachweis in menschlichen blutzellen. *Acta Haematol* 41:49–54, 1969.
77. Ghoos Y, Vantrappen G: The cytochemical localization of lysozyme activity in leukocytes. *Histochem J* 2:11–16, 1970.
78. Mason DY, Taylor CR: The distribution of muramidase (lysozyme) in human tissues. *J Clin Pathol* 28:124–132, 1975.
79. Mason DY: Intracellular lysozyme and lactoferrin in myeloproliferative disorders. *J Clin Pathol* 30:541–546, 1977.
80. Pinkus GS, Said JW: Profile of intracytoplasmic lysozyme in normal tissues, myeloproliferative disorders, hairy cell leukemia, and other pathologic processes. An immunoperoxidase study of paraffin sections and smears. *Am J Pathol* 89:351–366, 1977.
81. Carbone A, Michean C, Cailland J-M, et al: A cytochemical and immunohistochemical approach to malignant histiocytosis. *Cancer* 47:2862–2871, 1981.
82. Neiman RS, Barcos M, Berard CW, et al: Granulocytic sarcoma: A clinicopathologic study of 61 biopsied cases. *Cancer* 48:1426–1437, 1981.
83. Pulford KAF, Rigney EM, Michlem KJ, et al: KP1: A new monoclonal antibody that detects a monocyte/macrophage-associated antigen in routinely processed tissue sections. *J Clin Pathol* 42:414–421, 1989.
84. Falini B, Flengh L, Pileri S, et al: PG-M1: A new monoclonal antibody directed against a fixative-resistant epitope on the macrophage-restricted form of the CD68 molecule. *Am J Pathol* 142:1359–1372, 1993.
85. Warnke RA, Pulford KAF, Pallesen G, et al: Diagnosis of myelomonocytic and macrophage neoplasms in routinely processed tissue biopsies with monoclonal antibody KP1. *Am J Pathol* 135:1089–1095, 1989.
86. Ratnam KV, Su WPD, Ziesmer S, et al: The value of immunohistochemistry in the diagnosis of leukemia cutis: A study of 54 cases using paraffin-section markers. *J Cut Pathol* 19:193–200, 1992.
87. Arai E, Su WPD, Roche PC, et al: Cutaneous histiocytic malignancy: Immunohistochemical re-examination of cases previously diagnosed as cutaneous "histiocytic lymphoma" and "malignant histiocytosis." *J Cut Pathol* 20:115–120, 1993.
88. Storr J, Dolan G, Coustan-Smith E, et al: Value of monoclonal anti-myeloperoxidase (MPO7) for diagnosing acute leukemia. *J Clin Pathol* 43:847–849, 1990.
89. Buccheri V, Shetty V, Yoshida N, et al: The role of an anti-myeloperoxidase antibody in the diagnosis and classification of acute leukemia: A comparison with light and electron microscopy cytochemistry. *Br J Haematol* 80:62–68, 1992.
90. Bollum FJ: Terminal deoxynucleotidyl transferase as a hematopoietic cell marker (review). *Blood* 54:1203–1215, 1979.
91. Janossy G, Hoffbrand AV, Greaves MF, et al: Terminal transferase enzyme assay and immunological membrane markers in the diagnosis of leukaemia: A multiparameter analysis of 300 cases. *Br J Haematol* 44:221–234, 1980.
92. Kalwinsky DK, Weathered WH, Dahl GV, et al: Clinical utility of initial terminal deoxynucleotidyl transferase determinations in childhood acute leukemias. *Cancer Res* 41:2877–2881, 1981.
93. Kung PC, Long JC, McCaffrey RP, et al: Terminal deoxynucleotidyl transferase in the diagnosis of leukemia and malignant lymphoma. *Am J Med* 64:788–794, 1978.
94. Bertazzoni U, Brusamolino E, Isernia P, et al: Prognostic significance of terminal transferase and adenosine deaminase in acute and chronic myeloid leukemia. *Blood* 60:685–692, 1982.
95. Marks SM, Baltimore D, McCaffrey R: Terminal transferase as a predictor of initial responsiveness to vincristine and prednisone in blastic chronic myelogenous leukemia. *N Engl J Med* 298:812–814, 1978.
96. McCaffrey R, Lillquist A, Sallan S, et al: Clinical utility of leukemia cell terminal transferase measurements. *Cancer Res* 41:4814–4820, 1981.
97. Folds JD, Bollum FJ, Dean L, et al: Simultaneous evaluation for terminal deoxynucleotidyl transferase and myeloperoxidase in leukemia. *Am J Hematol* 12:391–396, 1982.
98. McGraw TP, Folds JD, Bollum FJ, et al: Terminal deoxynucleotidyl transferase–positive acute myeloblastic leukemia. *Am J Hematol* 10:251–258, 1981.
99. Bradstock KF, Janossy G, Hoffbrand AV, et al: Immunofluorescent and biochemical studies of terminal deoxynucleotidyl transferase in treated acute leukemia. *Br J Haematol* 47:121–131, 1981.
100. Hecht T, Forman SJ, Winkler US, et al: Histochemical demonstration of terminal deoxynucleotidyl transferase in leukemia. *Blood* 58:856–858, 1981.
101. Stass SA, Dean L, Peiper SC, et al: Determination of terminal deoxynucleotidyl transferase on bone marrow smears by immunoperoxidase. *Am J Clin Pathol* 77:174–176, 1982.
102. Hoyer LW, de los Santos RP, Hoyer JR: Antihemophilic factor antigen: Localization in endothelial cells by immunofluorescent microscopy. *J Clin Invest* 52:2757–2764, 1973.
103. Piovella F, Nalli G, Malamani GD, et al: The ultrastructural localization of factor VIII-antigen in human platelets, mega-

103. ...karyocytes and endothelial cells utilizing a ferritin-labelled antibody. *Br J Haematol* 39:209–213, 1978.
104. Innes DJ Jr, Mills Se, Walker GK: Megakaryocytic leukemia: Identification utilizing anti-factor VIII immunoperoxidase. *Am J Clin Pathol* 77:107–110, 1982.
105. Piovella F, Ascari E, Sitar GM, et al: Immunofluorescent detection of factor VIII–related antigen in human platelets and megakaryocytes. *Haemostasis* 3:288–295, 1974.
106. Guarda LG, Silva EG, Ordonez NG, et al: Factor VIII in Kaposi's sarcoma. *Am J Clin Pathol* 76:197–200, 1981.
107. Nadji M, Morales AR, Ziegles-Weissman J, et al: Kaposi's sarcoma: Immunohistologic evidence of an endothelial origin. *Arch Pathol Lab Med* 105:274–275, 1981.
108. Fortwengler HP Jr, Jones D, Espinosa E, et al: Evidence for endothelial cell origin of vinyl chloride–induced hepatic angiosarcoma. *Gastroenterology* 80:1415–1419, 1981.
109. Burgdorf WHC, Mukai K, Rosai J: Immunohistochemical identification of factor VIII–related antigen in endothelial cells of cutaneous lesions of alleged vascular nature. *Am J Clin Pathol* 75:167–171, 1981.
110. Sehested M, Hou-Jesen K: Factor VIII–related antigen as an endothelial cell marker in benign and malignant diseases. *Virchows Arch (Pathol Anat)* 391:217–225, 1981.
111. Neiman RS: Erythroblastic transformation in myeloproliferative disorders: Confirmation by an immunohistologic technique. *Cancer* 46:1636–1640, 1980.
112. Shar ST Jr, Roche PC, Schmer G, et al: Immunohistochemical identification of mast cells in paraffin- and epon-embedded tissues using platelet factor 4. *J Histochem Cytochem* 30:185–188, 1982.
113. Walls AF, Bennett AR, McBride HM, et al: Production of monoclonal antibodies specific for human mast cell tryptase. *Clin Exp Allergy* 20:581–589, 1990.
114. Walls AF, Jones DB, Williams JH, et al: Immunohistochemical identification of mast cells in formaldehyde-fixed tissue using monoclonal antibodies specific for tryptase. *J Pathol* 162:119–126, 1990.
115. LaMantia K, Conklyn M, Quagliata F, et al: Immunologic studies of 5' nucleotidase in normal and chronic lymphocytic leukemia lymphocytes. *Blood* 46:1042, 1975.
116. Lopes J, Zucker-Franklin D, Silber R: Heterogeneity of 5' nucleotidase activity in lymphocytes in chronic lymphocytic leukemia. *J Clin Invest* 52:1297–1300, 1973.
117. De Lellis RA, Sternberger LA, Mann RB, et al: Immunoperoxidase technics in diagnostic pathology: Report of a workshop sponsored by the national Cancer Institute. *Am J Clin Pathol* 71:483–488, 1979.
118. Pinkus GS: Diagnostic immunocytochemistry of paraffin-embedded tissues. *Hum Pathol* 13:411–415, 1982.
119. Nadji M, Tabei SZ, Castro A, et al: Prostatic specific antigen: An immunohistologic marker for prostatic neoplasms. *Cancer* 48:1229–1232, 1981.
120. Mitchell DP, Gusterson BA: Simultaneous demonstration of keratin and mucin. *J Histochem Cytochem* 30:707–709, 1982.
121. Chang TK, Li CY, Smithson WA: Immunocytochemical study of small round cell tumors in routinely processed specimens. *Arch Pathol Lab Med* 113:1343–1348, 1989.
122. Hachitanda Y, Tsuneyoshi M, Enjoji M: An ultrastructural and immunohistochemical evaluation of cytodifferentiation in neuroblastic tumors. *Mod Pathol* 2:13–19, 1989.
123. Gould VE, Lee I, Wiedenmann B, et al: Synaptophysin: A novel marker for neurons, certain neuroendocrine cells, and their neoplasms. *Hum Pathol* 17:979–983, 1986.
124. Schmidt RA, Cone R, Haas JE, et al: Diagnosis of rhabdomyosarcomas with HHF35, a monoclonal antibody directed against muscle actins. *Am J Pathol* 131:19–28, 1988.
125. Azumi N, Ben-Ezra J, Battifora H: Immunophenotypic diagnosis of leiomyosarcomas and rhabdomyosarcomas with monoclonal antibodies to muscle-specific actin and desmin in formalin-fixed tissue. *Mod Pathol* 1:469–474, 1988.
126. Wick MR, Swanson PE, Manivel JC: Placental-like alkaline phosphatase reactivity in human tumors: An immunohistochemical study of 520 cases. *Hum Pathol* 18:946–954, 1987.
127. Gown AM, Vogel AM, Hoak D, et al: Monoclonal antibodies specific for melanocytic tumors distinguish subpopulations of melanocytes. *Am J Pathol* 123:195–203, 1986.
128. Ordonez NG, Xiaolong JI, Hickey RC: Comparison of HMB-45 monoclonal antibody and S-100 protein in the immunohistochemical diagnosis of melanoma. *Am J Clin Pathol* 90:385–390, 1988.
129. Bonetti F, Pea M, Martignoni G, et al: False-positive immunostaining of normal epithelia and carcinoma with ascites fluid preparations of antimelanoma monoclonal antibody HMB45. *Am J Clin Pathol* 95:454–459, 1991.
130. Harris JP, South MA: Secretory component: A glandular epithelial cell marker. *Am J Pathol* 105:47–53, 1981.
131. Leong AS-Y, Milios J. An assessment of the efficacy of the microwave antigen-retrieval procedure on a range of tissue antigens. *Appl. Immunohistochem* 1(4):267–274, 1993.
132. Shi S-R, Key ME, Kalra KL. Antigen retrieval in formalin-fixed, paraffin-embedded tissues: an enhancement method for immunohistochemical staining based on microwave oven heating of tissue sections. *J Histochem Cytochem* 39:741–748, 1991.
133. Gown AM, deWever N, Battifora H. Microwave-based antigenic unmasking. A revolutionary new technique for routine immunohistochemistry. *Appl Immunohistochem* 1(4):256–266, 1993.
134. Beckstead JH. Improved antigen retrieval in formalin-fixed, paraffin-embedded tissues. *Appl Immunohistochem* 2(4):274–281, 1994.
135. Shi S-R, Imam A, Young L, et al. Antigen retrieval immunohistochemistry under the influence of pH using monoclonal antibodies. *J Histochem Cytochem* 43:193–201, 1995.
136. Cuevas EC, Bateman AC, Wilkins BS, et al. Microwave antigen retrieval in immunocytochemistry: a study of 80 antibodies. *J Clin Pathol* 47:448–452, 1994.

Chapter 5
SURFACE MARKERS

Surface markers are cell-specific antigens and receptors present on the cell membrane (Table 5-1). They can be visualized by binding to particulate materials (e.g., red blood cells and yeast cells) specific for a receptor or with specific antibodies conjugated with either an enzyme indicator or a fluorochrome. The immunologic techniques used for this purpose are both sensitive and specific (Table 5-2). They can be used in conjunction with many cytochemical markers to further increase the accuracy of cell identification. The drawbacks of these immunologic techniques are that fresh cell suspensions are needed and that the procedures are time-consuming. However, the advent of flow cytometry has greatly facilitated the performance of surface marker studies. Further automation of monoclonal antibody staining may finally reduce the testing time to a reasonable level.

Techniques involving the use of monoclonal antibodies for accurate identification of human blood cells have become prevalent.[1,2] These techniques were first employed to demonstrate the various T-cell subsets (Figure 5-1), but they have now been extended to B cells, monocytes, granulocytes, and others (Figure 5-2). The following sections present brief discussions of some early used markers; some of them (e.g., surface and cytoplasmic immunoglobulins and HLA-DR) are still very useful; others (e.g., human T-lymphocyte antigen, sheep erythrocyte rosette receptor and Fc receptor) have been replaced by monoclonal antibodies; and still others (e.g., mouse erythrocyte receptor) have become obsolete. However, these markers are of historic significance in the evolution of monoclonal antibodies.

SURFACE IMMUNOGLOBULIN

Surface immunoglobulin (SIg) is a useful cell marker for the identification of B lymphocytes. The most frequently used technique for the study of SIg in cell suspensions has been immunofluorescence. For tissue sections, the immunoperoxidase stain is used, but it is limited to frozen sections. Other techniques include rosette formation with erythrocytes, inert particles, and bacteria coated with immunoglobulin. However, these techniques are no longer used in clinical laboratories.

Demonstration of SIg is useful not only for the identification of B cells but also for the recognition of clonality. The latter is useful for substantiating the diagnosis of lymphoid neoplasms, as well as for identifying lymphoma cells in peripheral blood or for detecting tumor dissemination. Therefore, polyvalent immunoglobulin antiserum and monospecific antisera against the immunoglobulin heavy chains, IgG (γ), IgM (μ), IgA (α), and IgD (δ), as well as the κ and λ light chains, should be used. Monoclonality of SIg was originally defined as follows:

1. The κ to λ ratio is 3:1 or more, or the λ to κ ratio is 2:1 or more.
2. The ratio of the predominant heavy chain to the sum of other heavy chains is 3:1 or more.
3. The monoclonal population exceeds 75% of the total B-cell population.[3]

However, since the heavy chain gene may switch after immunoglobulin gene rearrangement,[4] the ratio of heavy chains is less reliable and is not tested in many laboratories. In addition, when the tumor and the normal populations differ in phenotype and/or size, the flow cytometric techniques can distinguish these two populations by "gating" and the cutoff of 75% is no longer required.[5] Nevertheless, the total percentage of B cells should be at least 20% to make calculation of the light chain ratio reliable.

The presence of a monoclonal pattern is usually indicative of neoplasia. A polyclonal pattern, on the other hand, is more suggestive of a benign disorder. Under most circumstances, a polyclonal pattern seen in a lymphoid neoplasm is caused by technical problems.[5] These include the following:

TABLE 5-1. Surface Markers for Human Blood Cells

Markers	T Cell	B Cell	Null Cell	Plasma Cell	Monocyte	Granulocyte	Erythroblast	Platelet
SIg	−	+	−	−	−	−	−	−
Fc receptor	±	+	±	−	+	+	−	−
Complement receptor	±	+	−	−	+	+	+	−
HLA-DR	±	+	±	−	+	+	+	−
MER	−	±	−	−	−	−	−	−
Epstein-Barr virus receptor	−	+	−	−	−	−	−	−
Sheep erythrocyte receptor	+	−	−	−	−	−	−	−
Human T-lymphocyte antigen	+	−	−	−	−	−	−	−
Common ALL antigen	−	−	+	−	−	−	−	−

ALL = acute lymphoblastic leukemia; HLA-DR = Ia-like antigen.

Note: + indicates presence of the marker on the cell surface; − indicates absence of the marker; ± indicates that in a population of cells, some have the marker and some do not.

1. Samples are not representative (sampling error). For example, a lymph node sample may have been taken from an area with very limited tumor cell infiltrate.
2. When tumor cells are few, the pattern seen represents the normal population, which is polyclonal, as in the early phase of leukemia or lymphoma.
3. The immunoglobulin antisera may react with the Fc receptor, not the surface immunoglobulin.[1,2,5] This problem can be avoided by the routine use of F(ab)2 antiserum, which binds specifically to surface immunoglobulins.
4. The patient's own serum immunoglobulin may adsorb nonspecifically to the surface of lymphocytes or may combine specifically with the Fc receptor of lymphocytes or macrophages.[1,2,5] This is more likely to occur when hypergammaglobulinemia is present. This problem can be solved by thoroughly washing the test lymphocytes, together with enzymatic stripping of the adsorbed immunoglobulin or incubation of the test lymphocytes at 37°C for 1 to 24 hr, so that cytophilic immunoglobulin will be shed from the lymphocytes. Furthermore, double staining with a light chain (κ or λ) and a B-cell antibody (e.g., CD19) may circumvent the problem of nonspecific adsorption of cytophilic immunoglobulin by excluding cells which are light chain positive but B-antigen negative.[2]

TABLE 5-2. Cell Specificity and Clinical Applications of Surface Markers Other Than Monoclonal Antibodies

Surface Markers	Cell Specificity	Clinical Application
SIg	B cells	B-CLL, B-ALL, B lymphomas
Fc receptor	B cells, monocytes	
Complement receptor	B cells, monocytes	
HLA-DR	Null cells, B cells, activated T cells, granulocytes, monocytes	Marker for null ALL, uALL, B-CLL, B lymphomas
MER	B cells	B-CLL, PLL
Epstein-Barr virus receptor	B cells	
Sheep erythrocyte receptor	T cells	T-ALL, T-CLL
Human T-lymphocyte antigen	T cells	T-ALL, T-CLL
Common ALL antigen	CALL lymphoblasts	CALL

ALL = acute lymphoblastic leukemia; CALL = common acute lymphoblastic leukemia; CLL = chronic lymphocytic leukemia; HLA-DR = Ia-like antigen; PLL = prolymphocytic leukemia; uALL = unclassified or undifferentiated acute lymphoblastic leukemia.

The SIg in most lymphoid neoplasms is IgM, with or without the coexistence of IgD.[4,5] IgD seldom exists alone, and its presence may indicate a mature lymphocyte in an antigen-dependent stage. Surface IgG is much less frequently seen than surface IgM, and surface IgA is rarely found in lymphoid neoplasms except in intestinal lymphoma. One study showed that surface IgG_2 was more frequently seen on normal lymphocytes, but surface IgG_3 and IgG_4 were common in human lymphoblastoid cell lines.[6] Of the light chains, κ is expressed more frequently than λ.

The intensity of immunofluorescence correlates with the amount of SIg and is helpful in the differential diagnosis. Aisenberg[7] has stated that follicular center cells stain more brightly than medullary cord cells. Thus, tumors derived

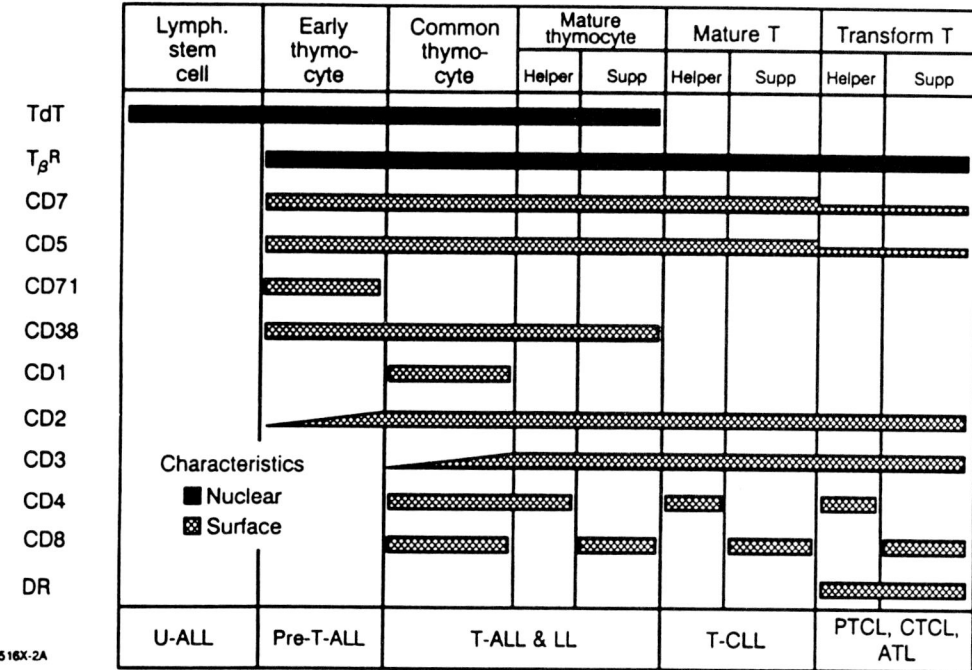

FIGURE 5-1. Major Immunogenotypic and Immunologic Characteristics in Stages of T-Lymphocyte Differentiation and Corresponding Neoplastic Diseases. $T\beta^R$ = rearrangement of the Tβ receptor gene; TdT = terminal deoxynucleotidyl transferase; DR = HLA-DR, Ia-like antigen; CD = cluster of differentiation; ALL = acute lymphocytic leukemia; ATL = adult T-cell leukemia/lymphoma; CLL = chronic lymphocytic leukemia; CTCL = cutaneous T-cell lymphoma; LL = lymphoblastic lymphoma; PTCL = peripheral T-cell lymphoma; u-ALL = undifferentiated acute lymphocytic leukemia.

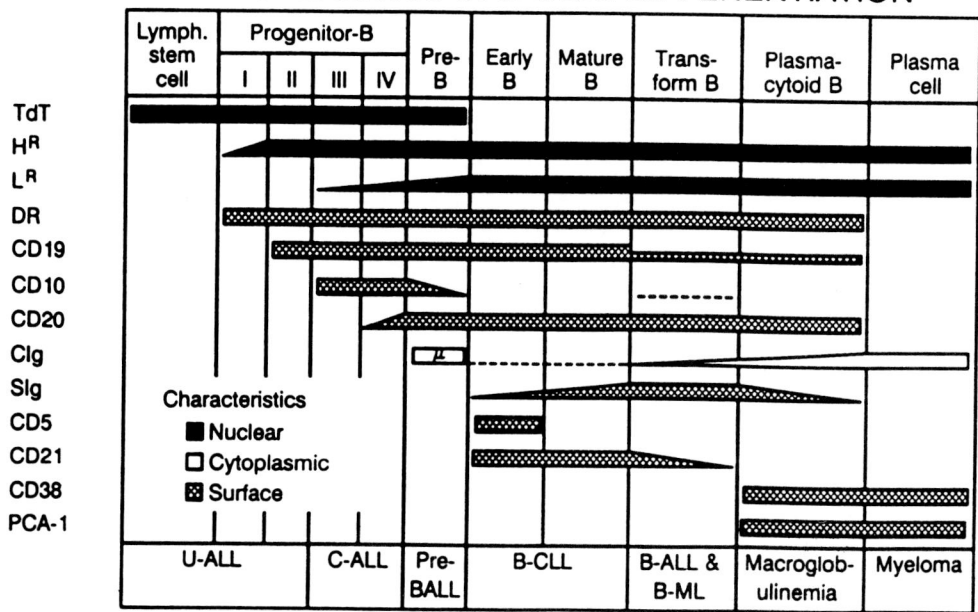

FIGURE 5-2. Major Immunogenotypic and Immunologic Characteristics in Stages of B-Lymphocyte Differentiation and Corresponding Neoplastic Diseases. TdT = terminal deoxynucleotidyl transferase; H^R = heavy chain gene rearrangement; L^R = light chain gene rearrangement; DR = HLA-DR, Ia-like antigen; CD = cluster of differentiation; ALL = acute lymphocytic leukemia; CLL = chronic lymphocytic leukemia; c-ALL = common acute lymphocytic leukemia; ML = malignant lymphoma; u-ALL = undifferentiated acute lymphocytic leukemia.

from medullary cord cells (such as chronic lymphocytic leukemia [CLL] and its lymphoma counterpart, small lymphocytic lymphoma) stain faintly, but other B-cell lymphomas display a wide range of brightness. On the other hand, Warnke and Rouse emphasize that only the germinal center B cells fail to express substantial levels of SIg under normal condition. Therefore, when a large population of B cells (defined by monoclonal antibodies) expresses no SIg, it is highly suggestive of lymphoma rather than hyperplasia. The frequency of SIg-negative, B lineage antigen-positive B-cell lymphoma is approximately 10% to 20% among B-cell lymphomas.[4,8,9] Most of the mediastinal lymphomas of the non-T-cell type belong to this category.[10]

When antiserum reacts to SIg, the immune complex thus formed is first evenly distributed; it then becomes patchy, then capped, and finally internalized.[5] Routine SIg studies are usually performed at 4°C, and sodium azide is added to the lymphocyte–antiserum mixture to prevent capping. However, the capping phenomenon, manifested as localization of immunofluorescence on one pole of the lymphocyte, is also helpful in distinguishing and subclassifying the B-cell subsets.[7,11] When lymphocytes are further incubated with antiserum at 37°C for 15 to 30 min after the routine procedure, the follicular center cells are usually positive and the medullary cord cells are negative for capping. For instance, capping is seldom seen in CLL cells[12] or in B-immunoblastic lymphomas.[13] Capping of IgM in lymphomas is associated with the presence of complement receptor.

CYTOPLASMIC IMMUNOGLOBULIN

Although cytoplasmic immunoglobulin (CIg) is not a surface marker, immunofluorescence staining for CIg performed on cell suspensions or smears is frequently included in surface marker studies. The meaning of a positive CIg result in a tissue section is different from that in a cell suspension. In tissue sections, CIg can be identified in all mature and immature B cells, whereas in cell suspensions CIg is demonstrated only in pre-B cells and plasma cells.[5] In multiple myeloma, testing for CIg is needed only when the tumor cells are nonsecretory or morphologically atypical.[5] When a biclonal or triclonal gammopathy is present, it is of academic interest to see whether the myeloma proteins are from the same or different clones of tumor cells. From a practical point of view, the major application of CIg in cell suspensions or smears is to identify pre-B-cell neoplasms, which can be seen in ALL[14] or CML in lymphoblast crisis.[15] Pre-B cells contain a small amount of μ chain without a light chain. Plasma cells contain abundant CIg, which can be any class or type of immunoglobulin.

FC RECEPTOR

The Fc receptor for the Fc fragment of immunoglobulins includes IgG, IgM, IgA, and IgE, but each receptor can react to only a single class of immunoglobulin. Although the Fc receptor is traditionally classified as a B-cell marker, it is also present in subpopulations of T cells and null cells; macrophages; granulocytes; cells from the liver, kidney, and breasts; and various neoplastic cells.[16] Therefore, the presence of Fc receptors has no discriminatory value.

Fc receptors were used to delineate T-cell subsets. T cells that react with IgG-Fc (Tγ cells) have been reported to have suppressor cell function, whereas those that react with IgM-Fc (Tμ cells) show helper cell function.[17] Although this concept is controversial, since the Tγ cells can be of macrophage origin, the Fc receptor certainly plays a role in immunoregulation, antigen localization, and mediation of antibody-dependent cellular cytotoxicity.[18,19] A T-lymphoma variant, erythrophagocytic Tγ lymphoma, which mimics malignant histiocytosis, has been described.[20] Its erythrophagocytic activity is assumed to be mediated by the Fc receptor. Since CD4 and CD8 monoclonal antibodies, which may identify T-helper cells and T-suppressor cells, respectively, are now available, EA rosetting for the IgM-Fc and IgG-Fc receptors is no longer used. This type of lymphoma has now been named *hepatosplenic γδ T-cell lymphoma* and is considered a separate clinical entity.[21–23] However, Tγ lymphocytes are not confined to T-suppressor cells. CD16 (the Fc receptor of IgG) is frequently demonstrated on tumor cells in the so-called Tγ lymphoproliferative disorder, which can be T-suppressor, T-helper, or natural killer cells.[24,25]

COMPLEMENT RECEPTOR

Complement receptors are mainly for the split products of C3 (C3b, C3d) and C4 (C4b); however, receptors for C1q, C8, and C2 inhibitor are also present on the cell membrane of B lymphocytes.[26,27] Similar to the Fc receptor, complement receptors have no value for cell type identification because they are present in a small population of a variety of cells: T cells, null cells, monocytes, neutrophils, eosinophils, and erythrocytes.[26,27] Nevertheless, the monocytes and granulocytes have only C3b,[28] and CLL cells have receptors for C3d but not for C3b.[29] This difference was used to distinguish normal B cells from morphologically normal-looking CLL cells. In some follicular lymphomas, complement receptors may be completely absent.[11]

The EAC-rosette technique was most commonly used for the detection of complement receptors. In this technique, erythrocytes are coated with immunoglobulin (antibody) and complement; after incubation, the antibody/complement-coated erythrocytes may form rosettes around the complement receptor-positive cells. Recently, monoclonal antibodies specific for a few complement receptors have become available, such as CD11b for C3bi receptor and CD21 for C3d receptor, and have replaced the EAC-rosette technique. However, antibodies for most complement receptors are still not available.

HLA-DR

HLA-DR, the Ia-like antigen, is a glycoprotein composed of a heavy chain and a light chain.[1] In the mouse, these proteins are controlled by genes in the I region of the H2 complex and are therefore called the *Ia antigens* (I region–associated antigens). The equivalent molecules in humans are termed *HLA-DR antigens* because there is no I region on human chromosomes. Its other name—p23,30—refers to the molecular weight of HLA-DR. HLA-DR is present on B cells, monocytes, activated T cells, null cells, and precursor cells of the myeloid and erythroid systems. The so-called null cells are mostly B cells at the earliest stage of differentiation when HLA-DR is present but the mature B-cell antigens are not.[30] Although HLA-DR alone is not specific enough to be used as a particular cell marker, it is still helpful in distinguishing small B cells from small T-cell neoplasms.[31,32] When both HLA-DR and SIg were studied on the same B-cell tumors, either the percentage of the HLA-DR-positive cells was within 10% of the SIg-positive cells or the percentage of HLA-DR-positive cells greatly exceeded that of the SIg-positive cells.[33] The latter group may represent B-cell tumors derived from primitive B cells.

MOUSE ERYTHROCYTE RECEPTOR

The mouse erythrocyte receptor (MER) has been demonstrated in lymphocytes. Spontaneous MER is seen in approximately 7% to 8% of peripheral blood lymphocytes. These lymphocytes have been proved to be B cells by double-labeling (SIg and MER) experiments.[34] The MER is separate from the Fc and complement receptors and appears earlier than the other two in lymphoid ontogeny. However, only a subpopulation of B cells possesses MER, and MER has not been demonstrated in T cells, monocytes, neutrophils, and eosinophils.[34,35] This largely neglected marker is highly specific for B-cell CLL. It is, however, also positive in prolymphocytic leukemia and sometimes in small lymphocytic lymphoma.[35,36] The availability of CD5 and CD23, which are characteristic of B-cell CLL, has largely replaced the role of MER testing.[37]

RECEPTOR FOR EPSTEIN-BARR VIRUS

The receptor for Epstein-Barr virus is present on essentially all B lymphocytes but not on thymocytes and T cells.[38] When the Epstein-Barr virus binds to this receptor, it can trigger polyclonal B-cell proliferation both in vivo and in vitro and is probably the basis of malignant transformation of B cells in vivo, as in Burkitt's lymphoma.[39] However, because Epstein-Barr virus is oncogenic, this receptor is not routinely used in clinical laboratories as a B-cell marker. Monoclonal antibody for CD21 is associated with Epstein-Barr virus receptor, and its use will make the old technique obsolete.

SHEEP ERYTHROCYTE ROSETTES

Human T cells possess a special receptor for sheep erythrocytes and will form spontaneous rosettes with them. The rosette thus formed is usually referred to as an *E-rosette* to distinguish it from the *EA-rosette*, which forms in response to Fc receptor, and the *EAC-rosette*, which forms in response to complement receptor. The E-rosette is specific for the T-cell lineage, including thymocytes and mature T cells. It is not present on B cells, monocytes, neutrophils, and, of course, null cells, which by definition are negative for both SIg and E-rosettes.

The E-rosette test is usually performed at 4°C, but further incubation at 37°C helps to distinguish normal T cells and T-cell neoplasms. For instance, at 37°C, E-rosettes formed with peripheral T cells dissociate, but those formed with thymocytes remain stable.[40] Similarly, malignancies of thymic origin, such as T-cell lymphoblastic lymphoma, form heat-stable rosettes[40,41] and neoplasms of peripheral T-cell origin, such as CLL and Sézary syndrome, form heat-labile rosettes.[42]

The availability of a monoclonal antibody (CD2) that reacts to the sheep erythrocyte receptor on the surface of T cells has made the E-rosette technique obsolete. CD2 is now used routinely with flow cytometry to identify E-rosette-positive T cells.

HUMAN T-LYMPHOCYTE ANTIGEN

Human T cells possess cell-specific antigens—human T-lymphocyte antigen (HTLA)—against which specific antisera can be prepared. The earlier HTLA antiserum was the fetal brain antiserum, which cross-reacted with HTLA[43]. T-cell-specific heteroantisera have also been prepared against thymus, peripheral T cells, lymphocytes from cases of agammaglobulinemia, and T-cell ALL.[44] These heteroan-

TABLE 5-3. Classification of T-lineage ALL

Group	Antigen							
	CD1	CD2	cCD3	sCD3	CD4	CD5	CD7	CD8
1	−	+	+	−	−	+	+	−
2	+	+	+	−	+	+	+	+
3	−	+	+	+	±	+	+	±

cCD3 = cytoplasmic CD3; sCD3 = surface membrane CD3.

tisera to T lymphocytes are heterogeneous, and their specificity for the T cells may not be the same. Their heterogeneity is proved by the fact that many different T-cell-specific antigens have been demonstrated by techniques using monoclonal antibodies.

Monoclonal antibodies have revolutionized this field by precisely pinpointing the various developmental stages and different functional subsets of T cells. The systematic application of a monoclonal antibody system divides T cells into five stages and two subsets[45,46] (Figure 5-1). Each stage has several differentiation antigens, although some of them appear in more than one stage. Based on the presence or absence of different T-cell antigens (CD1a, CD2, CD3, CD4, CD5, CD7, and CD8), as defined by monoclonal antibodies, Foon and Todd[30] classified T-lineage ALL into three groups. This classification has been further modified by dividing CD3 into cytoplasmic and membrane CD3 (Table 5-3).[46]

COMMON ALL ANTIGEN (CD10) AND THE NULL-CELL MARKERS

The *null cell* is so named because it lacks the classic T-cell and B-cell markers. However, more and more cell markers are being discovered on null cells. Therefore, terms like *non-T, non-B cell* or *third population cell* are being advocated as a substitute for *null cell.* However, since the discovery of natural killer cell as the third population of lymphocytes, the above terms are no longer appropriate for the description of null cell.

The common ALL antigen (CALLA) was considered a relatively specific marker for null cells, but it is mainly present in ALL and seldom found on normal null cells.[47] Patients who have null-cell ALL that expresses CALLA usually have a good prognosis.[48,49] However, cells from patients who have pre-B-cell ALL have also been found to express CALLA, and these patients appear to have a worse prognosis than the null-cell group.[50] In fact, CALLA can be demonstrated in most B-cell ALL and occasional T-cell ALL cases.

Nadler et al.[51] included CALLA as a marker for the classification of non-T ALL, which was later modified by Foon and Todd.[30] Gene rearrangement analysis and immunologic staining with B-cell-restricted monoclonal antibodies have proved that most of the non-T ALLs are indeed B-lineage ALLs (Table 5-4). Only a small number of cases are considered unclassified.[46]

MONOCLONAL ANTIBODIES

The cell surfaces of the human blood cells contain certain cell-specific antigens that can be recognized by specific monoclonal antibodies produced by the hybridoma technique. This technique is based on the fusion of mouse spleen cells with myeloma cells of certain genetic characteristics (no antibody production and lacking hypoxanthine phosphoribosyl transferase [HPRT]) to form somatic cell hybrids.[52] When a single cultured myeloma cell is fused with an antibody-forming cell (spleen cell from an immunized mouse), the resulting hybrid grows continuously in culture and produces highly specific monoclonal antibodies.

Theoretically, the production of monoclonal antibodies is unlimited because the hybrids can be subcloned indefinitely and the hybridoma cells can be frozen for storage.[52] When needed, monoclonal antibodies can be harvested from the supernatant of the culture medium, from the ascitic fluid, or from the serum of animals receiving the hybridoma cell inoculation.

TABLE 5-4. Classification of B-lineage ALL

Group	Antigen					
	HLA-DR	CD10	CD19	CD20	Cμ	SIg
1	+	−	−	−	−	−
2	+	−	+	−	−	−
3	+	+	+	−	−	−
4	+	+	+	+	−	−
5	+	+	+	+	+	−
6	+	±	+	+	−	+

Cμ = cytoplasmic μ chain; SIg = surface membrane immunoglobulin.

TABLE 5-5. Reactions of Monoclonal Antibodies to Various Human Blood Cells

Antigen	Monoclonal Antibody	T Cell	B Cell	NK Cell	Plasma Cell	Monocyte	Granulocyte	Erythroblast	Megakaryocyte
CD1a	Leu-6, OKT6, T6	+	−	−	−	−	−	−	−
CD2	Leu-5, OKT11, T11	+	−	−	−	−	−	−	−
CD3	Leu-4, OKT3, T3	+	−	−	−	−	−	−	−
CD4	Leu-3, OKT4, T4	+	−	−	−	−	−	−	−
CD5	Leu-1, OKT1, T1	+	−°	−	−	−	−	−	−
CD7	Leu-9, OKT16, 3A1	+	−	+	−	−	−	−	−
CD8	Leu-2, OKT8, T8	+	−	−	−	−	−	−	−
CD10	CALLA, OKBcALLa, J5	−	±	−	−	−	−	−	−
CD11b	Leu-15, OHM1, Mo1	±	−	+	−	+	+	−	−
CD11c	Leu-M5, S-HCL3	−	−†	+	−	+	+	−	−
CD13	Leu-M7, OKM13, My7	−	−	−	−	+	+	−	−
CD14	Leu-M3, OKM14, My4, Mo2	−	−	−	−	−	−	−	−
CD15	Leu-M1, My1	−	−	−	−	+	+	−	−
CD16	Leu-11	−	−	+	−	−	−	−	−
CD19	Leu-12, OKpanB, B4	−	+	−	−	−	−	−	−
CD20	Leu-16, B1	−	+	−	−	−	−	−	−
CD21	CR2, OKB7, B2	−	+	−	−	−	−	−	−
CD22	Leu-14, OKB22, B3, S-HCL1	−	+	−	−	−	−	−	−
CD23	Leu-20, B6	−	±	−	−	−	−	−	−
CD25	IL-2, OKT26a, Tac	±	±	−	−	−	−	−	−
CD30	Ki-1, Ber-H2	±	±	−	−	−	−	−	−
CD33	Leu-M9, My9	−	−	−	−	+	+	−	−
CD38	Leu-17, OKT10, T10	+	−	−	+	−	−	−	−
CD41	GPIIb/IIIa, J15	−	−	−	−	−	−	−	+
CD45	HLe-1, LCA	+	+	+	−	+	+	−	−
CD45RO	UCHL1	+	±	−	−	±	±	−	−
CD56	Leu-19, NKH-1	−	−	+	−	−	−	−	−
CD57	Leu-7, HNK-1	−	−	+	−	−	−	−	−
CD68	KP1, PG-M1	−	−	−	−	+	+	−	−
CD74	LN2	−	+	−	−	+	−	−	−
CDw75	LN1	±	+	−	−	−	−	−	−
—	HLA-DR, Ia	±	+	−	−	+	+	−	−
—	PCA-1	−	−	−	+	±	±	−	−
—	RC82.4	−	−	−	−	−	−	+	−
—	Glycophorin	−	−	−	−	−	−	+	−

°CD5 also reacts with B cells from CLL.
†CD11c also reacts with B cells from hairy cell leukemia.

Since the first monoclonal antibodies to human T-cell subsets were reported in 1979, numerous monoclonal antibodies were produced. Some monoclonal antibodies are highly specific to a certain cell lineage and are called "lineage restricted". The antibodies that react strongly to one cell lineage but may also cross-react with other cell types are called "lineage associated". These antibodies react to antigens of B cells, T cells, natural killer cells, monocytes/macrophages, granulocytes, megakaryocytes and nucleated erythrocytes. Since so many monoclonal antibodies exist, only the commonly used ones are listed in Tables 5-5 and 5-6. Because many monoclonal antibodies may react to the same epitope, standardization is needed to group similar antibodies together. This problem was addressed at the First International Workshop on Leukocyte Differentiation Antigens held in Paris in November 1982. As a result, 160 monoclonal antibodies were grouped by specificity into T-cell, B-cell, and monocyte-granulocyte categories.

TABLE 5-6. Cell Specificity and Clinical Applications of Monoclonal Antibodies

Cluster Designation	Monoclonal Antibodies	Cell Specificity	Clinical Application
CD1a	Leu6, OKT6, T6	Thymocyte, Langerhans cells	T-ALL, T lymphoma, histiocytosis X
CD2	Leu5, OKT11, T11	E-rosette receptor	T-ALL, T-CLL, T lymphoma
CD3	Leu4, OKT3, T3	T cell receptor complex	T-ALL, T-CLL, T lymphoma
CD4	Leu3, OKT4, T4	Helper-inducer T cell	Identification of T subset
CD5	Leu1, OKT1, T1	T cell, B cell from CLL	T-ALL, T lymphoma, B-CLL
CD7	Leu9, OKT16, 3A1	T cell, receptor for IgM-Fc	T-ALL, T lymphoma
CD8	Leu2, OKT8, T8	Cytotoxic-suppressor T cell	Identification of T subset
CD10	CALLA, OKBcALLa, J5	Immature B cell and T cell (rare)	ALL, B lymphoma
CD11b	Leu15, OKM1, Mo1	Monocyte, granulocyte, NK cell, T-suppressor cell	AML
CD11c	LeuM5, S-HCL3	Monocyte, B cell from hairy cell leukemia	AML, HCL
CD13	LeuM7, OKM13, My7	Monocyte, granulocyte	AML
CD14	LeuM3, OKM14, My4, Mo2	Monocyte	AML
CD15	LeuM1, My1	Monocyte, granulocyte, Reed-Sternberg cell	Hodgkin's disease
CD16	Leu11	NK cell, granulocyte, macrophage	NK-cell disorders
CD19	Leu12, OKpanB, B4	B cell	B-ALL, B-CLL, B lymphoma
CD20	Leu16, B1	B cell	B-ALL, B-CLL, B lymphoma
CD21	CR2, OKB7, B2	Follicular dendritic cell, B cell, C3d receptor	B lymphoma
CD22	Leu14, OKB22, B3, S-HCL1	B cell	B lymphoma, HCL
CD23	B6, Leu20	B cell	B-CLL
CD25	IL-2, OKT26a, Tac	IL-2 receptor on T cell (Tac antigen)	Hairy cell leukemia, human T-cell leukemia
CD30	Ki-1, Ber-H2	Reed-Sternberg cell, T or B cell from lymphoma	Ki-1 anaplastic lymphoma, Hodgkin's disease
CD33	LeuM9, My9	Monocyte, granulocyte	AML
CD34	HPCA-1, My10	Precursors of hematopoietic cells	Acute leukemia
CD38	Leu17, OKT10, T10	Plasma cell, activated T and B cells	Multiple myeloma
CD41	J15	GPIIb/IIIa antigen on platelet and megakaryocyte	Megakaryocytic leukemia
CD42a & 42b	HPL14, AN51, 10P42	Platelet GPIX and GPIb	Megakaryocytic leukemia
CD43	MT-1, Leu 22, L60	T cell, some B cells, granulocytes	T-lymphoma
CD45	HLe-1, LCA	All leukocytes	Lymphomas, leukemias
CD45RA	MT-2	T cell, some B cells	Follicular lymphoma
CD45RO	UCHL1	T subset, B subset, monocyte, granulocyte	T lymphoma
CD56	Leu19, NKH-1	NK cell	NK-cell disorders
CD57	Leu7, HNK-1	NK cell, T subset	NK-cell disorders
CD61	10P61, VI-PL2	Platelet GPIIIa	Megakaryocytic leukemia
CD68	KP1, PG-M1	Monocyte, histiocyte	Monocytic and histiocytic neoplasms
CD71	Transferrin receptor, OKT9, T9	Activated T and B cells, macrophages, proliferating cells	Acute leukemias and lymphomas
CD74	LN2	B cell, monocyte	B lymphoma
CDw75	LN1	B cell, T subset	B lymphoma
CD103	HML-1, B-ly7	B-cell	HCL
	FMC7	B cell	HCL, prolymphocytic leukemia
	HLA-DR	B cell, activated T cell, monocyte, granulocyte	B-cell neoplasms
	PCA-1	Plasma cell, monocyte (weak), granulocyte (weak)	Multiple myeloma
	RC-82.4	Erythroblast	Erythroleukemia
	Glycophorin	Erythroid series	Erythroleukemia
	TCR-1, βF-1, WT31	T cell	T-lymphoma, T-leukemia
	TCR-δ1, TCS-1, antiδ	T cell	T-lymphoma, T-leukemia

Abbreviations: ALL = acute lymphoblastic leukemia, AML = acute myelogenous leukemia, CLL = chronic lymphocytic leukemia, HCL = hairy cell leukemia.

TABLE 5-7. Immunophenotyping of AML

FAB Group	CD13	CD33	CD14	CD15	HLA-DR
M1	+	+	−	−	+
M2	+	+	−	+	+
M3	+	+	−	+	−
M4	+	+	<45%°	+	+
M5	+	+	>50%	+	+

°Percentage of positively stained cells in myeloid series.

Over 1,000 monoclonal antibodies have been produced since then.[53-56] The nomenclature for the antigens recognized by these antibodies is designated *CD* for *cluster of differentiation,* followed by a number. This effort at standardization helped to eliminate the early confusion and greatly facilitated scientific exchange. In the Fifth International Workshop on Leukocyte Differentiation Antigens held in Boston in 1993, the last cluster designation was CDw130.[57]

Monoclonal antibodies help identify not only cell lineages but also developmental stages. Thus, a specific diagnosis can sometimes be achieved. This is especially apparent in the diagnosis of B-cell neoplasms. For instance, the existence of CD5 (normally a T-cell marker) on the surface of a B-cell population is highly indicative of CLL or mantle cell lymphoma.[37,58]

In a normal cell population, the positive percentages of surface markers of the same cell lineage should be identical. When one or more surface markers are selectively lost in a cell population, this is called an *aberrant phenotype* and is usually indicative of a neoplasm.[59,60] This finding is especially helpful for the diagnosis of T-cell neoplasms because no special markers in T cells, like SIg in B cells, can identify clonality. In T-cell lymphoblastic leukemia, for instance, the percentage of CD7-positive cells is much higher than that of CD3-positive cells, whereas in the normal T-cell population, the percentages of CD7-positive cells and CD3-positive cells are identical. Conversely, the percentage of CD7-positive cells is much lower than that of CD3-positive cells and CD5-positive cells in peripheral T-cell lymphoma.

In cases of acute myeloblastic leukemia (AML), the diagnosis is usually determined by morphology and cytochemistry. However, cytochemistry can be negative in as many as 22% of cases of AML.[61] In those cases, monoclonal antibody staining may be helpful. Several markers are useful for the classification of AML[61,62]:

1. The percentages of the monocyte-associated antigens, CD14 (My4, Leu-M3) and CD11c (Leu M5), are higher in myeloid leukemias with monocytic components (M5 and M4).
2. CD15 (Leu M1, My1) is negative only in M1.
3. HLA-DR is negative only in M3.

Combined use of these myelomonocytic monoclonal antibodies can help classify AML, as shown in Table 5-7.

REFERENCES

1. Knowles DM, Chadburn A, Inghirani G: Immunophenotypic markers useful in the diagnosis and classification of hematopoietic neoplasms. In Knowles DM (ed): *Neoplastic Hematopathology.* Baltimore, Williams & Wilkins, 1992, pp 73–167.
2. Stetler-Stevenson M, Medeiros LJ, Jaffe ES: Immunophenotypic methods and findings in the diagnosis of lymphoproliferative diseases. In Jaffe ES (ed): *Surgical Pathology of the Lymph Nodes and Related Organs,* ed 2. Philadelphia, WB Saunders, 1995, pp 22–57.
3. Taylor CR: Results of multiparameter studies of B-cell lymphomas. *Am J Clin Pathol* 72(Suppl):687–698, 1979.
4. Sun T, Susin M: A practical approach to immunophenotyping of lymphomas. Comparison of immunohistologic and immunocytologic techniques. *Ann Clin Lab Sci* 17:14–26, 1987.
5. Sun T: *Color Atlas/Text of Flow Cytometric Analysis of Hematologic Neoplasms.* New York, Igaku-Shoin, 1993.
6. Simmons JG, Fuller CR, Buchanan PD, et al: Distribution of surface, cytoplasmic and secreted IgG subclasses in human lymphoblastoid cell lines and normal peripheral blood lymphocytes. *Scand J Immunol* 14:1–13, 1981.
7. Aisenberg AC: Cell surface markers in lymphoproliferative disease. *N Engl J Med* 304:331–336, 1981.
8. Warnke RA, Rouse RV: Limitations encountered in the application of tissue section immunodiagnosis to the study of lymphomas and related disorders. *Hum Pathol* 16:326–331, 1985.
9. Picker LJ, Weiss LM, Medeiros JF, et al: Immunophenotypic criteria for the diagnosis of non-Hodgkin's lymphoma. *Am J Pathol* 128:181–201, 1987.
10. Lamarre L, Jacobson JO, Aisenberg AC, et al: Primary large cell lymphoma of the mediastinum. *Am J Surg Pathol* 13:730–739, 1989.
11. Godal T, Lindmo T, Marton PF, et al: Immunological subsets in human B-cell lymphomas. *Scand J Immunol* 14:481–492, 1981.
12. Liebes L, Quagliata F, Silber R: The anomalous capping behavior of chronic lymphocytic leukemia lymphocytes: Studies with an antilymphocyte antiserum. *Clin Immunol Immunopathol* 10:222–232, 1978.
13. Habeshaw JA, Catley PF, Stansfeld AG, et al: Surface phenotyping, histology and the nature of non-Hodgkin lymphoma in 157 patients. *Br J Cancer* 40:11–34, 1979.
14. Brouet JC, Preud'homme JL, Penit C, et al: Acute lymphoblastic leukemia with pre–B cell characteristics. *Blood* 54:269–273, 1979.
15. LeBien TW, Hozier J, Minowada J, et al: Origin of chronic

15. myelocytic leukemia in a precursor of pre–B-lymphocytes. *N Engl J Med* 301:144–147, 1979.
16. Stein H: The immunologic and immunochemical basis for the Kiel classification. In Lennert K (ed): *Malignant Lymphoma Other Than Hodgkin's Disease*. New York, Springer-Verlag, 1978, pp 529–657.
17. Moretta L, Webb S, Grossi CE, et al: Functional analysis of two human T-cell subpopulations: Help and suppression of B-cell responses by T cells bearing receptors of IgM or IgG. *J Exp Med* 146:184–200, 1977.
18. Andersson B, Skoglung AC, Ronnholm M, et al: Functional aspects of IgM and IgG Fc receptors on murine T lymphocytes. *Immunol Rev* 56:1–50, 1981.
19. Fridman WH, Rabourdin-Combe C, Neauport-Sautes C, et al: Characterization and function of T cell Fcγ receptor. *Immunol Rev* 56:51–88, 1981.
20. Kadin ME, Kamoun M, Lamberg J: Erythrophagocytic Tγ lymphoma: A clinicopathologic entity resembling malignant histiocytosis. *N Engl J Med* 304:648–653, 1981.
21. Sun T, Brody J, Susin M, et al: Extranodal T-cell lymphoma mimicking malignant histiocytosis. *Am J Hematol* 35:269–274, 1990.
22. Farcet J-P, Gaulard P, Marolleau J-P, et al: Hepatosplenic T-cell lymphoma: Sinusal/sinusoidal localization of malignant cells expressing the T-cell receptor γδ. *Blood* 75:2213–2219, 1990.
23. Mastovich S, Ratech H, Ware RE, et al: Hepatosplenic T-cell lymphoma. An unusual case of γδ T-cell lymphoma with a blast-like terminal transformation. *Hum Pathol* 25:102–108, 1994.
24. Berliner N: T-gamma lymphocytosis and T-cell chronic leukemias. *Hematol/Oncol Clin North Am* 4:473–487, 1990.
25. Loughran TP: Clonal diseases of large granular lymphocytes. *Blood* 82:1–14, 1993.
26. Frank MM: Complement in the pathophysiology of human disease. *N Engl J Med* 316:1525–1530, 1987.
27. Williams LW, Burks AW, Steele RW: Complement, function and clinical relevance. *Ann Allergy* 60:293–301, 1988.
28. Reynolds HY, Atkinson JP, Newball HH: Receptors for immunoglobulin and complement on human alveolar macrophages. *J Immunol* 114:1813–1819, 1975.
29. Mann RB, Jaffe ES, Berard CW: Malignant lymphomas: A conceptual understanding of morphologic diversity. *Am J Pathol* 94:104–191, 1979.
30. Foon KA, Todd RF III: Immunologic classification of leukemia and lymphoma. *Blood* 68:1–31, 1986.
31. Li CY, Ziesmer SC, Yam LT, et al: Practical immunocytochemical identification of human blood cells. *Am J Clin Pathol* 81:204–212, 1984.
32. Li CY: Immunocytochemical techniques for identifying leukemias. *Mayo Clin Proc* 59:185–188, 1984.
33. Halper JP, Knowles DM, Wang CY: Ia-antigen expression by human malignant lymphomas: Correlation with conventional lymphoid markers. *Blood* 55:373–382, 1980.
34. Gupta S, Good RA, Siegal FP: Rosette formation with mouse erythrocytes, II: A marker of human B and non-T lymphocytes. *Clin Exp Immunol* 25:319–327, 1976.
35. Stathopoulos A, Elliott EV: Formation of mouse or sheep red blood cell rosettes by lymphocytes from normal and leukemic individuals. *Lancet* 1:600–602, 1974.
36. Koziner B, Kepin S, Passe S, et al: Characterization of B-cell leukemias: A tentative immunomorphological scheme. *Blood* 56:815–823, 1980.
37. Boumsell L, Coppin H, Pham D, et al: An antigen shared by a human T-cell subset and B-cell chronic lymphocytic leukemia cells. *J Exp Med* 152:229–234, 1980.
38. Greaves MF, Brown G, Rickinson A: Receptors for Epstein-Barr virus on human B lymphocytes. *Clin Immunol Immunopathol* 3:514–525, 1975.
39. DeWaele M, Thielemans C, Van Camp BKG: Characterization of immunoregulatory T cells in EBV-induced infectious mononucleosis by monoclonal antibodies. *N Engl J Med* 304:460–462, 1981.
40. Borella L, Sen L: E receptors on blasts from untreated acute lymphoblastic leukemia (ALL): Comparison of temperature dependence of E rosettes formed by normal and leukemic lymphoid cells. *J Immunol* 114:187–190, 1975.
41. Melvin S: Comparison of techniques for detecting T-cell acute lymphocytic leukemia. *Blood* 54:210–215, 1979.
42. Siegal FP, Filippa DA, Koziner B: Surface markers in leukemias and lymphomas. *Am J Pathol* 90:451–460, 1978.
43. Brown G, Greaves MF: Cell surface markers for human T and B cells. *Eur J Immunol* 4:302–310, 1974.
44. Collins RD, Waldron JA, Glick AD: Results of multiparameter studies of T-cell lymphoid neoplasms. *Am J Clin Pathol* 72(Suppl):699–707, 1979.
45. Reinherz EL, Schlossman SF: Derivation of human T-cell leukemias. *Cancer Res* 41:4767–4770, 1981.
46. Deegan MJ: Membrane antigen analysis in the diagnosis of lymphoid leukemias and lymphomas: Differential diagnosis, prognosis as related to immunophenotype and recommendation for testing. *Arch Pathol Lab Med* 113:606–618, 1989.
47. Janossy G, Hoffbrand AV, Greaves MF, et al: Terminal transferase enzyme assay and immunological membrane markers in the diagnosis of leukemia: A multiparameter analysis of 300 cases. *Br J Haematol* 44:221–234, 1980.
48. LeBien TW, McKenna RW, Abramson CS, et al: Use of monoclonal antibodies, morphology and cytochemistry to probe the cellular heterogeneity of acute leukemia and lymphoma. *Cancer Res* 41:4776–4780, 1981.
49. Peiper SC, Stass SA: Markers of cellular differentiation in acute lymphoblastic leukemia. *Arch Pathol Lab Med* 106:3–8, 1982.
50. Pullen DJ, Falleta JM, Crist WM, et al: Southwest Oncology Group experience with immunological phenotyping in acute lymphocytic leukemia of childhood. *Cancer Res* 41:4802–4809, 1981.
51. Nadler LM, Korsmeyer SJ, Anderson KC, et al: B-cell origin of non–T cell acute lymphoblastic leukemia. *J Clin Invest* 74:332–340, 1984.
52. Kennett RH, McKearn TJ, Bechtol KB (eds): *Monoclonal Antibodies: Hybridomas. A New Dimension in Biological Analysis*. New York, Plenum Press, 1980.

53. Bernard A, Boumsell L, Dausset J, et al (eds): *Leucocyte Typing I.* Berlin, Springer-Verlag, 1984.
54. Reinherz EL, Haynes BF, Nadler LM, et al (eds): *Leucocyte Typing* II. New York, Springer-Verlag, 1986.
55. McMichael AJ, Beverley PCL, Cobbold S. et al (eds): *Leucocyte Typing III.* Oxford, Oxford University Press, 1987.
56. Knapp W, Dorken B, Gilles WR, et al (eds): *Leucocyte Typing IV.* New York, Oxford University Press, 1990.
57. Pinto A, Gattei V, Soligo O, et al: New molecules burst at the leukocyte surface: A comprehensive review based on the 5th International Workshop on Leukocyte Differentiation Antigens, Boston, U.S.A. 3-7 November 1993, *Leukemia* 8:347–358, 1994.
58. Harris NL, Jaffe ES, Stein H, et al: A revised European–American classification of lymphoid neoplasms: A proposal from the International Lymphoma Study Group. *Blood* 84:1361–1392, 1994.
59. Sun T, Ngu, Henshall J, et al: Marker discrepancy as a diagnostic criterion for lymphoid neoplasms. *Diagn Clin Immunol* 5:393–399, 1988.
60. Weiss LM, Crabtree GS, Rouse RV, et al: Morphologic and immunologic characterization of 50 peripheral T-cell lymphomas. *Am J Pathol* 118:316–324, 1985.
61. Neame PB, Soamboonsrup P, Browman GP, et al: Classifying acute leukemia by immunophenotyping: A combined FAB–immunologic classification of AML. *Blood* 68:1355–1362, 1986.
62. Krause JR, Penchansky L, Contis L, et al: Flow cytometry in the diagnosis of acute leukemia. *Am J Clin Pathol* 89:341–346, 1988.

Chapter 6
FLOW CYTOMETRY

The flow cytometer, hailed as a new product or technical revolution, is not as new as it appears. The concept of flow cytometry has been around for about 50 years. The best-known example is the Coulter counter, which has been extensively used in clinical laboratories for more than 20 years. However, it has become apparent only recently, with the availability of a great variety of monoclonal antibodies, that flow cytometry has become an indispensable instrument for rapid processing of large numbers of specimens. The outbreak of the acquired immunodeficiency syndrome (AIDS) accelerated the acceptance of the flow cytometer as a routine laboratory instrument because of the tremendous demands for testing the helper/suppressor T-cell ratios as a screening technique for this disease. Nevertheless, since many monoclonal antibodies are cell lineage or developmental stage specific for blood cells, flow cytometry has been promptly adopted by hematology/oncology laboratories as a tool for routine clinical use.[1-18]

Flow cytometry, compared to manual techniques, has the advantages of being more efficient, sensitive, accurate, and reproducible. It once took a technician 2 days to perform a T- and B-cell panel, including a sheep erythrocyte rosetting technique, SIg staining, and one or two special stains, such as TdT and CALLA. With flow cytometry, several specimens can be simultaneously processed with a panel of 10 or more antibodies (monoclonal and polyclonal) and be completed within 1 or 2 days. Flow cytometry usually counts 3,000–5,000 cells for the study of one marker compared to 100–200 cells counted in the manual technique. Therefore, the increased sensitivity of flow cytometry allows the detection of small numbers of abnormal cells and is more accurate than the manual technique in computing the percentage of a specific group of cells. The major merit of flow cytometry, however, is its ability to measure multiple parameters simultaneously; thus, it may further subclassify or characterize the cells better than a single marker. Through its sorting mechanism, flow cytometry can collect a special group of cells for further studies. The major limitations of flow cytometry at this stage are the high cost of the instrument, the special skill required to operate it, and the lack of a morphologic record. The failure to distinguish a normal cell from a tumor cell morphologically leads to the indiscriminate counting of both populations, resulting in a wrong conclusion when the tumor cells are in the minority. However, with the use of more parameters simultaneously, the distinction between normal and abnormal cells is more easily achieved.

BASIC PRINCIPLES OF FLOW CYTOMETRY

Although various types of flow cytometers are available commercially, they all consist of essentially the same basic units: a fluid transport system, an optical system, an electronic system, and a computer system.

Fluid Transport System

A specimen consisting of a single cell suspension is sucked into the instrument and transported to the flow chamber by means of differential air pressure of a vacuum. Once in the flow chamber, the specimen is surrounded by a cell–free stream of sheath fluid, forming a laminar flow configuration (Figure 6-1). The outer sheath fluid forces the cells in the specimen to line up in single file. When cells flow through the sensing areas (or measurement region) one at a time, electrical or optical signals are generated.

Optical System

Electric signals are generated when cells suspended in an electrical-conducting medium change the electrical resistance of the fluid as they pass through a light beam in the sensing area. The signal generated is proportional to the cell volume (the Coulter principle). This principle is used in flow cytometers which contain the mercury-cadmium arc lamp (such as the FACS Analyzer, Becton Dickinson). However, most instruments use lasers as the light source, and optical signals are generated. The most fre-

Flow Cytometry

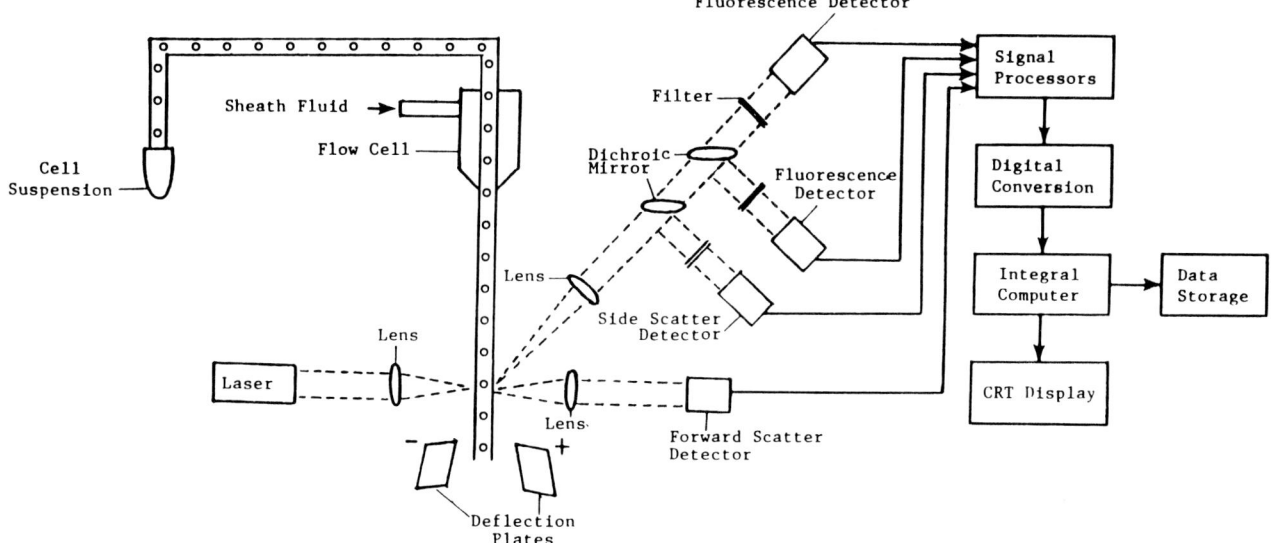

FIGURE 6-1. Basic structure of a flow cytometer. (From Sun T: *Color Atlas/Text of Flow Cytometric Analysis of Hematologic Neoplasms.* New York, Igaku-Shoin, 1993)

quently used optical signals are forward angle (2°–10°) and right angle (90°) light scatter (Figure 6-2). The former is proportional to cell size, and the latter is related to cell structures such as cytoplasmic granularity and nuclear structure. Lasers can deliver intense, coherent, monochromatic light, resulting in low divergence and high brightness of the signals generated. The use of small, air-cooled lasers instead of large, water-cooled ion lasers has permitted the development of smaller, less expensive, easier to install flow cytometers such as the FACScan (Becton-Dickinson) and Profile (Coulter).

Fluorescent Signals: The ability of a flow cytometer to detect fluorescent signals is its most versatile function. Fluorochrome-labeled cells absorb incident light from the laser or the mercury arc lamp and emit a long wavelength

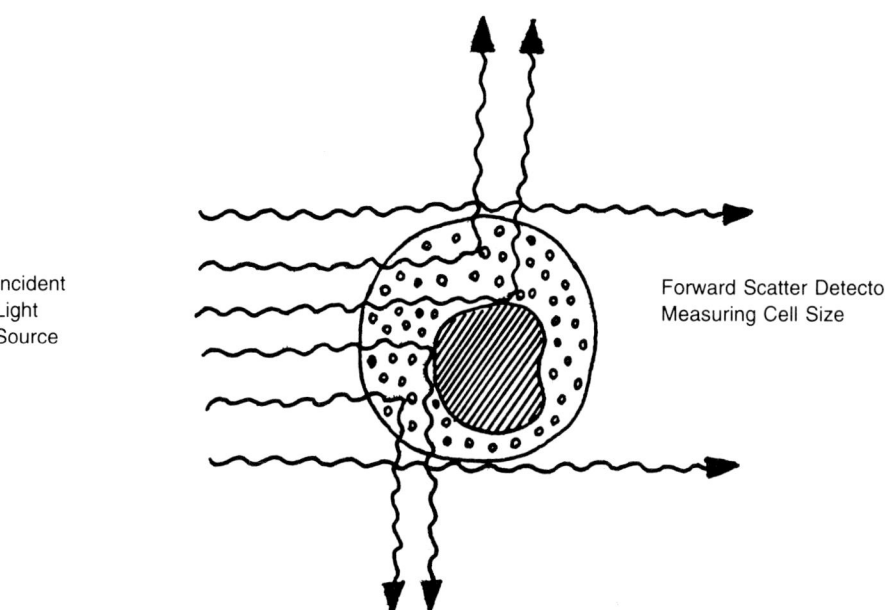

FIGURE 6-2. Relationship of light scatter and cell size/structure. (From the same source as Figure 6-1).

TABLE 6-1. Wavelength and Color of Fluorochromes

Fluorochrome	Excitation Max. (nm)	Emission Max. (nm)	Color
Propidium iodide	488	620	Red
Peridinin chlorophyll (per CP)	488	670	Red
Fluorescein (FITC)	494	517	Green
R-phycoerythrin (PE)	495	576	Orange
Rhodamin (RDI)	545	575	Orange
Texas Red (Tx Red)	596	615	Red
Phycocyanin (PC)	620	655	Red
Allophycocyanin (APC)	620	660	Red
CY5	633	670	Red

which is called *fluorescence*. The color of the light emitted is a function of its wavelength (Table 6-1). As long as the wavelengths emitted from a fluorochrome do not overlap each other entirely, the same specimen can be labeled with two or three fluorochromes. The spectrum of the wavelength of the light source determines what kind of fluorochrome combination can be used (Table 6-2). For three-color immunofluorescent analysis, a dual-laser system was required at this stage. However, the discovery of newer dyes may now allow a single-laser system to perform three- to four-color analysis.

A series of optics are used to direct fluorescence to detectors. The dichroic mirrors selectively split the light beam, allowing certain wavelengths to pass through and reflecting others. The filters selectively block some wavelengths above or below a certain spectral point.

Electronic System

The optical signals are transformed into a computer printout of graphs and statistics through multiple steps. The optical signal first enters the photomultiplier tube, where it is converted to an electronic signal (voltage pulse). The analog signal is digitized in the analog-to-digital converter. Finally, the pulse height analyzer analyzes the digital information and quantifies it for computer display.

TABLE 6.2 Wavelength of the Light Source and Choice of Fluorochrome Combination

Light Source	Excitation Wavelength	Fluorochrome Combination
Mercury arc lamp	485, 546	FITC, PE, RDI
Argon ion laser	488	FITC, PE, RDI
Dye laser	600	Tx Red, APC
Krypton-ion laser	568, 647	APC
Helium-neon laser	633	APC

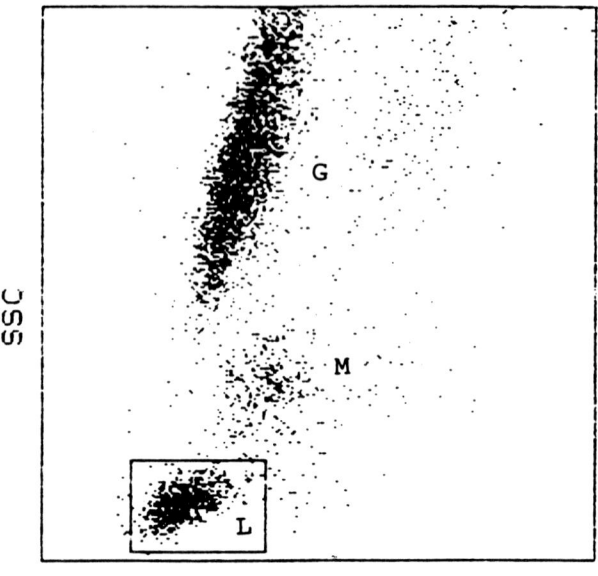

FIGURE 6-3. Scattergram of lysed whole blood sample showing groups of lymphocytes (L), monocytes (M), and granulocytes (G).

Computer System

The flow cytometer can be interphased to an external computer that performs three important functions:

1. *List mode storage*: The information on all parameters measured can be stored permanently on a floppy disk or temporarily on a hard disk. All data can be combined and analyzed later and printed in graphic form as a permanent record.
2. *Gating*: Gating consists of isolating electronically a special group of cells for analysis, avoiding the difficult task of purifying the cell population by biological means. Depending on the software capability, several gates can be set so that information can be gathered on several populations of cells.
3. *Graphic display*: The computer can provide graphic displays in several forms.

Scattergram (dot-plot, cytogram): This is a graphic display of two related parameters. For instance, when forward-angle light scatter plots against right-angle light scatter, a dot-plot is formed, each dot representing a single cell. On the basis of cell size (forward angle) and cytoplasmic granularity (right angle), the scattergram usually shows three distinct groups of cells in peripheral blood samples—the lymphocytes, monocytes, and granulocytes—in order of increasing size and granularity (Figure 6-3). In lymph node specimens, the distinction between a group of large

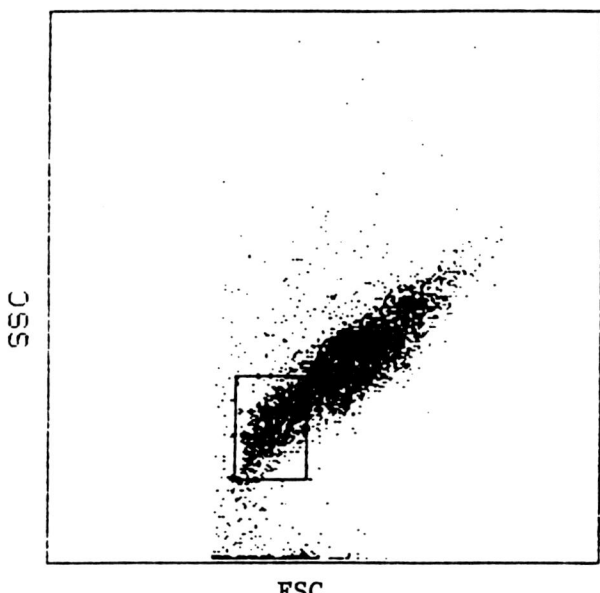

FIGURE 6-4. Scattergram of a lymph node suspension showing two groups of lymphoid cells. The large cells are lymphoma cells and the small cells (gated) are reactive lymphocytes in this case.

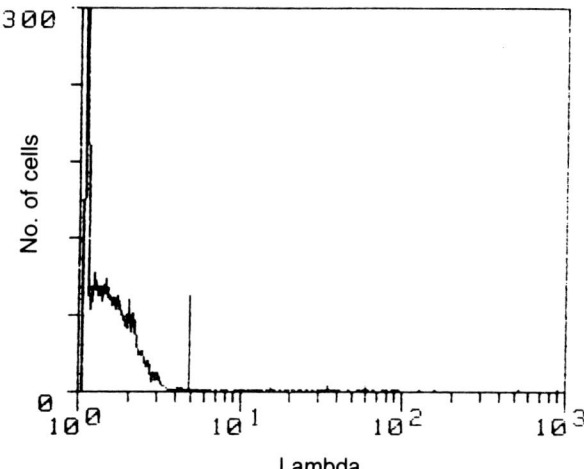

FIGURE 6-6. Single histogram of the same case as Figure 6-5 showing only λ antigen-negative population.

cells and a group of small cells frequently helps to separate lymphoma cells from reactive lymphoctyes (Figure 6-4).

Single Histogram: This graph is usually used to display number of cells (y-axis) versus fluorescence intensity (x-axis). When cells are stained with a fluorochrome-labeled antibody, a single histogram provides the percentages of positive and negative populations (Figures 6-5 and 6-6). A negative control should be used to determine the cutoff point between these two populations. When DNA stain is used, the single histogram can demonstrate the percentage of cells in different stages of the cell cycle and determine the ploidy of chromosomes compared to a normal control.

Contourgram (contour map, contour histogram, two-dimensional plot): The contourgram computes the percentage of cell groups, as determined by two parameters (e.g., two monoclonal antibodies or DNA and RNA contents) (Figure 6-7). This is useful for further classification of subpopulations. When the cutoff points of these two

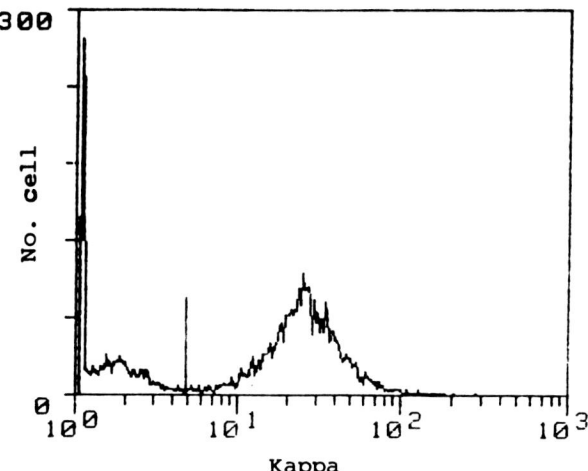

FIGURE 6-5. Single histogram of a lymphoma case showing κ antigen-negative (left) and -positive (right) populations.

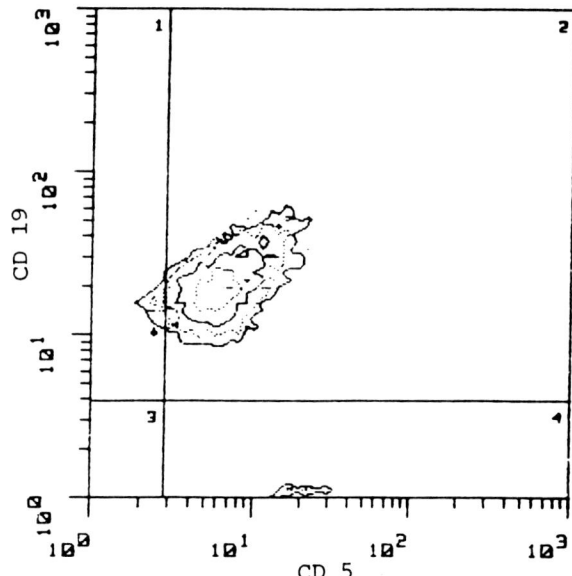

FIGURE 6-7. Contourgram of a case of CLL showing CD19+ and CD5+ population in quadrant 2.

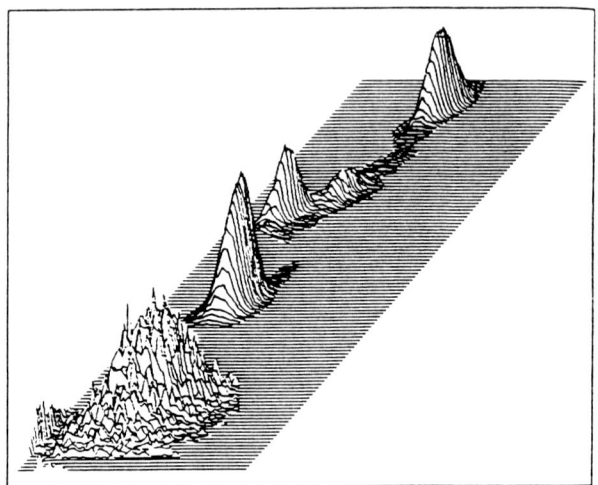

FIGURE 6-8. A composite isometric plot combining individual two-parameter light scatter histograms of platelets, red cells, lymphocytes, monocytes, and granulocytes. (From Marti GE: Diagnostic flow cytometry in hematology: The leukemias. *Pathol Immunopathol Res* 5:416–436, 1986).

parameters are determined, the contourgram can be divided into four quadrants, and the percentages of the four subpopulations are readily computed.

Isometric Plot (three-dimensional isometric curve): The isometric plot is most frequently used for DNA/RNA analysis (Figure 6-8). When three-color immunofluorescent analysis becomes popular, the isometric plot will be more frequently used for monoclonal antibody studies.

Cell Sorter

For cell sorting, the stream of cell suspension first passes through an ultrasonically vibrating nozzle so that the stream can be broken up into evenly spaced droplets. The droplets containing the cells of interest are selectively charged electrically and then deflected as they fall through an electromagnetic field formed by two deflection plates. The selected cells thus alter their paths and are collected in a separate container, while the uncharged droplets fall vertically into a waste container. The cells separated in this way are usually viable and 95% pure. The cell sorter is undoubtedly a useful tool in research laboratories. However, it is not an absolute necessity for a clinical laboratory.

MONOCLONAL ANTIBODY PANEL

The availability of cell lineage and stage-specific monoclonal antibodies has greatly enhanced the progress of diagnostic hematology. Furthermore, because a large number

TABLE 6-3. Monoclonal Antibody Panels for Hematologic Neoplasms

1. Lymphoma
   B cell: SIg, CD10, CD19, CD20. T cell: CD3, CD5, CD7. MHC-II antigen: HLA-DR. Granulocyte: CD13, CD33 (to rule out granulocytic sarcoma).
2. Hodgkin's disease
   B cell: SIg, CD20 (to rule out B-cell lymphoma). T cell: CD3, CD4, CD8 (helper cell is predominant in Hodgkin's disease); (CD15 and CD30 may identify Reed-Sternberg cells, but are not useful in FCM).
3. Chronic lymphocytic leukemia
   B cell: SIg, CD19, CD20. T cell: CD3, CD5, CD7. Special combination: CD20-CD5, CD3-CD5 (to identify CD5-positive B cells).
4. T-gamma lymphoproliferative disorder
   T cell: CD2, CD3, CD4, CD5, CD7, CD8. NK cell: CD16, CD56, CD57.
5. Hairy cell leukemia
   AP, TRAP. B cell: SIg, CD19, CD20. T cell: CD3. Special combination: CD22-CD11c. Special marker: CD25.
6. Acute lymphoblastic leukemia
   CD10 (CALLA), TdT. B cell: SIg, Cμ, CD19, CD20. T cell: CD3, CD5, CD7. Special combination: CD3-CD7 (to identify T-cell marker discrepancy), CD10-CD19 (to identify CALLA-positive B cells).
7. Macroglobulinemia (diagnosed by immunochemical technique; FCM not recommended) CIg and lymphoma panel.
8. Myeloma (diagnosed by immunochemical technique, FCM not recommended) CIg, PC-1, PCA-1, CD38.
9. Sézary syndrome
   CD3, CD4, CD8, AP, TRAP, PAS.
10. Acute myeloblastic leukemia
    MPO, Combo. Myeloid: CD13, CD33. Monocytoid: CD11c, CD14. Megakaryocyte: CD41, CD61. Erythroid: antiglycophorin, HLA-DR (absent in M3), CD13 (absent in M1), CD34 (to mark immature cells).

AP = acid phosphatase; CIg = cytoplasmic immunoglobulin; Cμ = cytoplasmic μ chain; Combo = combined chloroacetate esterase and α-naphthyl butyrate esterase; MPO = myeloperoxidase; SIg = surface immunoglobulin; TRAP = tartrate-resistant acid phosphatase
Source: Sun T: *Color Atlas/Text of Flow Cytometric Analysis of Hematologic Neoplasms.* New York, Igaku-Shoin, 1993.

of monoclonal antibodies are commercially available, the demand for rapid processing with a highly efficient instrument like a flow cytometer becomes apparent. However, the high cost of monoclonal antibodies prohibits their indiscriminate use as a standard panel under various conditions. Therefore, special panels are tailored for various types of hematologic neoplasms (Table 6-3). The application of these special panels is detailed in Chapter 5.

In addition, the possibility of measuring double-stained cells by flow cytometry provides the opportunity for further characterization or classification of a cell population and sometimes leads to a definitive diagnosis. For example, CD5+, CD19+, (or CD20+) cells are usually from CLL (or its equivalent), and simultaneous B-cell antigen–and monocyte antigen (CD11c)–positive cells are most likely from hairy cell leukemia.

Another special feature of flow cytometry is its determination of clonal excess. This can be accomplished either by comparing directly the curves generated by the entire κ- and λ-bearing B-cell populations[19] or by comparing the proportion of κ- and λ-bearing cells at certain levels of fluorescent intensity (e.g., every 10 channels)[20]. However, it requires a data analysis system, such as the Komogorov-Smirnov test,[21] to compare the curves. Determination of clonal excess is useful when the B-cell tumor population is a minority group or when peripheral blood is examined for the detection of residual disease.[22]

DNA/RNA ANALYSIS

The Cell Cycles

All tissues consist of three different cell populations.[23] The first population of cells is called *cycling cells*, which divide continuously from one mitosis to the next. The second population comprises cells that leave the cell cycle to die after a certain number of divisions. The third population of cells leaves the cell cycle transiently and becomes inactive until some microenvironmental factors stimulate its reentry to the cell cycle.

The cell cycle is divided into different phases (Figure 6-9).[8,23] The inactive phase is designated G0 (gap 0). The first phase in the active cycle is termed G1 (gap 1). It is followed by the S (synthesis)-phase, in which DNA is actively synthesized. The final period is the G_2 (gap 2) phase,

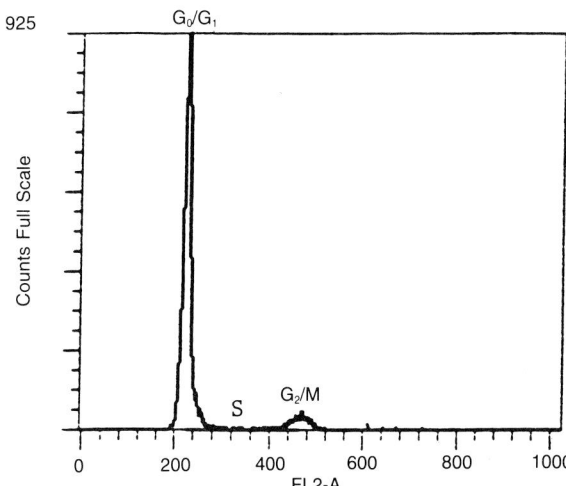

FIGURE 6-10. DNA cell cycle analysis of a lymph node showing the G_0/G_1 peak, S-phase, and G_2/M peak. (From the same source as Figure 6-1).

which occurs between the completion of DNA synthesis and mitosis (M-phase).

Recent evidence indicates that there is a second cell cycle, which regulates the growth of cell size. The increase in cell mass is mainly the result of synthesis of protein and RNA, which constitute about one-half of the dry weight of the cell.

On the basis of the above theoretical background, DNA/RNA analysis has been used as part of the workup panel for hematologic neoplasms as well as for solid tumors. The fact that DNA/RNA analysis can be performed on archival materials makes it an ideal tool for both prospective and retrospective studies.[24–26]

Ploidy

A normal cell contains two sets of chromosomes; therefore, a normal DNA content is designated *diploidy*. Because the DNA content in G_0/G_1 phase is constant, any change of DNA quantity in G_0/G_1 cells is considered abnormal, or *aneuploidy* (Figure 6-10). When the DNA content is higher than the normal control, it is called *hyperdiploidy*; when it is lower, *hypodiploidy*. When the quantity of DNA is two times as high as that of the normal control, it is termed *tetraploidy*. Aneuploidy represents quantitative changes in chromosomes, such as trisomy (hyperdiploidy) and deletions (hypodiploidy). In specimens in which adequate metaphase cannot be obtained for karyotyping, ploidy analysis is more sensitive to detect chromosomal abnormalities.[27] However, the flow cytometric method is unable to detect balanced translocations, partial chromosome deletions, or inversion.[28]

Aneuploidy is not present only in malignancy; it can

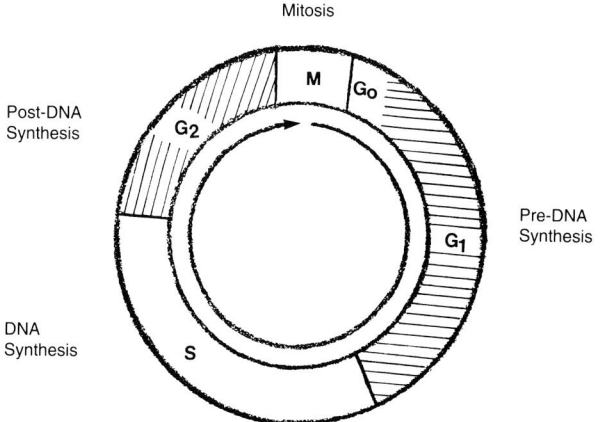

FIGURE 6-9. Cell populations and the phases of the cell cycle. (From the same source as Figure 6-1).

also be demonstrated in benign conditions, such as colon adenoma and atypical ductal proliferations in the breast.[24] However, these benign lesions may in fact be premalignant. In hematology, premalignant conditions such as angioimmunoblastic lymphadenopathy, myelodysplastic syndrome, and benign monoclonal gammopathy may also show aneuploidy.[28]

Conversely, not all tumor cells are aneuploid. Aneuploidy is more frequently demonstrated in high-grade than in low-grade malignancies, thus generally predicting a poor prognosis. However, exceptions to this rule exist; for instance, in neuroblastoma,[29] medulloblastoma,[30] and squamous cell carcinomas of the head and neck,[32] DNA aneuploidy may indicate a favorable prognosis. Most early studies were done on non-Hodgkin's lymphomas.[26,32-43] Relatively few studies were done on leukemias.[11,44-51]

When lymphomas are classified by the Working Formulation, the frequency of aneuploidy is lower in the low-grade tumors than in the intermediate and high-grade lymphomas.[32-25] The intermediate and high-grade lymphomas, on the other hand, may or may not show a statistically significant difference in the frequency of aneuploidy. Similar results were obtained by comparison with other classifications.[36-38] However, the correlation between aneuploidy and prognosis in lymphomas is controversial; several studies showed no correlation between these two parameters.[37,41,52] In terms of immunologic classification, aneuploidy was found to be more common in B-cell lymphomas than in T-cell lymphomas in one large series,[38] but this finding was challenged by another study.[35] Among B-cell lymphomas, the large-cell variety is more commonly aneuploid than the small-cell type.[35-38] When the lymphoma cell population is aneuploid, DNA analysis can be used to detect bone marrow or peripheral blood involvement by the malignant clone.[36] Since no monoclonal antibody can define T-cell monoclonality, double staining with T-cell antibody and DNA stain to mark an aneuploid population is the only means for direct flow cytometric identification of T-cell neoplasms.[28]

In a large study series of leukemias, it was found that the frequencies of aneuploidy in cases of ALL (25%) and of acute myeloblastic leukemia (27%) were extremely close.[11] Andreef et al. concurred with this finding.[44] Several studies of pediatric ALL showed that those with aneuploidy had longer remission than those with diploidy,[48,49,51] but one study found no difference between these two groups.[50] Cases of CLL, hairy cell leukemia, and the remission phase of CML seldom showed aneuploidy.[4,11] However, during blast crisis, 50% of CML cases showed aneuploidy.[11]

Many arbitrary factors affect the percentage of aneuploidy in lymphomas and leukemias. For instance, criteria for aneuploidy differ in various studies. The criteria, as summarized by Shackney et al.[38] included (1) multiple G_1 peaks; (2) a single G_1 peak in the normal position with an increased coefficient of variation (CV), i.e., increased width of the peak; and (3) a single G_1 peak in an abnormal position with a normal CV. The DNA stain (e.g., propidium iodide vs. mithramycin) and the techniques for cell preparation and staining may affect the position of the G_1 peak and its CV, thus causing false aneuploidy. Merkel et al. maintained that when the CV of the G_1 peak is greater than 5%, a near-diploid stemline may be obscured.[52] Braylan et al. used double staining of cells for κ or λ light chains and DNA[40]; thus, the ploidy of a monoclonal population was more accurately defined.

Some studies showed no correlation between ploidy and period of survival[37,41,52] because the DNA content in G_1 phase does not represent proliferative activity.

S-Phase

Several investigations have demonstrated that the percentage of cells in S-phase correlates well with [3H]thymidine labeling index.[36,39] Therefore, the S-phase is representative of proliferative activity and is a better indicator of the prognosis than ploidy in terms of survival.[36,39,41] Braylan et al.[39] used 5%, and Roos et al.[41] used 4% as the cutoff point of S-phase cells for the distinction between a poor and a good prognosis. As with ploidy, the percentage of cells in S-phase is proportional to the grade of malignancy.[32-34,36,38,40] High-grade lymphomas, for instance, usually have a high S-phase. MacCartney et al. found that a low-grade lymphoma with a high S-phase is more likely to transform into high-grade lymphoma than a low-grade lymphoma with a low S-phase.[42] Some studies used %S + G_2M (cutoff point of 20%) as an index for proliferative activity and found results similar to those that used %S alone.[35,53]

RNA Index

RNA content reflects the cell mass. The increase in RNA content in the cell cycle is a good indicator of cell growth. The meaning of the RNA index of the G_1 phase may vary in different clinical settings. In non-Hodgkin's lymphoma, the RNA index of the G_1 phase may correlate with the grade of malignancy, cell size, proliferative activity of tumor cells, and survival.[35,36] One study showed that double-stranded RNA was the only nucleic acid parameter that was able to distinguish reactive lymphadenopathy from low-grade lymphoma.[35] The RNA index may also be used to distinguish lymphoblastic and myeloblastic leukemias, with higher RNA values being found in the latter group.[11,44] The same principle can be used to distinguish lymphoblastic and myeloblastic transformation of CML.[50] In multiple myeloma, the RNA index can be applied to measure the differentiation of tumor cells.[54] A low index means early differentiation and a poor prognosis.

PITFALLS OF FLOW CYTOMETRIC STUDIES

The major pitfall of flow cytometry is the lack of correlation between cell morphology and cell markers. The parameters that a flow cytometer uses to distinguish cell populations are cell size, cytoplasmic granularity, immunophenotype (e.g., T cell or B cell), intensity of surface immunoglobulin staining, double labeling (e.g., C19 and CD5 for cells of CLL), and DNA/RNA content. Therefore, when the tumor cells and their normal counterparts are of the same phenotype and size, they cannot be distinguished. In our experience, this situation most frequently occurs in a follicular B-cell lymphoma with a large number of interfollicular B cells. Occasionally, when a diffuse, small cleaved-cell lymphoma is intermingled with normal small B cells, the result of the flow cytometric study will also be distorted. Since the clonality of B cells is determined by the κ/λ surface immunoglobulin ratio, a diluted tumor cell population inevitably shows a polyclonal pattern. Fortunately, the reactive lymphoid population in a B-cell lymphoma is usually composed of small T lymphocytes, so that a monoclonal pattern is often obtained. In large-cell lymphomas, the reactive population (usually small cells) can be easily separated by gating. However, when the tumor cells are in the minority, even they differ from the normal population in phenotype; the cell surface κ/λ ratio of this small population is not reliable. Our requirement is a minimum of 20% B cells or a κ/λ ratio of 15%:5% for the establishment of monoclonality.[55]

In addition to low tumor cell:normal cell ratio, other sample problems can cause false-negative results.[56] For lymphomas, the most common problem is sampling error. Therefore, an imprint from the lymph node should be routinely performed to make sure that the specimen contains the suspected tumor cell population. Specimens containing large necrotic or fibrotic areas of large numbers of degenerated or dead cells also provide unsatisfactory results. The spleen specimen is particularly problematic because autolysis takes place rapidly once the spleen is removed from the patient. Therefore, a spleen specimen should be processed within 1 hr after splenectomy.

There are many technical problems that affect clonal analysis. The most significant problem is usually instrument calibration. Adjustment of the photomultiplier tube is crucial. Using an isotypic, species-specific negative control as a standard, a cutoff point of cursor position is set by photomultiplier tube manipulation. For instance, if the monoclonal antibody used is mouse derived and the antibody is IgG, then mouse IgG immunoglobulin of no spe-

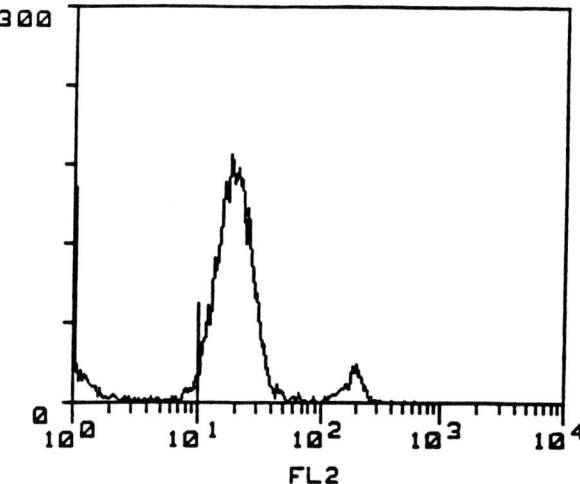

FIGURE 6-11. A histogram of a peripheral blood specimen stained with CD33 showing a granulocyte peak and a monocyte peak. This is an example of optimal adjustment of the photomultiplier tube. (From the same source as Figure 6-1).

cific antibody function is used as the negative control. The cursor is then set at the point where the autofluorescent peak of the mouse IgG ends. Any fluorescence recorded beyond the cutoff point is considered positive. Figure 6-11 illustrates a single histogram showing two CD33+ peaks. CD33 is a myelomonocyte marker; therefore, these two peaks represent granulocytes and monocytes, respectively. When the photomultiplier tube is underadjusted, the cursor deviates to the left and the granulocyte peak is mistaken for a negative peak (Figure 6-12). When the photomulti-

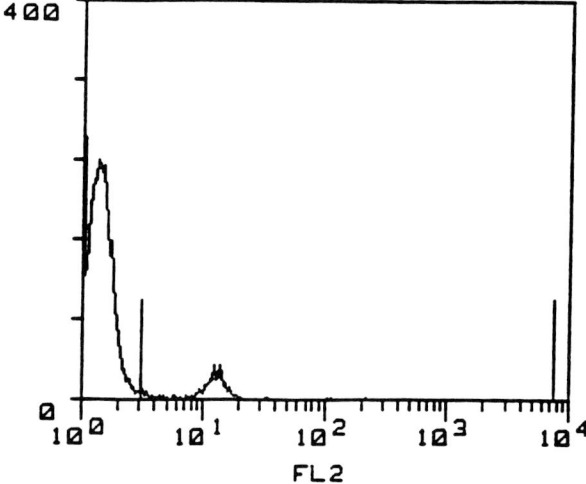

FIGURE 6-12. A histogram of the same specimen as Fig 6-11. The granulocyte peak has become negative because of underadjustment of the photomultiplier tube. (From the same source as Figure 6-1).

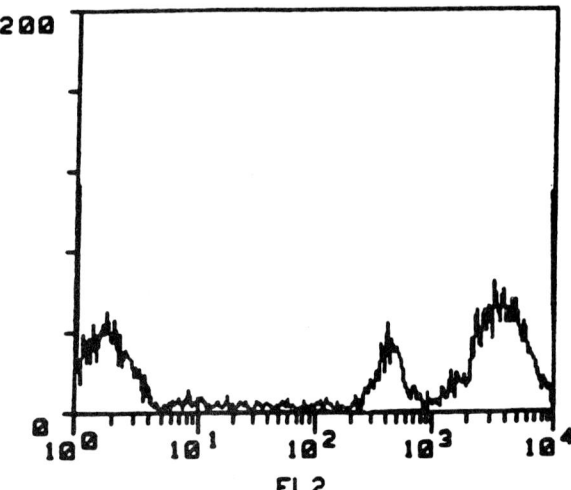

FIGURE 6-13. A histogram of a lymph node cell suspension with CD19 showing one negative and two positive populations in a case of mixed small- and large-cell lymphoma. (From the same source as Figure 6-1).

plier tube is overadjusted, a strongly positive peak may be off the screen (Figures 6-13 and 6-14).

When double labeling (two-color analysis) is desired, two fluorochromes, such as fluorescein and phycoerythrin, are used. Although both fluorochromes are excited at 488 nm, they emit at different wavelengths. However, the spectra of these emissions overlap. Therefore, electronic adjustment must be made to correct spectral overlap, a procedure known as *electronic compensation*. The compensation phe-

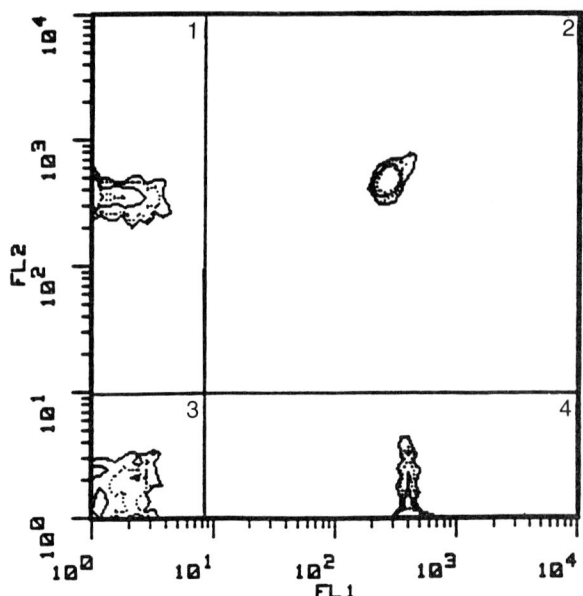

FIGURE 6-15. A contourgram of a double-stained specimen showing one cell population in each of the four quadrants, representing optimal compensation. (From the same source as Figure 6-1).

nomenon is best illustrated in a contourgram. Figure 6-15 shows a contourgram depicting a specimen double-stained by CD3 (y-axis) and CD4 (x-axis). Four distinct populations are demonstrated in four quadrants, representing optimal compensation. Figure 6-16 shows that the population in

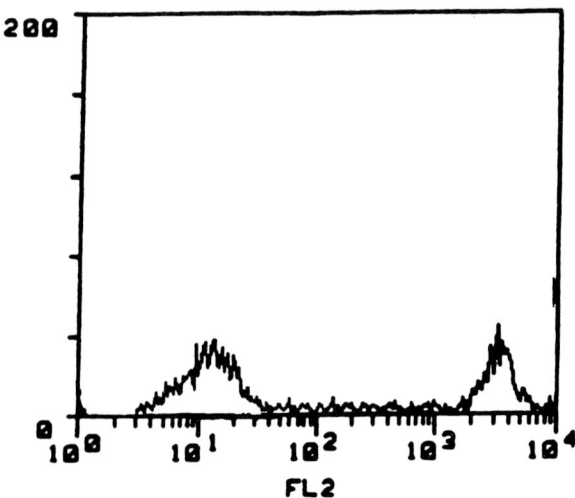

FIGURE 6-14. A histogram of the same case as Fig. 6-13. The strongly positive population has disappeared from the screen because of overadjustment of the photomultiplier tube. (From the same source as Figure 6-1).

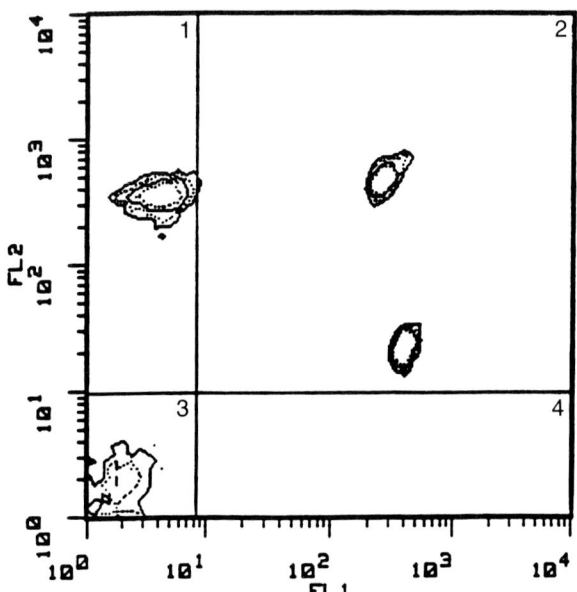

FIGURE 6-16. A contourgram of the same specimen as Fig. 6-15 showing the population originally in quadrant 4 of slide 9 moves to quadrant 2, representing spectral overlap (i.e., no compensation). (From the same source as Figure 6-1).

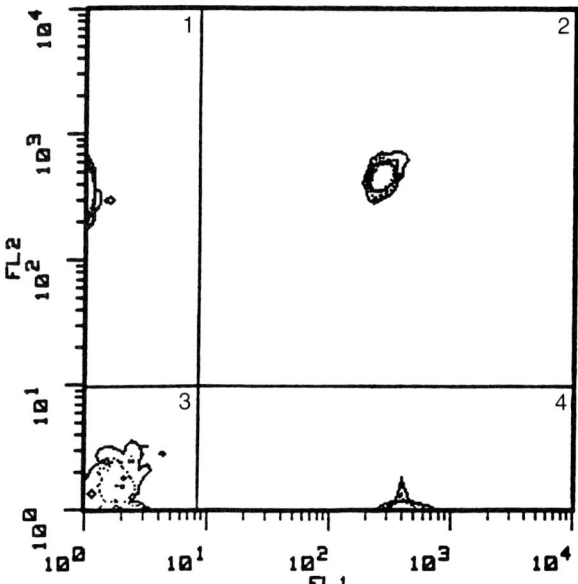

FIGURE 6-17. A contourgram of the same specimen as Fig. 6-15 showing near-disappearance of the cell populations in quadrants 1 and 4, representing overcompensation. (From the same source as Figure 6-1).

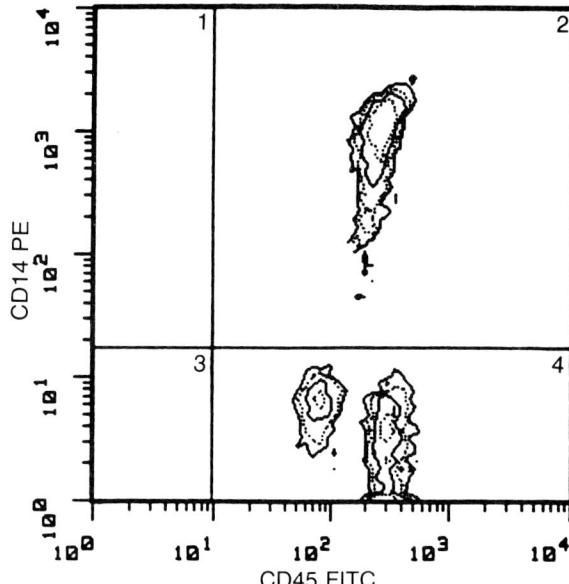

FIGURE 6-18. A contourgram of a peripheral blood specimen stained with a monocyte marker, CD14 (y-axis), and a panleukocyte marker, CD45 (x-axis), showing the monocyte population in quadrant 2 and the granulocyte (left) and lymphocyte (right) populations in quadrant 4. (From the same source as Figure 6-1).

quadrant 4 of Figure 6-15 moves to quadrant 2, representing spectral overlap or no compensation. Undercompensation may sometimes cause false-positive results concerning the double-labeled population. By contrast, when it is overcompensated, the populations in quadrants 1 and 4 may disappear, as illustrated in Figure 6-17. These examples indicate that optimal compensation is a very important prerequisite in double-labeling situations.

From a diagnostic point of view, correct gating is most important. To check if the gating is correct, double staining of the sample with panleukocyte antibody (CD45) and monocyte antibody (CD14) is mandatory (Figure 6-18). The countourgram indicates if the gated population is pure (i.e., only lymphocytes are counted).

The major reagent problem is inappropriate antibody dilution, which leads to undesirable results (i.e., false-negative or weakly positive results in a positive case). Ideally, each new batch of antibody should be titered before use. Monoclonal antibodies are generally used for flow cytometry, except for anti-immunoglobulin antibodies, for which polyclonal antibody should be used. SIg have many epitopes; therefore, polyclonal antibodies are more likely to react positively than monoclonal antibodies. A neoplasm, for instance, may not show a certain epitope of the immunoglobulin that is specific for a monoclonal antibody.

Other potential problems can usually be avoided by using standard procedures.[57] For instance, the patient's immunoglobulin may adhere to the surface of his or her own lymphocytes. This is known as *cytophilic immunoglobulin*, and it may cause aberrant results with anti-immunoglobulin antibodies. By incubating the lymphocytes in phosphate-buffered saline or RPMI medium (Rosewell Park Memorial Institute medium; GIBCO, Grand Island, NY) at 37°C for 1 hr, the cytophilic immunoglobulin will be shed and can be washed from the cell surface.

The Fc receptor is present on the surface of lymphocytes and monocytes. If the antibody used contains the Fc fragment, false-positive results may be obtained. Therefore, an ideal antibody should contain only the Fab fragment.

A capping phenomenon is frequently seen in SIg reactions because the anti-Ig–SIg immune complex can be internalized, leading to false-negative results. The use of sodium azide as a preservative for antibody reagent and as an additive to phosphate-buffered saline diluent may prevent this problem.

Furthermore, phagocytosis of immunoglobulin by monocytes or macrophages may give rise to false-positive resutls for SIg. Pretreatment to separate the phagocytic cells from lymphocytes may eliminate this problem.

Finally, the patient's conditions, such as medications and biological factors, may also cause some artifacts in immunophenotyping by flow cytometry (Table 6-4). For details, the reader is referred to *Clinical Application of Flow Cytometry: Quality Assurance and Immunophenotyping of Peripheral Blood Lymphocytes*, issued by the

TABLE 6-4. Potential Sources of Artifacts in Immunophenotyping by FCM

Case	Effect	Resulting Artifact
Medications or Drugs		
1. Zidovudine (AZT)	Increased granulocyte fragility	Decreased light scatter resolution; increased granulocyte contamination of mononuclear preparations
2. Some antibodies (e.g., cephalosporins)	Increased cellular autofluorescence	False-positives if appropriate negative control is not used
3. Some chemotherapeutic agents (e.g., daunorubicin)	Increased cellular autofluorescence	False-positives if appropriate negative control is not used
4. Nicotine	Increased lymphocyte margination, decreased lymphocyte counts	Lowered absolute values for lymphocyte subsets
5. Corticosteroids	Decreased CD4 levels	Overestimation of disease-related alterations
6. Anti–human lymphocyte antibodies (e.g., OKT3) or soluble CD4	Lymphocytopenia, modulation, or blocking of cell surface receptors	Decreased labeling with antibody reagent
Biological factors		
1. Reticulocytosis	Incomplete red cell lysis, increased contamination of mononuclear preps	Decreased light scatter resolution: RBC contamination of lymphocyte gates
2. Strenuous exercise	Increased lymphocyte margination, decreased lymphocyte counts	Lowered absolute values for lymphocyte subsets
3. Diurnal variation	Variable absolute lymphocyte count	Variable absolute subset values
4. Specimen age and holding conditions	Variable granulocyte preservation and/or leukocyte viability	Increased granulocyte contamination of lymphocyte gates; false-positive nonspecific staining of dead cells

Permission to use portions of H42-T (*Clinical Applications of Flow Cytometry: Quality Assurance and Immunophenotyping of Peripheral Blood Lymphocytes; Tentative Guideline*) has been granted by the National Committee for Clinical Laboratory Standards. The current H42 edition may be obtained from NCCLS, 771 E. Lancaster Avenue, Villanova, PA 19085, U.S.A.

The above statement is required by the NCCLS to be "included prominently with the reproduced and excerpted text".

National Committee for Clinical Laboratory Standards (NCCLS) in May 1992.[58]

diploid population may become aneuploid and the S-phase may increase progressively.[34,59]

SUMMARY

Flow cytometer is a high-speed, sensitive tool which enables busy clinical laboratories to perform large-scale studies on lymphomas and leukemias routinely. The skillful application of monoclonal antibody panels may help to diagnose and classify hematologic neoplasms earlier and more accurately than manual techniques. Furthermore, it may detect a small population of lymphoma cells in the blood or bone marrow by virtue of their monoclonality or aneuploidy.[10,36] The combined analysis of DNA content, S-phase, and RNA index in tumors can be used to grade the tumors more objectively and predict the prognosis in terms of survival and of transformation of lymphomas from low grade to high grade.[27,32,43] On the other hand, when a low-grade lymphoma transforms into a high grade-variety, a

REFERENCES

1. Melamed MR, Lindmo T, Mendelsohn ML (eds): *Flow Cytometry and Sorting*, ed 2. New York, Wiley-Liss, 1990.
2. Grogan WM, Collins JM: *Guide to Flow Cytometry Methods*. New York, Marcel Dekker, 1990.
3. Coon JS, Weinstein RS (eds): *Diagnostic Flow Cytometry*. Baltimore, Williams & Wilkins, 1991.
4. Laerum OD, Bjerknes R (eds): *Flow Cytometry in Hematology*. London, Academic Press, 1992.
5. Shapiro HM: *Practical Flow Cytometry*, ed 3. New York, Alan R Liss, 1995.
6. Riley RS, Mahin EJ, William R: *Clinical Application of Flow Cytometry*. New York, Igaku-Shoin, 1993.
7. Bauer KD, Daque RE, Shankey TV (eds): *Clinical Flow Cytometry: Principles and Application*. Baltimore, Williams & Wilkins, 1993.

8. Karen DF (ed): *Flow Cytometry in Clinical Diagnosis*. Chicago, American Society of Clinical Pathologists Press, 1993.
9. Sun T: *Color Atlas/Text of Flow Cytometric Analysis of Hematologic Neoplasms*. New York, Igaku-Shoin, 1993.
10. Ault KA: Clinical applications of fluorescence-activated cell sorting techniques. *Diagn Immunol* 1:2–10, 1983.
11. Barlogie B, Mclaughlin P, Alexanian R: Characterization of hematologic malignancy by flow cytometry. *Analy Quant Cytol Histol* 9:147–155, 1987.
12. Braylan RC: Flow cytometry. *Arch Pathol Lab Med* 107:1–6, 1983.
13. Colvin RB, Preffer FI: New technologies in cell analysis by flow cytometry. *Arch Pathol Lab Med* 111:628–632, 1987.
14. Coon JS, Landay AL, Weinstein RS: Biology of disease: Advances in flow cytometry for diagnostic pathology. *Lab Invest* 57:453–479, 1987.
15. Marti GE: Diagnostic flow cytometry in hematology: The leukemias. *Pathol Immunopathol Res* 5:416–436, 1986.
16. Parker JW: Flow cytometry in the diagnosis of hematologic diseases. *Ann Clin Lab Sci* 16:427–442, 1986.
17. Shapiro HM: Technical developments in flow cytometry. *Hum Pathol* 17:649–651, 1986.
18. Wunderlich J: Fluorescence flow cytometry and immunology applied to cancer. *Analy Quant Cytol Histol* 9:133–137, 1987.
19. Ault KA: Detection of small numbers of monoclonal B-lymphocytes in the blood of patients with lymphoma. *N Engl J Med* 300:1401–1405, 1979.
20. Ligler FS, Smith RG, Keltman JR, et al: Detection of tumor cells in the peripheral blood of nonleukemia patients with B-cell lymphoma: Analysis of "clonal excess." *Blood* 55:792–800, 1980.
21. Young IT: Proof without prejudice: Use of the Kolmogorov-Smirov test for the analysis of histogram from flow systems and other sources. *J Histochem Cytochem* 25:935–941, 1977.
22. Berliner N, Ault KA, Martin P, et al: Detection of clonal excess in lymphoproliferative disease by kappa/lambda analysis: Correlation with immunoglobulin gene DNA rearrangement. *Blood* 67:80–85, 1986.
23. Baserga R: The cell cycle. *N Engl J Med* 304:453–459, 1981.
24. Herman CJ, Walloch J: DNA analysis of solid tumors: Practical value: In Coon JS, Weinstein RS (eds): *Diagnostic Flow Cytometry*. Baltimore, Williams & Wilkins, 1991, pp 135–146.
25. Hyder D, Schnitzer B: Analysis of hematopoietic/lymphoreticular malignancies. In Kren D (ed): *Flow Cytometry in Clinical Diagnosis*. Chicago, American Society of Clinical Pathologists Press, 1989, pp 179–212.
26. Frierson HF Jr: Flow cytometric analysis of ploidy in solid neoplasms: Comparison of fresh tissues with formalin-fixed paraffin-embedded specimens. *Hum Pathol* 19:290–294, 1988.
27. McIntire TL, Goldey SH, Benson NA, et al: Flow cytometric analysis of DNA in cells obtained from deparaffinized formalin-fixed lymphoid tissues. *Cytometry* 8:474–478, 1987.
28. Barlogie B, Raber M, Schumann J, et al: Flow cytometry in clinical cancer research. *Cancer Res* 43:3982–3997, 1983.
29. Oppedal BR, Storm-Mathisen I, Lie SO, et al: Prognostic factors in neuroblastoma. Clinical, histopathologic and immunoclinical features and DNA ploidy in relation to prognosis. *Cancer* 62:772–780, 1988.
30. Tomita T, Yasue M, Englehard HH, et al: Flow cytometric DNA analysis of medulloblastoma. Prognostic implication of aneuploidy. *Cancer* 61:744–749, 1988.
31. Goldsmith MM, Cresson DH, Arnold LA, et al: DNA flow cytometry as a prognostic indicator in head and neck cancer. *Otolaryngol Head Neck Surg* 96:307–318, 1987.
32. Christensson B Tribukait B, Linder IL, et al: Cell proliferation and DNA content in non-Hodgkin's lymphoma: Flow cytometry in relation to lymphoma classification. *Cancer* 58:1295–1304, 1986.
33. Diamond LW, Nathwani B, Rappaport H: Flow cytometry in the diagnosis and classification of malignant lymphoma and leukemia. *Cancer* 50:1122–1135, 1982.
34. Juneja SK, Sooper IA, Hodgson GS, et al: DNA ploidy patterns and cytokinetics of non-Hodgkin's lymphoma. *J Clin Pathol* 39:987–992, 1986.
35. Crigley J, Barlogie B, Butler JJ, et al: Heterogeneity of non-Hodgkin's lymphoma probed by nucleic acid cytometry. *Blood* 65:1090–1096, 1985.
36. Andreeff M, Hansen H, Cirrincione C, et al: Prognostic value of DNA/RNA flow cytometry of B-cell non-Hodgkin's lymphoma: Development of laboratory model and correlation with four taxonomic systems. *Ann NY Acad Sci* 468:368–386, 1986.
37. Morgan DR, Williamson JMS, Quirke P, et al: DNA content and prognosis of non-Hodgkin's lymphoma. *Br J Cancer* 54:643–649, 1986.
38. Shackney SE, Levine AM, Fisher RI, et al: The biology of tumor growth in the non-Hodgkin's lymphomas: A dual parameter flow cytometry study of 220 cases. *J Clin Invest* 73:1201–1214, 1984.
39. Braylan RC, Diamond LW, Powell ML, et al: Percentage of cells in the S-phase of the cell cycle in human lymphoma determined by flow cytometry. *Cytometry* 1:171–174, 1980.
40. Braylan RC, Benson NA, Nourse VA: Cellular DNA of human neoplastic B-cells measured by flow cytometry. *Cancer Res* 44:5010–5016, 1984.
41. Roos G, Dige U, Linner P, et al: Prognostic significance of DNA analysis by flow cytometry in non-Hodgkin's lymphoma. *Hematol Oncol* 3:233–242, 1985.
42. MacArtney JC, Canplejohn RS, Alder J, et al: Prognostic importance of DNA flow cytometry in non-Hodgkin's lymphomas. *J Clin Pathol* 39:542–546, 1986.
43. Andreeff M: Flow cytometry of lymphoma. In Melamed MR, Lindmo T, Mendelsohn ML (eds): *Flow Cytometry and Sorting*, ed 2. New York, Wiley-Liss, 1990, pp 725–743.
44. Andreeff M, Assing G, Cirrincione C: Prognostic value of DNA/RNA flow cytometry in myeloblastic and lymphoblastic leukemia in adults: RNA content and S-phase predict remission duration and survival in multivariate analysis. *Ann NY Acad Sci* 468:387–406, 1986.
45. Andreeff M, Darzynkiewicz Z, Sharpless TK, et al: Discrimination of human leukemia subtype by flow cytometric analysis of cellular DNA and RNA. *Blood* 55:282–293, 1980.

46. Barlogie B, Keating MJ, McCredie KB, et al: Biological and prognostic implications of bone marrow DNA and RNA cytometry in adult acute leukemia. *Blood* 60 (Suppl 1):120a, 1982.
47. Hiddemann W, Wormann B, Gohde W, et al: DNA aneuploidies in adult patients with adult myeloid leukemia. *Cancer* 57:2146–2152, 1986.
48. Look AT, Melvin SL, Williams DL, et al: Aneuploidy and percentage of S-phase cells determined by flow cytometry correlate with cell phenotype in childhood acute leukemia. *Blood* 60:959–967, 1982.
49. Look AT, Roberson PK, Williams DL, et al: Prognostic importance of blast cell DNA content in childhood acute lymphoblastic leukemia. *Blood* 65:1079–1086, 1985.
50. Andreeff M: Flow cytometry of leukemia. In Melamed MR, Lindomo T, Mendelsohn ML (eds): *Flow Cytometry and Sorting*, ed 2. New York, Wiley-Liss, 1990, pp 725–743.
51. Hiddemann W, Woermann B, Ritter J, et al: Frequency and clinical significance of DNA aneuploidy in acute leukemia. *Ann NY Acad Sci* 468:227–240, 1986.
52. Merkel DE, Dressler LG, McGuire WL: Flow cytometry, cellular DNA content and prognosis in human malignancy. *J Clin Oncol* 5:1690–1703, 1987.
53. Bauer KD, Merkel DE, Winte JN, et al: Prognostic implications of ploidy and proliferative activity in diffuse large cell lymphomas. *Cancer Res* 46:3173–3178, 1986.
54. Barlogie B, Alexanian R, Gehan EA, et al: Marrow cytometry and prognosis in myeloma. *J Clin Invest* 72:853–861, 1983.
55. Sun T, Susin, M: A practical approach to immunophenotyping of lymphomas: Comparison of immunohistologic and immunocytologic techniques. *Ann Clin Lab Sci* 17:14–26, 1987.
56. Sun T, Susin M: Pitfalls in flow cytometric studies of hematologic disorders. ASCP Check Sample, Hematology No. H91-3, American Society of Clinical Pathologists, Chicago, 1991.
57. Parker JW: Immunologic basis for the redefinition of malignant lymphomas. *Am J Clin Pathol* 72(Suppl):670–686, 1979.
58. National Committee for Clinical Laboratory Standards: *NCCLS Tentative Guideline: Clinical Applications of Flow Cytometry: Quality Assurance and Immunophenotyping of Peripheral Blood Lymphocytes*. NCCLS document H42-T, vol 12, no. 6. Vilanova, Pa.: NCCLS, May 1992.
59. Winberg CD, Sheibani K, Krance R, et al: Peripheral T-cell lymphoma: Immunologic and cell kinetic observations associated with morphological progression. *Blood* 66:980–989, 1985.

Chapter 7

IMMUNOGENOTYPING AND POLYMERASE CHAIN REACTION

Immunophenotyping by monoclonal antibodies with flow cytometric analysis has undoubtedly made a great contribution to the diagnosis and classification of lymphoid neoplasms. However, there are several shortcomings in immunophenotyping.[1-7] First, immunophenotyping, even with the use of flow cytometry, is not sensitive enough to make a preliminary diagnosis when the tumor cells are in the minority. For instance, calculation of the κ/λ ratio requires at last 20% B cells to make the results reliable.[8] Even then, if a large number of normal B lymphocytes are present, the result will be distorted. Second, the light chain ratio is the only parameter used to identify the clonality of B lymphocytes. When a B-cell tumor bears no SIg (e.g., SIg-negative B-cell lymphoma), then the clonality of the population tested cannot be established. In addition, other cell lineage–associated antigens may not be expressed in some tumors (e.g., non-T, non-B ALL). Third, there is no marker to enable the identification of the clonality of T-cell neoplasms by immunophenotyping. Although some tumors may show a phenotype of a T-helper cell (e.g., Sézary syndrome) or of a T-suppressor cell (e.g., T-suppressor cell CLL), the finding of a high percentage of T-helper or T-suppressor cells does not necessarily indicate monoclonality. In patients with acquired immunodeficiency syndrome (AIDS) or other viral infections (e.g., cytomegalovirus infection), the percentage of T-suppressor cells can reach 95% or more. In Hodgkin's disease, on the other hand, 90% or more T-helper cells can be present in a lymph node.[8] Finally, immunophenotyping by flow cytometry requires a fresh specimen and that by immunostaining requires a frozen block. Many important markers, such as SIg or helper/suppressor T-cell markers, cannot be detected in paraffin sections.

Advances in molecular biology have made immunogenotyping of lymphoid neoplasms possible, and this new technique overcomes the above-mentioned disadvantages of immunophenotyping. Immunogenotyping, usually referred to as *Southern blot hybridization* or *gene rearrangement analysis*, can be performed on as few as 2 μg of DNA, the equivalent of about 0.2 mg of wet tissue.[2] There is no need for fresh tissue, as required by flow cytometric studies. DNA analysis can be done at leisure by the technologists since the specimen is frozen. Under favorable conditions, a specimen can be used for DNA study even after being stored at 4°C for 3–4 months.[4] The comparison of cytometric immunophenotyping and immunogenotyping is presented in Table 7-1.

Since gene rearrangement is an analysis at the DNA level, it can identify the cell lineage even if this is not expressed phenotypically. It is particularly useful for the determination of T-cell clonality because flow cytometry cannot identify T-cell tumors unless there is selective loss of T-cell antigens.[9] In addition, immunogenotyping is an extremely sensitive test; as few as 1–5% of tumor cells in the population analyzed can be detected by this technique.[1,2,6] However, gene rearrangement analysis is time-consuming; it takes at least 1 week to complete the test. Furthermore, radioisotopes remain the most frequently used label for DNA probes, as other labels, such as fluorophores and enzymes, are still not sensitive enough to demonstrate gene rearrangement in a small population of cells. Therefore, use of the immunogenotyping technique is mainly confined to large medical centers. However, this is a highly promising technique and, with further improvement, is expected to be widely used in clinical laboratories.

STRUCTURE AND REARRANGEMENT OF ANTIGEN RECEPTOR GENES

Immunoglobulin molecules are composed of two identical heavy chains and two identical light chains. The five classes of heavy chains—IgG, IgA, IgM, IgD, and IgE—are all encoded by the same heavy chain gene located on chromosome 14.[6,7] The light chains have two types, κ and λ; they are encoded by two different genes located on chromosomes 2

TABLE 7-1. Comparison of Cytometric Immunophenotyping and Immunogenotyping

	Immunophenotyping	Immunogenotyping
Specimen requirement	Fresh	Fresh/frozen
Minimal specimen size	0.5 mg	0.2 mg
Time for test	2 days	7 days
Resulting analysis	Quantitative	Qualitative
Scope of diagnosis	Mainly B-cell tumors	Both B- and T-cell tumors
Reliable detectable level of clonal cell population	20%	5%
Identification of secondary/recurrent tumor	Using anti-idiotype monoclonal antibodies	Comparing rearranged bands
Monitoring course of disease	Quantifying percentage of clonal population	Visualizing rearranged bands

and 22, respectively. These genes are arranged in their germline configuration as discontinuous segments of DNA.

The heavy chain gene contains four regions: C (constant), V (variable), J (joining), and D (diversity). (Figure 7-1 and Table 7-2). Both light chain genes contain only three regions: C, V, and J. The heavy chain gene has about 100–200 V_H segments, 10 D segments, and 6 J_H segments.[10] The light chain gene has about 40–80 V_L segments and 4–5 J_L segments.[10] During differentiation of the B cell, a series of gene rearrangements takes place (Figure 7-2).

The B cell randomly selects a particular $V_H/D/J_H$ and V_L/J_L combination to encode for the variable region of the antibody, while C_H and C_L encode for the constant region. During normal B-cell differentiation, the heavy chain gene is first rearranged, followed by the κ light chain gene. If κ gene rearrangement fails to produce the κ light chain protein, the λ gene will be rearranged.[1-7]

The T-cell receptor (TCR) is a heterodimer consisting of two polypeptide chains. The majority of T cells carry the α/β heterodimer on their cell membrane, while the minority bears the γ/δ receptor.[6,11] Although α and δ chain genes do not belong to the same receptor, they are both located on the same locus of chromosome 14. The β and γ chain genes are located on the long and short arms of chromosome 7, respectively. The composition of TCR genes is presented in Table 7-2. During normal T-cell development, the δ and γ chain genes are probably rearranged at about the same time, followed by the β chain gene; the α chain gene is the last one to be rearranged.

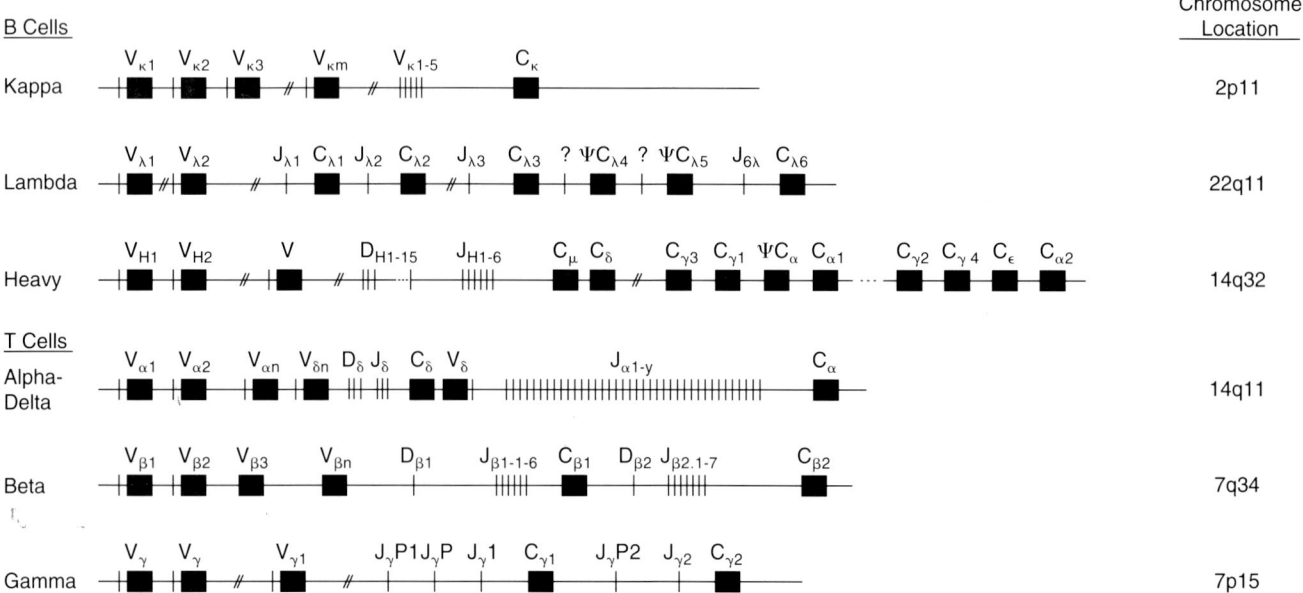

FIGURE 7-1. Germline genomic organizations and chromosomal locations of the human immunoglobulin genes IgH, Igκ, and Igλ and the T-cell receptor genes α, β, γ, and δ. V = variable; D = diversity; J = joining segments; C = constant-region genes. (From Griesser H, Tkachuk D, Reis MD, et al: Gene rearrangements and translocations in lymphoproliferative diseases. *Blood* 73:1404, 1989)

TABLE 7-2. Composition of Immunoglobulin in Heavy Chain, Light Chain, and TCR Genes and Number of Segments

	Heavy Chain	κ Chain	λ Chain	TCRα	TCRβ	TCRγ	TCRδ
Locus	14q32	2p12	22q11	14q11	7q34	7p15	14q11
V segments	100–200	40–80	40	50–100	75–100	8	4
D segments	10	0	0	0	2	0	2
J segments	6	5	4	50–100	13	2	3
C segments	9	1	4	1	2	2	1

SOUTHERN BLOT HYBRIDIZATION

Any specimens containing lymphoid tissue can be used for Southern blot hybridization.[12] DNA is isolated from the specimens by phenol-chloroform extraction and ethanol precipitation. The DNA extract is then subjected to restriction endonuclease digestion (Figure 7-3). The most commonly used restriction enzymes are Bam HI, Eco RI and Hind III. Each of these enzymes cuts DNA at predetermined sites defined by specific short sequences of base pairs. After digestion, the restriction fragments are size fractionated by electrophoresis in 0.8% agarose gels. The DNA is then treated with base to become single-stranded and transferred to nitrocellulose or nylon membrane by direct printing under pressure. The DNA electrophoretic pattern on the membrane is permanently immobilized by heating. Bands containing DNA of the gene fragment of interest are detected by a DNA probe, usually labeled with a radioisotope, ^{32}P. After hybridization, the membrane is rinsed and subjected to autoradiography. The image ob-

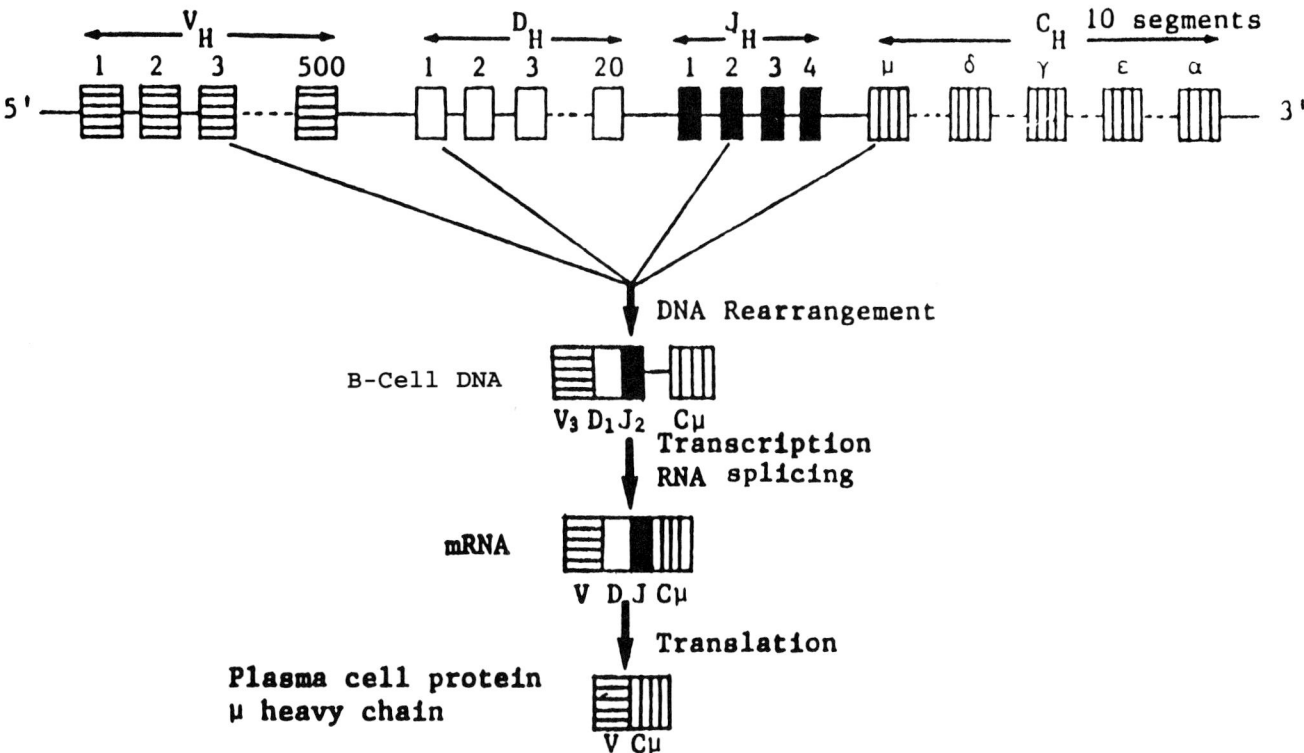

FIGURE 7-2. Immunoglobulin heavy chain gene rearrangement. The germline heavy chain genes include four regions: V, D, J, and C. Each region contains a certain number of segments. DNA rearrangement consists of the random selection of one segment from each region. The selected gene segments are transcribed into messenger RNAs (mRNA), which are, in turn, translated into proteins (immunoglobulins). (From Sun T: *Interpretation of Protein and Isoenzyme Patterns in Body Fluids.* New York, Igaku-Shoin, 1991, p 42)

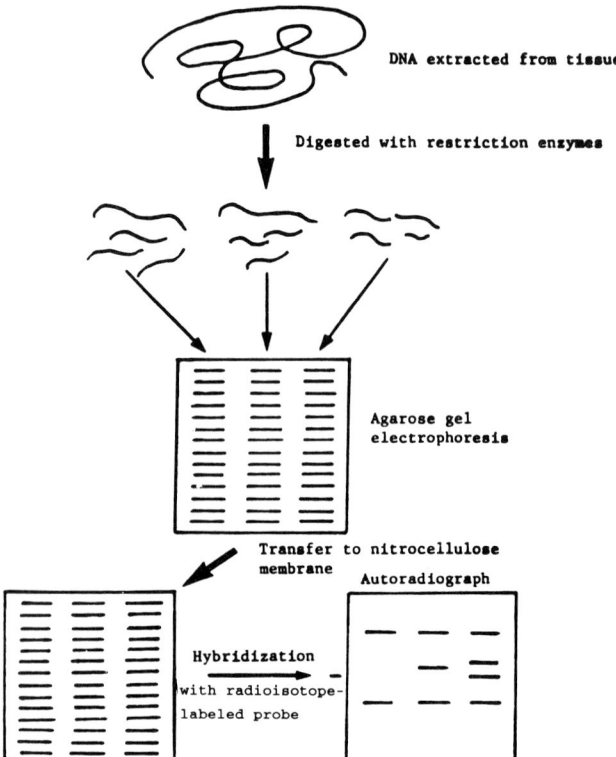

FIGURE 7-3. Southern blot hybridization procedure. DNA extracted from the specimen is first digested with restriction enzymes. The DNA fragments are size-fractionated by agarose gel electrophoresis. The DNA electrophoretic pattern on agarose is then transferred to nitrocellulose membrane to allow for hybridization with a radioisotope-labeled probe. The results are demonstrated by autoradiography.

tained on the x-ray film will show the germline and nongermline bands of the gene under study. Placenta tissue, fibroblasts, or normal lymphocytes are usually used as a negative control to show the germlines. A positive control to show a nongermline or rearranged band is also required. The presence of a band different from the germlines is considered a rearranged band.

GENE REARRANGEMENT IN LYMPHOID NEOPLASMS

The demonstration of rearranged band(s) by immunogenotyping in a lymphoid population indicates monoclonality and, under most circumstances, malignancy (Figures 7-4 and 7-5). Thus, DNA hybridization analysis becomes a very useful tool in distinguishing between lymphoid neoplasms and hyperplasia (Table 7-3).[6,13] This technique was instrumental in resolving the cell lineage of common ALL (non-T, non-B ALL)[14] and hairy cell leukemia[15,16] as being of B-cell origin. Some of the so-called histiocytic malignancies have been reclassified as T-cell neoplasms after DNA studies.[17-19] The unique advantage of this DNA technique is that the results of analysis are not affected by the coexistent nontumor populations, such as the dilution effect by the normal cells seen in immunophenotyping. Although the technique is complicated, when it is appropriately performed the results are highly reproducible. Thus, a recent study shows that the agreement of test results among 11 laboratories was 96% and the agreement in interpretation was greater than 95%.[20] In the same study, the cell lineage of 13 cases of lymphoid tumors could not be determined by phenotyping but was resolved in 10 of these cases by gene rearrangement analysis. On the other hand, only 97 of 100 phenotypically B-cell neoplasms and 32 of 36 phenotypically T-cell neoplasms showed corresponding gene rearrangement results. It seems that phenotyping and genotyping are complementary to each other; thus, genotyping still cannot totally replace phenotyping.

For a routine workup, immunophenotyping may identify most B-cell neoplasms without the need for genotypic confirmation. However, genotyping is much more frequently needed in the diagnosis of T-cell neoplasms than B-cell neoplasms.[21] Unfortunately, the successful rate of demonstrating gene rearrangement is lower in T-cell than in B-cell tumors.[22,23] With the availability of α, β, γ, and δ chain gene probes, the successful rate of TCR gene analysis is expected to be improved. The most commonly used probe for TCR gene rearrangement was the C region, but this has now been replaced by the J region of the TCR β chain gene. The limited number of V and J segments in the γ and δ chain genes (Table 7-2) sometimes cause false-positive results, as faint bands may be demonstrated.[1-3,6] This is because polyclonally rearranged bands are confined to a limited number (seven and eight bands); thus, the intensity of the bands may reach a detectable level. On the other hand, false-negative results may be obtained from the α chain gene probing because this gene is spread out over a large area of chromosome 14.[1,2,6,7]

While the demonstration of gene rearrangement in non-Hodgkin's lymphomas is generally accepted as a powerful tool for diagnosis, the existence of gene rearrangement in Hodgkin's disease is still controversial. DNA studies in Hodgkin's disease usually show no gene rearrangement. When the result is positive, partial rearrangement of the heavy chain gene is most commonly encountered and TCR gene rearrangement is seen in only a few cases.[4,24-30] However, in most cases, the rearrangement bands are faint, with only a few exceptions.[26,30] There are many possible explanations for these positive results: they may represent monoclonality of the Reed-Sternberg cells, small clones of

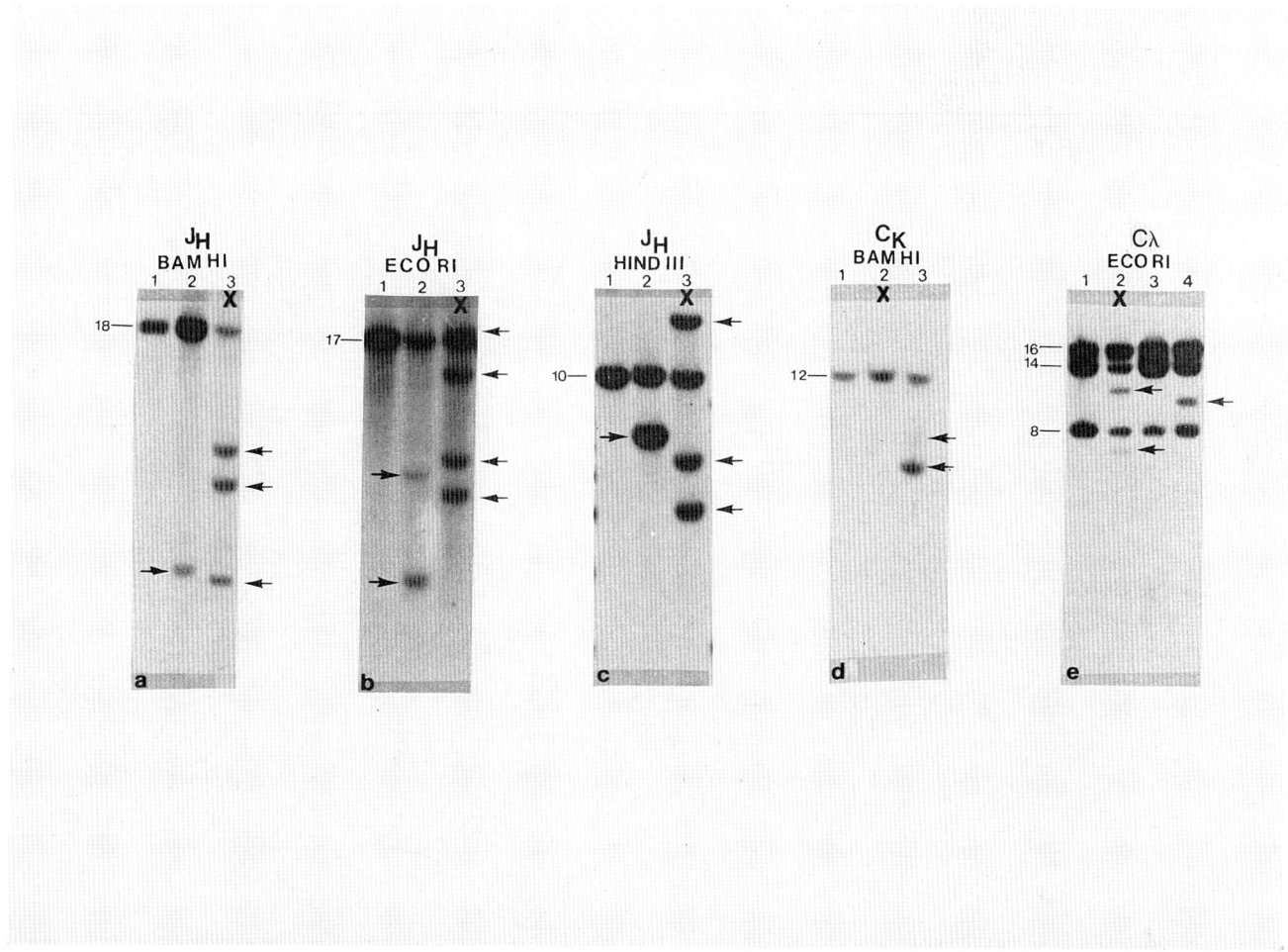

FIGURE 7-4. Southern blot hybridization analysis of the immunoglobulin heavy chain gene (J_H) and the κ and λ light chain genes (Cκ and Cλ) in a case of hairy cell leukemia. DNAs were digested with the restriction enzymes Bam HI, Eco RI and Hind III. In panel J_H, lane 1 is the negative control and lane 2 is the positive control. The lines marked by an X contain the patient specimen. The rearranged band is indicated by an arrow. In panel Cκ, lane 1 is the negative control and lane 3 is the positive control. In panel Cλ, lanes 1 and 3 are the negative control and lane 4 is the positive control. In the patient specimen, each enzyme revealed more than two rearranged heavy chain bands. Two rearranged λ light chain bands of unequal intensity were detected, but no κ light chain rearrangement was found. (From Sun T, Eisenberg A, Benn P, et al: Comparison of phenotyping and genotyping of lymphoid neoplasms. *J Clin Lab Anal* 3:156–162, 1989).

nonneoplasic cells, transformation of Hodgkin's disease to or from lymphomas, or misdiagnosis of a lymphoma as Hodgkin's disease. A definite answer will probably not be available until a pure culture of Reed-Sternberg cells is obtainable.

Another controversial entity is angioimmunoblastic lymphadenopathy (AILD). Minden and Mak found 9 of 11 AILD cases showing TCR β chain gene rearrangement; 4 of them had immunoglobulin heavy chain gene rearrangement and one had κ chain gene rearrangement.[31] In most other reports, only TCR gene rearrangements were detected.[32,33] Sklar considers AILD as a polyclonal disorder that predisposes to the development of T-cell lymphoma.[2]

GENE REARRANGEMENTS AS MARKERS OF CLONAL ORIGIN AND RECURRENT TUMORS

Gene rearrangement analysis not only can help establish a diagnosis of lymphoid neoplasms but can also identify the clonal origins of two or more coexistent tumors (e.g.,

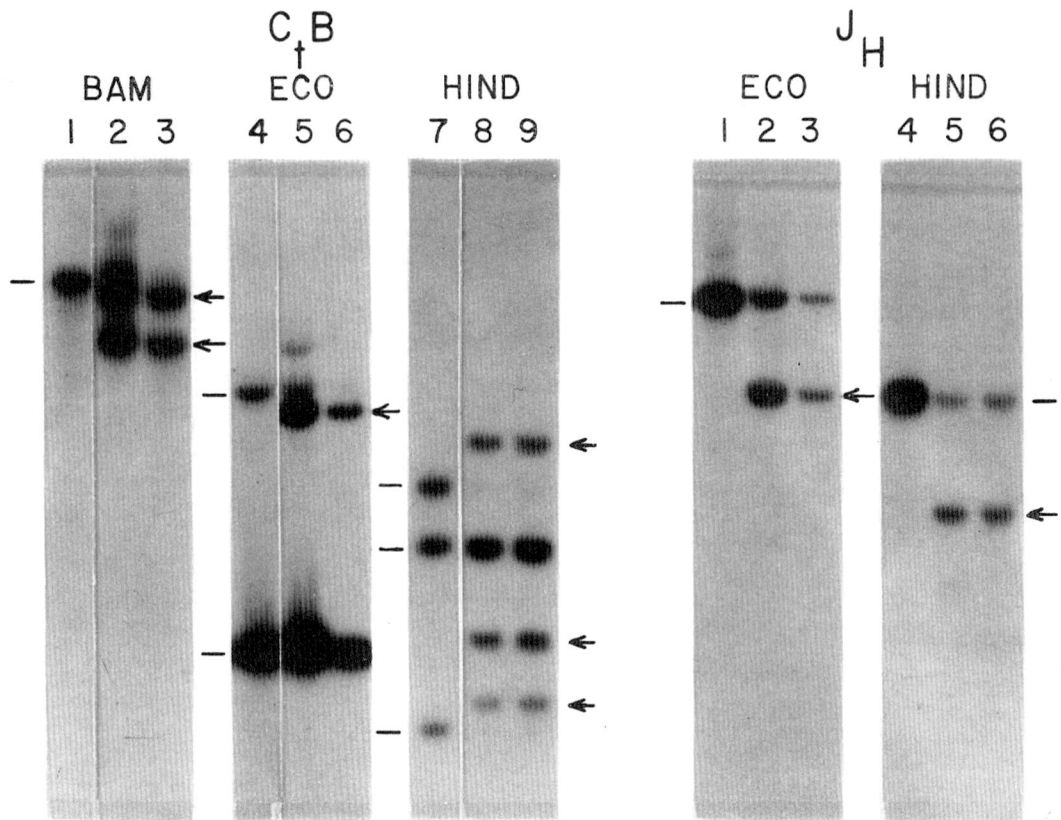

FIGURE 7-5. Southern blot hybridization analysis of the immunoglobulin heavy chain gene (J_H) and TCR β chain gene ($C_tβ$) in a case of T-cell ALL. Bigenotypic rearrangement is demonstrated. In panel $C_tβ$, lanes 1–3 were cut with Bam HI, lanes 4–6 were cut with Eco RI, and lanes 7 and 8 were cut with Hind III. In panel J_H, lanes 1–3 were cut with Eco RI and lanes 4–6 were cut with Hind III. Lanes 1, 4, and 7 are negative controls showing only germline bands. Lanes 2, 5, and 8 contain bone marrow specimen, and lanes 3, 6, and 9 contain pleural fluid specimen from the same patient. Germline bands are indicated by – and rearranged bands by arrows. Faint bands in lanes 2 and 5 in panel $C_tβ$ are due to partial digestion. (From the same source as Figure 7-4).

composite lymphoma)[34–36] or the relationship of two consecutively appearing tumors (e.g., Richter's syndrome).[37–41] Tumors of the same clonal origin should show identical rearranged bands. Nonidentical bands may indicate different clonal origins. It turns out that the components of CLL and large-cell lymphoma in Richter's syndrome can have the same clonal origin in some cases but different clonal origins in others.[37–41] The relationship of various components in a composite lymphoma is the same as in Richter's syndrome.[34–36] By the same token, the identity of rearranged bands may also help to determine the relationship between the primary tumor and its metastatic component or to distinguish a recurrent tumor from the emergence of a new, unrelated tumor.[1–7]

Lymphoma cells can also be detected in the peripheral blood by this technique despite the absence of morphologic evidence of hematogenous spread.[42]

GENE REARRANGEMENT IN NONNEOPLASTIC CONDITIONS

Although monoclonality, as demonstrated by gene rearrangement analysis, usually indicates malignancy, it can also be present in benign conditions. The better-known examples are the demonstration of immunoglobulin gene rearrangement in benign lymphoepithelial lesions in Sjögren's disease[43] and TCR gene rearrangement in lymphomatoid papulosis.[44] Gene rearrangement has also been

TABLE 7-3. Immunoglobulin and TCR Gene Rearrangement in Lymphoproliferative Disorders

Lymphoproliferative Disorder	IgH	IgL	TCRα	TCRβ	TCRγ	TCRδ
B-ALL	+	+	−	±	±	−
T-ALL	±	−	±	+	+	±
Non-T, Non-B ALL	+	−	±	±	±	±
B-CLL	+	+	−	±	±	−
T-CLL	−	−	±	+	+	+
Hairy cell leukemia	+	+	0	−	0	0
Sézary syndrome	±	−	0	+	0	0
ATL	−	−	±	+	+	+
B-cell lymphoma	+	+	−	±	±	−
T-cell lymphoma	−	−	±	+	+	±
Lennert's lymphoma	−	−	±	+	+	±
Ki-l lymphoma	±	−	±	±	+	±
Hodgkin's disease	±	−	±	±	±	−
AILD	±	−	±	+	+	±

Ki-l lymphoma = ki-l (CD30)-positive anaplastic large-cell lymphoma. IgH = heavy chain gene, IgL = light chain gene
+ = rearranged, − = germline, 0 = no data available

demonstrated in AIDS-related lymphadenopathy, lymphadenopathy-associated rheumatoid arthritis, posttransplant lymphoproliferative disorders, pityriasis lichenoids et varioliformis acuta, and systemic Castlemans disease.[1,6] It should be pointed out that most of these "benign" disorders may be premalignant conditions that are susceptible to transformation to neoplasms.[2] Indeed, the high incidence of malignant transformation in Sjögren's disease is well known,[45] and AIDS-related lymphadenopathy may also transform into lymphoma.[46]

CROSS-LINEAGE REARRANGEMENT, LINEAGE INFIDELITY, OR PROMISCUITY

When rearrangement is confined to immunoglobulin genes or TCR genes, the cell lineage of the tumor is clear-cut. When both immunoglobulin heavy chain and TCR genes are rearranged, the condition is called *lineage infidelity* or *promiscuity*. When immunoglobulin light chain is rearranged, however, the tumor should be classified as of B-cell origin, regardless of whether the TCR gene is rearranged. Rearrangement of TCR was reported in 25% of patients with non-T-cell ALL,[47] and rearrangement of the heavy chain gene was seen in 10% of patients with T-cell leukemias.[48,49] TCR or immunoglobulin gene rearrangements may also be demonstrated in about 50% of cases of myelogenous leukemia with TdT expression and in 10% of cases without TdT expression.[50] Non-T, non-B ALL, AILD, and CD30+ (ki-1) anaplastic large cell lymphoma show more frequent rearrangements in both T- and B-cell lineage than do other lymphoid tumors.[6] However, the rearranged bands in cross-lineage conditions are usually faint and represent partial (DJ segment) rearrangement. It is possible that tumor cells with a double lineage are derived from immature lymphoid cells at a stage of differentiation prior to lineage commitment; alternatively, they may be due to the presence of a common recombinase that can catalyze both immunoglobulin and TCR gene rearrangements.[1-3,6]

IDENTIFICATION OF CHROMOSOMAL TRANSLOCATION BY THE DNA HYBRIDIZATION TECHNIQUE

In addition to identifying the clonality and lineage of lymphoid tumors, the DNA hybridization technique can identify chromosomal translocations, which may occur after gene rearrangement.[1-3,6,51] Because of the translocation, the restriction enzyme site may change, thus affecting the length of the DNA fragments after digestion. Therefore, a rearranged band(s) can be demonstrated when a probe aiming at the breakpoint cluster region (BCR) or its equivalent is used. Chromosomal translocation has been seen in increasing numbers of lymphomas and leukemias; the better-known examples are t(8;14) in Burkitt's lymphoma, t(14;18) in follicular lymphoma, and t(9;22) in chronic myeloid leukemia. This topic will be discussed further in Chapter 8.

PROBLEMS WITH INTERPRETATION OF IMMUNOGENOTYPING RESULTS

Nongermline bands can be seen in several conditions that are not due to monoclonal gene rearrangements. As already mentioned, polyclonal TCR γ and δ chain gene rearrangements may manifest as faint nongermline bands because only limited probabilities exist for recombination in their V and J segments. Inherited polymorphisms in immunoglobulin and TCR genes may also produce nongermline bands, but identification of the same bands in nonlymphoid cells, such as polymorphs and fibroblasts, from the same patient may confirm the condition as inherited polymorphism rather than monoclonal gene rearrangement.[1-3,7] Partial digestion of DNA is the major technical cause of nongermline bands. The use of two or three restriction enzymes may eliminate this false-positive result.[1-3,7]

The detection of multiple rearranged bands or the emergence of new rearranged bands is another problem in the interpretation of immunogenotyping, especially when the test is used to determine the clonal origin of two different tumor components, such as composite lymphoma or Richter's syndrome.[34-41] The presence of multiple rearranged bands may give the false impression of the existence of more than one clone of tumor cells. However, this pattern is frequently due to secondary restructuring, such as heavy chain switching, DNA deletion, and point mutation.[1-3] Fortunately, when comparing two tumors of the same clonal origin, at least one rearranged band between the tumors is identical. In addition, light chain genes seldom, if ever, undergo secondary restructuring or postrearrangement changes; the rearranged bands of light chain genes between two tumors of the same origin are usually identical. A minor problem in the interpretation of light chain gene rearrangement is the demonstration of a nonproductive κ light chain gene (which should be normally deleted) when the λ light chain gene is rearranged.

False-negative results are usually due to technical problems, such as underloaded DNA, inappropriate digestion, underexposed autoradiography, or incorrect performance of other procedures. One nontechnical cause is comigration of the rearranged band with a germline. This condition occurs when the rearrangement introduces a new restriction enzyme site which produces a restriction fragment of approximately the same size as the germline.[1-3,7] This problem should be tackled with the use of additional restriction enzymes.

POLYMERASE CHAIN REACTION

Polymerase chain reaction (PCR) is an *in vitro* technique for enzymatic amplification of a DNA segment of interest.[52-57] It is composed of repetitive cycling of three simple reactions: DNA denaturation, primer annealing, and primer extension (Figure 7-6). All reactions take place in the same test tube at various temperatures. The finding of a heat-stable Taq DNA polymerase, isolated from the thermophilic bacterium *Thermus aquaticus*, has allowed the automation of the procedure, since heat-labile polymerase has to be replenished after each cycle. DNA denaturation is accomplished at high temperature (90°–95°C), which breaks the hydrogen bonds of the double-stranded DNA and produces the single-stranded DNA. Two single-stranded oligonucleotides (primers), synthesized to be complementary to known sequences of the target DNA, are added with polymerases and excess deoxyribonucleoside triphosphates (nucleotides) as the building blocks for new DNA synthesis. The second step is performed at a reduced temperature (45°–55°C) when the two primers anneal to the two single-stranded DNA molecules derived from the target DNA. In the third step, the polymerase catalyzes the synthesis of a complementary second strand of new DNA at 72°C, leading to the extension of each annealed primer. Two new single-stranded DNA copies are produced in the first cycle, but DNA increases geometrically in subsequent cycles. After the cycle is repeated 30 times, about 1 million copies of the target DNA segments are generated in 4 hr.

The amplified DNA can be detected by ethidium bromide staining of the DNA bands after agarose gel electrophoresis. When the amount of DNA after amplification is still too low to be detected by fluorescent staining, a Southern blot procedure has to be conducted, using radioisotope-labeled probes.

The major barrier to the use of PCR is the requirement of primer synthesis, which limits its application to DNA of known structure. PCR is a highly sensitive technique; it can detect as little as one DNA molecule in a sample. However, this great asset of PCR is also its disadvantage because it may generate false-positive results from carryovers of previously amplified DNA and from cross-contamination with true-positive samples. Therefore, scrupulous adherence to standard techniques and strict measures for quality assurance must be adopted when PCR is used.

PCR is most desirable for the diagnosis of lymphomas and leukemias with chromosomal translocations. For instance, for the diagnosis of follicular lymphoma with chromosome 14;18 translocation, two primers can be tailor-made to be complementary to the sequences flanking the selected segments (crossover sites or breakpoint cluster regions) in chromosomes 14 and 18, respectively. As a result, DNA molecules from the tumor cells carrying both chromosome 14 and chromosome 18 segments are amplified geometrically, while normal DNA molecules carrying either chromosome 14 or chromosome 18 segments are amplified arithmetically.[57] In the end, the DNA molecules

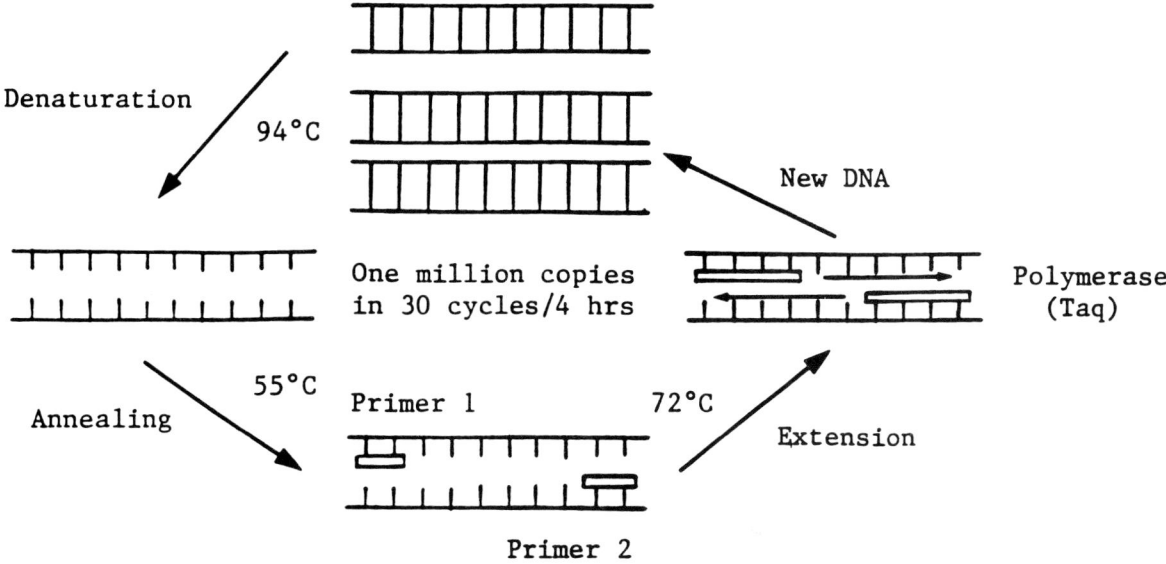

FIGURE 7-6. PCR. The first step is to denature the double-stranded DNA at 94°C to yield single-stranded DNA. At 55°C, the two primers anneal to the 5' and 3' ends of the single-stranded DNA, respectively. At 72°C, the polymerase catalyzes the extension of each annealed primer in the presence of excess nucleotides. Two copies of double-stranded DNA are thus formed. The cycle repeats 30 times, and 1 million copies of DNA are produced in 4 hr. (From Sun T: *Color Atlas/Text of Flow Cytometric Analysis of Hematologic Neoplasms.* New York, Igaku-Shoin, 1993, p 31.).

from tumor cells are selectively amplified and can be identified for diagnostic purposes. PCR is also useful for the detection of minimal residual disease in leukemias and lymphomas.[58,59]

IN SITU HYBRIDIZATION

The *in situ* hybridization technique is useful for the studies of lymphoid neoplasms at the DNA/RNA level.[1] This technique consists of applying appropriate probes (DNA, RNA, or oligonucleotide) to cytology smears, frozen sections, or paraffin sections. The probes are composed of single-stranded DNA or RNA which hybridize with the denatured DNA or RNA in the smears or sections. The result can be detected by autoradiography when the probes are labeled with radioisotopes, or by regular immunohistologic or immunocytologic techniques when linked to biotin. This technique has been used most frequently to detect viral DNA or RNA, such as the correlation of Epstein-Barr virus with lymphoproliferative disorders.[60] Another major application of *in situ* hybridization is in the detection of numerical and structural chromosomal abnormalities by using fluorochrome-labeled, chromosome-specific probes.[61] This technique is designated *fluorescent in situ hybridization (FISH)*. It is able to identify chromosomes at interphase directly in intact cells on smears or sections. The same principle can be applied to *RNA in situ hybridization (RISH)*.

SUMMARY

Immunogenotyping or gene rearrangement analysis is an excellent technique for the diagnosis and classification of lymphomas and leukemias. Its indications are as follows: (1) tumor cells fail to express a phenotype; (2) tumor cells are in minority not detectable by phenotyping; (3) a well-differentiated T-cell tumor that cannot be distinguished from a normal cell population in immunophenotyping; (4) no fresh specimen is available for phenotyping; (5) when the relationship of a primary and a secondary/recurrent tumor is to be determined; and (6) enumeration of existent clones in the tumor is desired. The major drawbacks of immunogenotyping are its time-consuming nature and high cost. Cross-lineage rearrangement of immunoglobulin and TCR genes does occur from time to time, but it is not a major problem for B-cell neoplasms when the light chain gene rearrangment is assessed. By contrast, the sensitivity of TCR gene rearrangement analysis for the diagnosis of T-cell neoplasms requires further improvement.

REFERENCES

1. Medeiros LJ, Bagg A, Cossman J: Molecular genetics in the diagnosis and classification of lymphoid neoplasm. In Jaffe ES (ed): *Surgical Pathology of the Lymph Node and Related Organs*, ed 2. Philadelphia, WB Saunders, 1995, pp 58–97.
2. Sklar J: Antigen receptor genes: Structure, function and techniques for analysis of their rearrangements. In Knowles DM

(ed): *Neoplastic Hematopathology.* Baltimore, Williams & Wilkins, 1992, pp 215–244.
3. Cossman J, Uppenkamp M, Sundeen J, et al: Molecular genetics and the diagnosis of lymphoma. *Arch Pathol Lab Med* 112:117–127, 1988.
4. Sun T, Eisenberg A, Benn P, et al: Comparison of phenotyping and genotyping of lymphoid neoplasms. *J Clin Lab Analy* 3:156–162, 1989.
5. Papadopoulos KP, Bagg A, Bexwoda WR, et al: The routine diagnostic utility of immunoglobulin and T-cell receptor gene rearrangements in lymphoproliferative disorders. *Am J Clin Pathol* 91:633–638, 1989.
6. Griesser H, Tkachuk D, Reis MD, et al: Gene rearrangements and translocations in lymphoproliferative diseases. *Blood* 73:1402–1415, 1989.
7. Willman CL, Griffith BB, Whittaker M: Molecular genetic approaches for the diagnosis of clonality in lymphoid neoplasms. *Clin Lab Med* 10:119–149, 1990.
8. Sun T, Sussin M: A practical approach to immunophenotyping of lymphomas: Comparison of immunohistologic and immunocytologic techniques. *Ann Clin Lab Sci* 17:14–23, 1987.
9. Sun T, Ngu M, Henshall J, et al: Marker discrepancy as a diagnostic criterion for lymphoid neoplasms. *Diagn Clin Immunol* 5:393–399, 1988.
10. Nossal GJV: Current concepts: Immunology—the basic components of the immune system. *N Engl J Med* 316:1320–1321, 1987.
11. Davis MM, Bjorkman PJ: T-cell antigen receptor genes and T-cell recognition. *Nature* 334:395–402, 1988.
12. Southern EM: Detection of specific sequences among DNA fragments separated by gel electrophoresis. *J Mol Biol* 98:503–517, 1975.
13. Piper MA, Unger ER: *Nucleic Acid Probes: A Primer for Pathologists.* Chicago, ASCP Press, 1989, p 100.
14. Korsmeyer SJ, Arnold A, Bakhshi A, et al: Immunoglobulin gene rearrangement and cell surface antigen expression in acute lymphocytic leukemias of T-cell and B-cell precursor origins. *J Clin Invest* 71:301–313, 1983.
15. Cleary ML, Wood GS, Warnke R, et al: Immunoglobulin gene rearrangements in hairy cell leukemia. *Blood* 64:99–104, 1984.
16. Korsmeyer SJ, Greene WC, Cossman J, et al: Rearrangement and expression of immunoglobulin genes and expression of Tac antigen in hairy cell leukemia. *Proc Natl Acad Sci USA* 80:4522–4526, 1983.
17. Weiss LM, Trela M, Turner R, et al: Frequent immunoglobulin and T-cell receptor gene rearrangements in "histiocytic" neoplasms. *Am J Pathol* 121:369–373, 1985.
18. Isaacson PG, Spencer J, Connolly CE, et al: Malignant histiocytes of the intestine: A T-cell lymphoma. *Lancet* 2:688–691, 1985.
19. Sun T, Brody J, Susin M, et al: Extranodal T-cell lymphoma mimicking malignant histiocytosis. *Am J Hematol* 35:269–274, 1990.
20. Cossman J, Zehnbauer B, Garrett CT, et al: Gene rearrangements in the diagnosis of lymphoma/leukemia: Guidelines for use based on a multi-institutional study. *Am J Clin Pathol* 95:347–354, 1991.
21. Knowles DM: Immunophenotypic and antigen receptor gene rearrangement analysis in T-cell neoplasia. *Am J Pathol* 134:761–785, 1989.
22. O'Connor NTJ, Wainscoat JS, Weatherall DJ, et al: Rearrangement of the T-cell receptor δ-chain in the diagnosis of lymphoproliferative disorders. *Lancet* 1:1295–1297, 1985.
23. Weiss LM, Picker LJ, Grogan TM, et al: Absence of clonal beta and gamma T-cell receptor gene rearrangements in a subset of peripheral T-cell lymphomas. *Am J Pathol* 130:436–442, 1988.
24. Knowles DM, Neri A, Pelicci PG, et al: Immunoglobulin and T-cell receptor δ-chain rearrangement analysis of Hodgkin's disease: Implications for lineage determination and differential diagnosis. *Proc Natl Acad Sci USA* 83:7942–7946, 1986.
25. Weiss LM, Strickler JG, Hu E, et al: Immunoglobulin gene rearrangements in Hodgkin's disease. *Hum Pathol* 17:1009–1014, 1986.
26. Griesser H, Feller AC, Mak TK, et al: Clonal rearrangements of T-cell receptor and immunoglobulin genes and immunophenotypic antigen expression in different subclasses of Hodgkin's disease. *Int J Cancer* 40:157–160, 1987.
27. Sundeen JT, Lipford E, Uppenkamp M, et al: Rearranged antigen receptor genes in Hodgkin's disease. *Blood* 70:96–103, 1987.
28. O'Connor NTJ, Crick JA, Gatter KC, et al: Cell lineage in Hodgkin's disease. *Lancet* 2:158, 1987.
29. Falk MH, Tesch H, Stein H, et al: Phenotype v immunoglobulin and T-cell receptor genotype of Hodgkin-derived cell lines: Activation of immature lymphoid cells in Hodgkin's disease. *Int J Cancer* 40:262–269, 1987.
30. Roth MS, Schnitzer B, Bingham EL, et al: Rearrangement of immunoglobulin and T-cell receptor genes in Hodgkin's disease. *Am J Pathol* 131:331–338, 1988.
31. Minden MD, Mak TW: The structure of the T-cell antigen receptor genes in normal and malignant T cells. *Blood* 68:327–336, 1986.
32. Weiss LM, Hu E, Wood GS, et al: Clonal T-cell populations in angioimmunoblastic lymphadenopathy and angioimmunoblastic lymphadenopathy-like lymphoma. *Am J Pathol* 122:392–398, 1986.
33. O'Connor NTJ, Crick JA, Wainscoat JS, et al: Evidence for monoclonal T-lymphocyte proliferation in angioimmunoblastic lymphadenopathy. *J Clin Pathol* 39:1229–1232, 1986.
34. Sklar J, Cleary ML, Theilemans K, et al: Biclonal B-cell lymphoma. *N Engl J Med* 311:20–27, 1984.
35. Sulak LE, Craig FE, Montiel MM, et al: Biclonal composite lymphoma (letter). *Arch Pathol Lab Med* 114:638, 1990.
36. Sun T, Susin M, Koduru P, et al: Phenotyping and genotyping of composite lymphoma with Ki-1 component. *Hematol Pathol* 6:179–192, 1992.
37. Sun T, Susin M, Desner M, et al: The clonal origin of two cell populations in Richter's syndrome. *Hum Pathol* 21:722–728, 1990.
38. Koduru PRK, Lichtman SM, Smilari TF, et al: Serial phenotypic, cytogenetic and molecular genetic studies in Richter's

39. Traweek ST, Liu J, Johnson RM, et al: High-grade transformation of chronic lymphocytic leukemia and low-grade non-Hodgkin's lymphoma: Genotypic confirmation of clonal identity. *Am J Clin Pathol* 100:519–526, 1993.
40. Cherepakhin V, Baird SM, Meisenholder GW, et al: Common clonal origin of chronic lymphocytic leukemia and high-grade lymphoma of Richter's syndrome. *Blood* 82:3141–3147, 1993.
41. Matolcsy A, Inghirami G, Knowles DM: Molecular genetic demonstration of the diverse evolution of Richter's syndrome (chronic lymphocytic leukemia and subsequent large cell lymphoma). *Blood* 83:1363–1372, 1994.
42. Horning SJ, Galli N, Cleary M, et al: Detection of non-Hodgkin's lymphoma in the peripheral blood by analysis of antigen receptor gene rearrangements: Results of a prospective study. *Blood* 75:1139–1145, 1990.
43. Fishleder A, Tubbs R, Hesse B, et al: Uniform detection of immunoglobulin-gene rearrangement in benign lymphoepithelial lesions. *N Engl J Med* 316:1118–1121, 1987.
44. Weiss LM, Wood GS, Trela M, et al: Clonal T-cell populations in lymphomatoid papulosis: Evidence of a lymphoproliferative origin for a clinically benign disease. *N Engl J Med* 315:475–479, 1986.
45. Hyjeh E, Smith WJ, Isaacson PG: Primary B-cell lymphoma of salivary glands and its relationship to myoepithelial sialadenitis. *Hum Pathol* 19:766–776, 1988.
46. Levy N, Nelson J, Meyer P, et al: Reactive lymphoid hyperplasia with single class (monoclonal) surface immunoglobulin. *Am J Clin Pathhol* 80:300–308, 1983.
47. Tawa A, Hozumi N, Minden M, et al: Rearrangement of the T-cell receptor β-chain gene in non-T-cell, non-B-cell acute lymphoblastic leukemia of childhood. *N Engl J Med* 313:1033–1037, 1985.
48. Kurosawa Y, von Bockner H, Hass W, et al: Identification of D segments of immunoglobulin heavy-chain genes and their rearrangement in T-lymphocytes. *Nature* 290:565–570, 1981.
49. Kuchingham GR, Rovigatti U, Mauer AM, et al: Rearrangements of immunoglobulin heavy chain genes in T-cell acute lymphoblastic leukemia. *Blood* 65:725–729, 1985.
50. Seremetis SV, Pelicci PG, Tabilia A, et al: High frequency of clonal immunoglobulin or T-cell receptor gene rearrangements in acute myelogenous leukemia expressing terminal deoxynucleotidyl transferase. *J Exp Med* 165:1703–1712, 1987.
51. McKeithan TW: Molecular biology of non-Hodgkin's lymphomas. *Semin Oncol* 17:30–42, 1990.
52. Eisenstein BI: The polymerase chain reaction: A new method of using molecular genetics for medical diagnosis. *N Engl J Med* 322:178–183, 1990.
53. Morgan GJ, Hughes T, Janssen JW, et al: Polymerase chain reaction for detection of residual leukemia. *Lancet* 1:928–929, 1989.
54. Cunningham D, Hichish T, Rosin RD, et al: Polymerase chain reaction for detection of dissemination in gastric lymphoma. *Lancet* 1:695–697, 1989.
55. Loh EY, Elliot JF, Cwirla S, et al: Polymerase chain reaction with single-sided specificity: Analysis of T-cell receptor δ chain. *Science* 243:217–220, 1989.
56. Dobrovic A, Trainor KJ, Morley AA: Detection of the molecular abnormality in chronic myeloid leukemia by use of the polymerase chain reaction. *Blood* 72:2063–2065, 1988.
57. Lee MS, Chang KS, Cabanillas F, et al: Detection of minimal residual cells carrying the t(14;18) by DNA sequence amplification. *Science* 237:175–178, 1987.
58. Negrin RS, Blume KG: The use of polymerase chain reaction for the detection of minimal residual malignant disease. *Blood* 78:255–258, 1991.
59. Gribben JG, Neuberg D, Barber M, et al: Detection of residual lymphoma cells by polymerase chain reaction in peripheral blood is significantly less predictive for relapse than detection in bone marrow. *Blood* 83:3800–3807, 1994.
60. Hamilton-Dutoit SJ, Pallesen G: Detection of Epstein-Barr virus small RNAs in routine paraffin sections using non-isotopic RNA/RNA in situ hybridization. *Histopathology* 25:101–111, 1994.
61. Anastasi J: Interphase cytogenetic analysis in the diagnosis and study of neoplastic disorders. *Am J Clin Pathol* 95(Suppl 1):s22–s28, 1991.

Chapter 8
CYTOGENETICS AND ONCOGENES

The diagnosis of lymphoid neoplasms by both immunophenotyping and immunogenotyping is based on the identification of monoclonality. However, monoclonality is not synonymous with malignancy. When there is no morphologic evidence to support the diagnosis of lymphoid neoplasms despite the demonstration of monoclonality, cytogenetic study plays an important role in making the final decision.[1,2] When a monoclonal population shows cytogenetic aberrations, the diagnosis of lymphoid malignancy is virtually established. Even if phenotyping or genotyping fails to demonstrate monoclonality, the detection of cytogenetic abnormality alone may indicate strongly, if not conclusively, malignancy or premalignancy. In fact, the detection of a structural chromosomal aberration in even two cells can be considered evidence of the presence of an abnormal clone.[1] The effects of abnormal cytogenetics on the prognosis of acute leukemias are well established, but its correlation with the prognosis of lymphomas is less conclusive.[1]

From the same clone of tumor cells, cytogenetic changes are constant, even though additional chromosomal aberration may appear as the disease progresses.[3] Thus, by comparing the karyotypes, the clonal origin of two or more tumors can be established.[4] By the same token, the relationship of a primary tumor and a secondary/recurrent tumor can also be determined. On the other hand, a remission is certain when a cytogenetic abnormality is no longer detectable in the tissues (blood, marrow, or lymph node) examined.[5]

However, the connection with a nonrandom (recurring) cytogenetic abnormality has been established in only a limited number of tumors, such as t(8;14) in Burkitt's lymphoma, t(9;22) in Philadelphia chromosome–positive CML, and t(14;18) in some follicular lymphomas. In most cases, the same kind of tumor may show various cytogenetic changes, and the same cytogenetic changes may appear in different kinds of tumors. In other words, under most circumstances, cytogenetic results can help to determine only the malignant or benign nature of a lesion, not a specific diagnosis. Another drawback of karyotyping is the requirement of a fresh specimen, which makes retrospective study impossible. Fortunately, chromosomal abnormalities can now be detected by molecular biological techniques such as Southern blotting and PCR, as noted in Chapter 7.

STRUCTURAL AND NUMERICAL ANOMALIES IN CHROMOSOMES

At present, much of what we know about the biological significance of chromosomal abnormalities and oncogenes in human tumors has come from studies of lymphomas and lymphoid leukemias.[1] Recent investigations have found that a high proportion of cases (90%) of non-Hodgkin's lymphomas show clonal chromosomal abnormalities, and many of these are nonrandom. These chromosomal abnormalities correlate well with immunophenotypes and histologic patterns.[1] More important, chromosomal studies have unveiled the possible mechanisms of tumorigenesis. Dewald et al. suggested that structural chromosomal abnormalities initiate malignant transformation and numerical chromosomal anomalies are associated with chromosome evolution, which is important in the progression of disease.[3] These authors emphasized that if only a numerical anomaly is detected in a tumor, subtle structural abnormalities may be overlooked because of inexperience or poor techniques.

In their Mayo Clinic series, 1352 chromosomal anomalies were found in 748 cases of hematologic neoplasms.[3] Among the 1352 anomalies, 769 were structural and 583 were numerical. The structural anomalies included 443 translocations, 268 deletions, 40 isochromosomes, 6 inversions, and 12 duplications of part of the long arm of chromosome 1. The numerical anomalies included 260 monosomies, 322 trisomies, and 1 near-haploid chromosome complement.

CHROMOSOMAL TRANSLOCATIONS AND ONCOGENES

Among the chromosomal abnormalities, translocation is by far the most important phenomenon, not only because it is the most frequent and consistent finding but also because of its biologic significance. It has been widely speculated that translocations related to malignancy bring together a growth-related gene, such as a proto-oncogene, a growth factor gene, or a growth factor receptor gene adjacent to an active, cell-specific gene.[1,6] As a result, there are excess products or abnormal products of a growth-related gene, leading to malignant transformation.

The most frequently studied genes are the proto-oncogenes at the translocation sites.[7-9] Proto-oncogenes are of normal cellular genes which are considered to be related to normal cellular proliferation and differentiation.[8] The prefix "c" (stands for cellular) is usually added to the name of the proto-oncogene to distinguish it from its viral oncogene counterpart, which is given the prefix "v" (e.g., *c-myc* vs. *v-myc*). A proto-oncogene may transform into an oncogene only after being activated, such as after chromosomal translocation. The most frequently encountered proto-oncogene at a translocation site is *c-myc*.[6,10] Molecular analyses of the recurring chromosomal abnormalities involving translocation have resulted in the discovery of several putative proto-oncogenes: gene without a viral oncogene homologue. These include *bcl-1*, *bcl-2*, *tcl-1*, *tcl-2*, *tcl-3*, and *tcl-4*.[1,2] It was further discovered that these proto-oncogenes are frequently juxtaposed to the immunoglobulin genes in B-cell tumors or to TCR genes in T-cell neoplasms.[6,10] Table 8-1 presents various lymphomas and leukemias that show chromosomal translocations. A few tumors are discussed further to exemplify the role of chromosomal changes in hematologic neoplasms.

Burkitt's Lymphoma

A consistent finding in Burkitt's lymphoma is the translocation between chromosome 8, where the *c-myc* proto-oncogene is located, and a chromosome where an immunoglobulin gene (heavy or light chain) is located (Figure 8-1). Approximately 75% to 90% of Burkitt's lymphomas show t(8;14) (q24;q32), in which the *c-myc* gene is translocated to chromosome 14 and juxtaposed to the heavy chain gene.[1,6] Less frequently, t(8;14) is also seen in small, non-cleaved cell, non-Burkitt's and large-cell immunoblastic lymphomas. The two variant translocations [t(2;8) and t(8;22)] occur in 10% to 25% of Burkitt's tumors.[1,5] In these settings, *c-myc* remains on chromosome 8, but part of the κ or λ light chain locus, respectively, moves adjacent to it. As a result of the translocation, *c-myc* comes under the control of a transcriptional enhancer of the immunoglobulin gene and is thus activated.[1,6,10] Constitutive (unregulated) *c-myc* expression may prevent cells from entering the resting state (G_0 phase) and differentiating, leading

TABLE 8-1. Chromosomal Translocation Observed in Lymphoid Neoplasms

Neoplasm	Proto-oncogene/Chromosome	Antigen receptor gene/Chromosome
B-ALL	*c-abl*/9q34	*bcr*/22q11
Burkitt's lymphoma/ALL	*c-myc*/8q24	IgH/14q32
Burkitt's lymphoma/ALL	*c-myc*/8q24	Igκ/2p12
Burkitt's lymphoma/ALL	*c-myc*/8q24	Igλ/22q11
T-ALL	*c-myc*/8q24	TCRα/14q11
T-ALL	*tcl-2*/11p13	TCRδ/14q11
T-ALL	*tcl-3*/10q24	TCRδ/14q11
T-ALL	*tcl-4*/9q32	TCRβ/7q34–36
T-ALL	*tcl-5*/1p32	TCRδ/14q11
T-ALL	*lyl-1*/19p13	TCRβ/7q34
T-ALL	*tal-1*/11p15	TCRδ/14q11
B-CLL	*bcl-1*/11q13	IgH/14q32
B-CLL	*bcl-3*/19q13	IgH/14q32
T-CLL	*c-myc*/8q24	TCRα/14q11
Mantle cell lymphoma	*bcl-1*/11q13	IgH/14q32
Follicular lymphoma	*bcl-2*/18q21	IgH/14q32
Immunoblastic lymphoma	*c-myc*/8q24	Igκ/2p12
Multiple myeloma	*bcl-1*/11q13	IgH/14q32

IgH = immunoglobulin heavy chain gene; Igκ = immunoglobulin κ light chain gene; Igλ = immunoglobulin λ light chain gene; TCR = T-cell receptor gene.

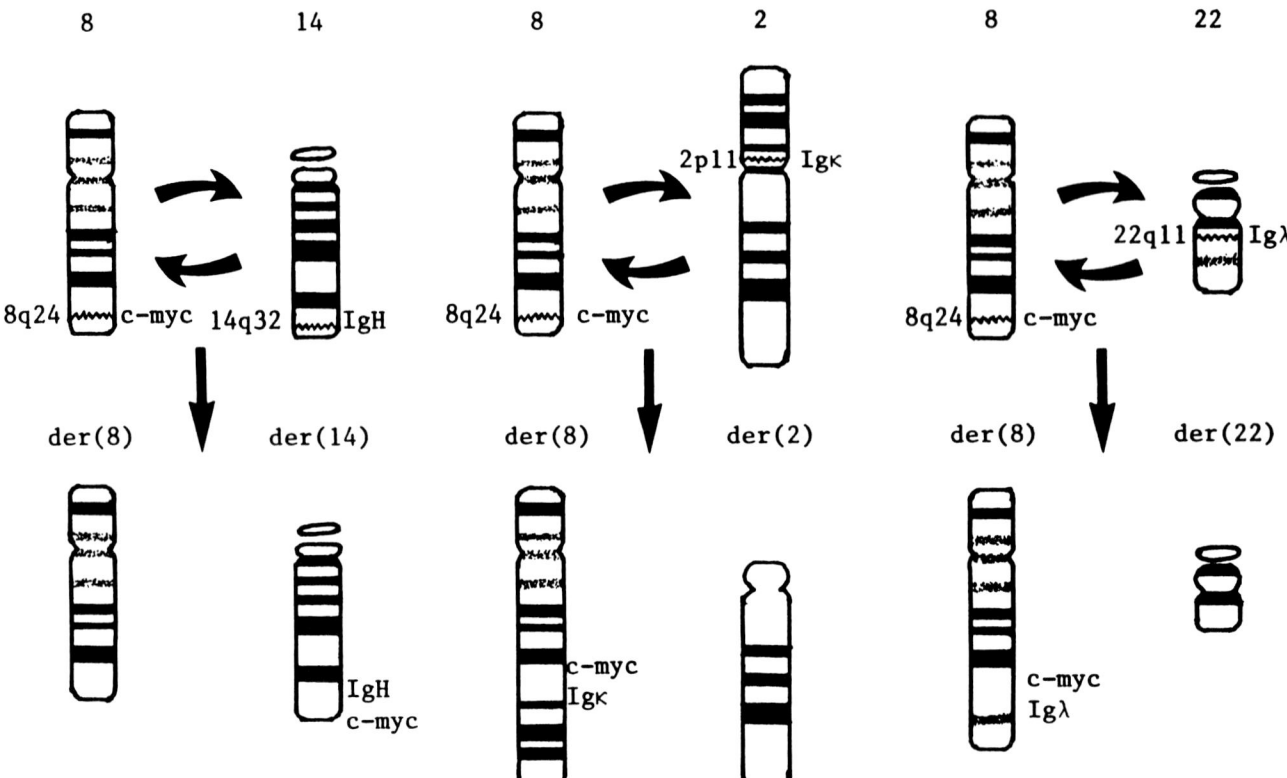

FIGURE 8-1. Diagrammatic illustration of three forms of chromosomal translocation in Burkitt's lymphoma. (From Sun T: *Color Atlas/Text of Flow Cytometer Analysis of Hematologic Neoplasms*, New York, Igaku-Shoin, 1993).

to continuing proliferation of undifferentiated cells.[10] The importance of the influence of the immunoglobulin genes is supported by an experiment showing that when the Burkitt's lymphoma derivative 14 chromosome is introduced into fibroblasts that have inactive immunoglobulin genes, transcription of *myc* is suppressed.[11]

Philadelphia Chromosome–Positive Chronic Myelogenous Leukemia (Ph′+ CML)

Ph′+ CML and some cases of Ph′− CML involve the translocation of another proto-oncogene, *c-abl*, from chromosome 9 to chromosome 22 [t(9;22) (q24;q11)] (Figures 8-2 and 8-3). However, the mechanism of tumorigenesis in CML differs from that in Burkitt's lymphoma. The translocation results in the fusion of *c-abl* and a restriction region on chromosome 22, called the *breakpoint cluster region (bcr)*, leading to the transcription of an aberrant hybrid *c-abl-bcr* RNA.[12] The final product is an abnormal protein with tyrosine kinase activity which enhances phosphorylation of tyrosine.[13] The abnormal degree of phosphorylation may disturb the normal process of transduction in the cell and cause a malignant or premalignant transformation.[7] Ph′+ acute lymphoblastic leukemia (Ph′+ ALL) also shows t(9;22), but the breakpoint of chromosome 22 in ALL differs from that in CML, so that different abnormal RNA and protein products are generated in Ph′+ ALL.[14] Even in Ph′+ CML cases, the breakpoint in chromosome 22 may vary. Some studies suggest that patients with breakpoints in 5′ subregions of *bcr* have a better prognosis than those with 3′ breakpoints.[15,16] Another study found no difference in prognosis, regardless of where the breakpoint was located.[17]

B-CELL TUMORS INVOLVING TRANSLOCATION OF PUTATIVE ONCOGENES AND THE HEAVY CHAIN GENE

In addition to Burkitt's lymphoma, chromosomal translocation is frequently seen in other B-cell tumors. The most frequently encountered pattern is t(14;18) (q32;q21), which is seen in 85% of follicular lymphomas and 20% of diffuse lymphomas.[10,18,19] Another translocation, t(11;14) (q13;q32), occurs in CLL, mantle cell lymphomas, and multiple myeloma.[20–22] The breakpoints on chromosomes 11 and 18 involve DNA sequences that are not homologues

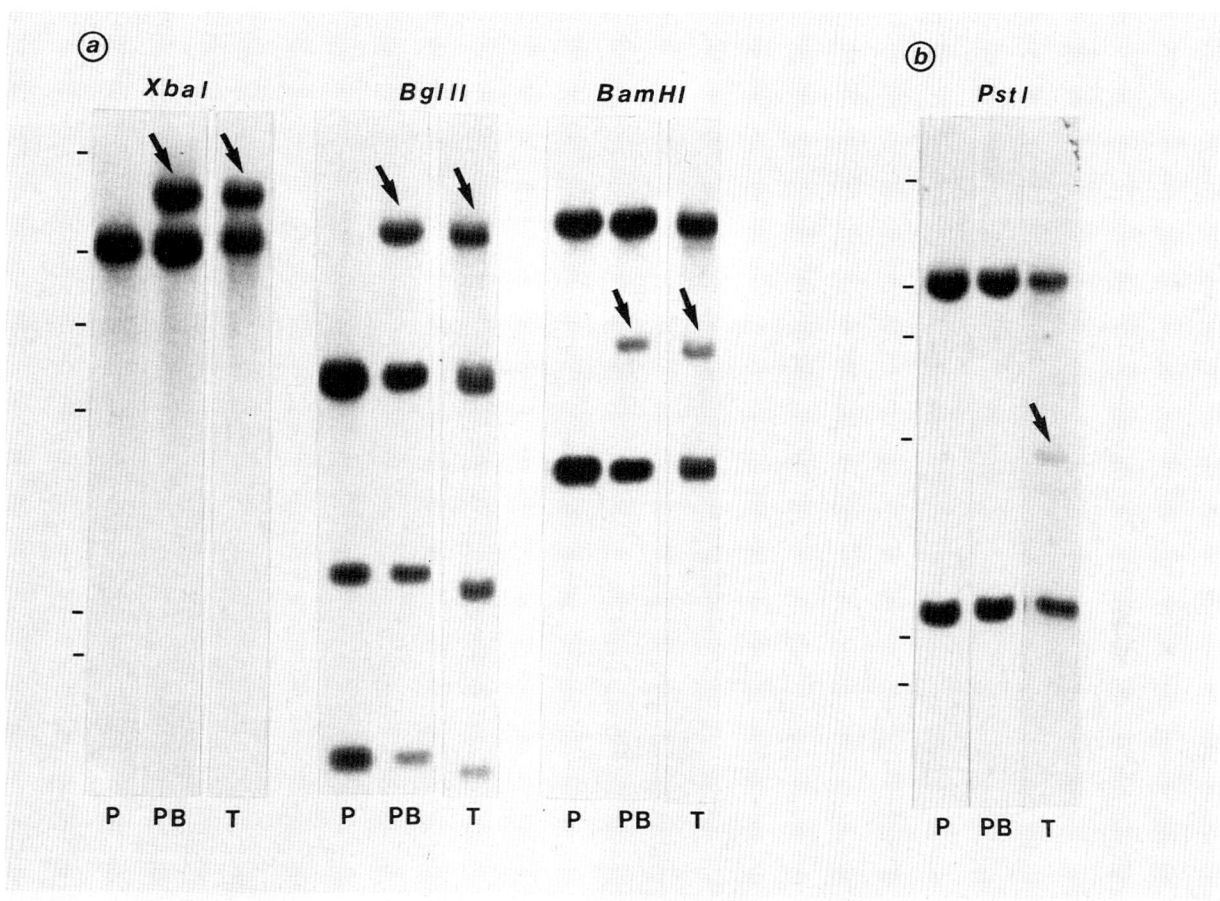

FIGURE 8-2. Southern blot analysis of DNA from peripheral blood (PB) and an extramedually tumor tissue (T) of a CML case using the Transprobe-I for the *bcr* gene, showing identical rearranged bands (arrows) after digestion with Xba I, Bgl III, and Bam HI. The identity of the two rearranged bands indicates that the extramedullary tumor is of CML origin. (From Sun T, Susin M, Koduru P, et al: Extramedullary blast crisis in chronic myelogenous leukemia. *Cancer* 68:605–610, 1991).

of any known viral oncogenes; they are therefore designated *bcl*-1 and *bcl*-2 (B-cell lymphoma/leukemia 1 and 2), respectively. The mechanism of malignant transformation in these two chromosomal abnormalities is due to deregulation of the proto-oncogenes, similar to the role of *c-myc* in the pathogenesis of Burkitt's lymphoma.[6] The supportive evidence for this hypothesis is the finding that the RNA transcript of the *bcl*-2 gene is higher in B-cell neoplasms with t(14;18) translocation than in those without it.[23] Recent studies also suggest that the t(11;14) and t(14;18) translocations occur during the process of V–D–J joining through the catalyzing action on the breakpoints by the same enzyme involved in V–D–J joining.[24]

In follicular lymphoma, the proto-oncogene *bcl*-2 (18q21) encodes for an inner mitochondrial membrane protein that plays a role in blocking programmed cell death (apoptosis).[25] Therefore, cells with abnormal expression of this protein remain in the G_0 stage and become immortalized lymphoma cells. In mantle cell lymphoma, the proto-oncogene *bcl*-1 (11q13) is juxtaposed to an immunoglobulin enhancer sequence located on chromosome 14. This translocation results in deregulation of a gene, *PRAD1*, linked to the *bcl*-1 locus.[26] *PRAD1* encodes for cyclin D1, a cell cycle protein. As a result of *PRAD1* activation, the G_1-S transition of the cell cycle is disturbed and the t(11;14) carrying cells cannot exit from the cell cycle, leading to lymphoid proliferation.[27]

T-Cell Lymphoma/Leukemia

T-cell neoplasms frequently have translocations involving band q11 of chromosome 14, the site of the TCR α chain and δ chain genes. Less frequently seen is the involvement of chromosome 7, where the TCR β chain (7q34-36) and γ chain (7p15) are located. The only known proto-oncogene found in T-cell tumors is *c-myc*, as seen in the t(8;14)(q24;q11) translocation.[28,29] However, several DNA sequences at the second chromosomal breakpoint

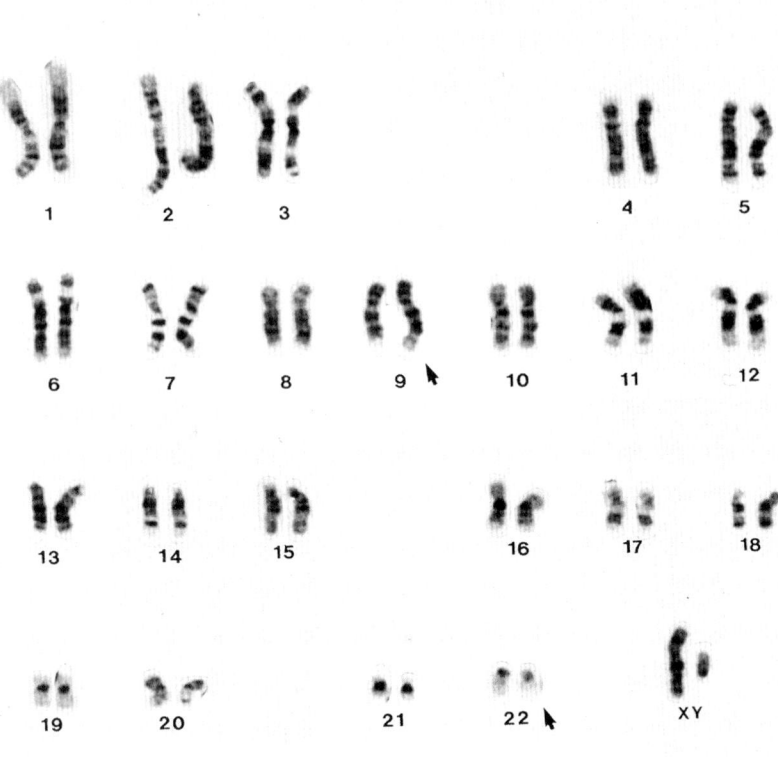

FIGURE 8-3. Trypsin-Giemsa-banded karyotype of leukemic cells from the bone marrow of a patient with CML showing 46, XY, t(9;22)(q34;q11). (Courtesy of Dr. P. Koduru, North Shore University Hospital–Cornell University Medical College).

have been isolated and designated putative proto-oncogenes *tcl*-1, *tcl*-2, *tcl*-3, and *tcl*-4. The proto-oncogene in t(11;14)(p13;q11), for instance, is *tcl*-2.[30] The pathogenesis of T-cell neoplasms may be similar to that of B-cell neoplasms in that the translocation may activate the proto-oncogenes by the promotor or enhancer of the TCR genes, leading to cellular proliferation and malignant transformation.[1] The mechanism of the inversion of chromosome 14 [inv(14)(q11;q32)] in T-cell tumor transformation is unclear, but it is interesting to see that the breakpoints involve both a T-cell receptor α chain gene (q11) and an immunoglobulin heavy chain gene (q32). The same chromosomal aberration is also found in B-cell tumors.[31] Another chromosomal translocation, t(7;14)(q34-36;q32), seen in T-cell neoplasms also involves the TCR and immunoglobulin heavy chain genes.[32]

Acute Myelogenous Leukemia (AML)

Chromosomal abnormalities, including translocation, deletion, inversion, and numerical changes, have been reported in AML.[2,33,34,35] Some chromosomal anomalies are associated with a subtype of AML, such as t(9;22)(q34;q11) in M1, t(8;21)(9q22;q22) in M2, t(15;17)(q22;q12) in M3, and t(9;11)(p22;q23 or q24) in M4 and M5. Other aberrations are specific for a certain syndrome, such as inv/del(16)(q22) in M4 with abnormal bone marrow eosinophils, t(6;9)(p23;q34) in AML with bone marrow basophilia, and inv(3)(q21q26) in AML with abnormal thrombopoiesis. The chromosomal translocation, t(15;17), in M3 is most specific, with a reported frequency of more than 90%. The identification of this chromosomal abnormality is especially helpful in the diagnosis of the M3 variants, as their morphologic diagnosis is sometimes difficult.[36] A hand-mirror variant of microgranular M3 was recently reported, with the diagnosis based on this particular translocation.[37]

The t(1;22)(p13;q13) karyotype in cases of acute megakaryoblastic leukemia (M7) is of interest in the demonstration of the N-ras oncogene in the breakpoint 1p13 and the c-sis oncogene at 22q13[38]. The c-sis gene encodes platelet-derived growth factor β, which plays an important role in the occurrence of myelofibrosis, an important clinical manifestation of acute megakaryoblastic leukemia.

Approximately 50% of patients with myelodysplasic syndrome (MDS) have a chromosomal abnormality.[39,40] Some abnormalities, such as monosomy 7 and 5q- anomaly, define a specific clinical entity.[41,42] MDS cases with cytogenetic abnormalities have a much higher incidence of leukemic transformation,[39,40] but chromosomal changes *per se* cannot distinguish MDS from leukemia.

PROGNOSTIC SIGNIFICANCE OF CHROMOSOMAL ABNORMALITIES

As mentioned before, numerical abnormalities may represent secondary changes and are more closely related to the prognosis. For instance, hyperdiploidy with more than 50 chromosomes accounts for one-fourth of childhood ALL, and patients with this abnormality have the most durable responses to treatment.[43] In this particular group of patients, trisomies can be detected in any chromosome, but chromosomes 4, 6, 10, 14, 17, 18, 20, 21 and X are more frequently involved. On the other hand, hypodiploidy usually predicts a poor prognosis in childhood ALL.[43] With the advent of flow cytometry, different ploidy groups can be easily identified. The chromosomal correlation with prognosis in the adult population differs from that in the pediatric population. For instance, one report found that a +5, +6, or +18 is related to shorter survival in patients with non-Hodgkin's lymphoma.[44] Some translocation patterns, such as t(8;14)(q24;q32), also indicate a poor prognosis.[45,46] The association with a favorable prognosis in lymphomas with t(14;18) is probably related to the predominance of a histologic type, follicular lymphoma, in those tumors.[45,46]

SUMMARY

Cytogenetic analysis is an important tool used to identify the benign or malignant nature of a lesion, thus guiding the treatment of patients. Although rarely used as a primary parameter for diagnosis, the demonstration of a nonrandom chromosomal anomaly is extremely helpful for the diagnosis of a particular tumor—especially its variants, which are sometimes difficult to recognize. The chromosomal pattern can also be used to identify secondary/recurrent tumors, as well as to determine the clonal origin of two different tumors. Molecular cytogenetic analysis using the new techniques, such as Southern blotting and PCR, greatly enhances the capacity of cytogenetics because of the sensitivity and specificity of these techniques. Thus, it has become the most promising means for early detection and long-term follow-up of hematologic neoplasms. The study of structural chromosomal changes, especially translocations, has started to unveil the mechanisms of malignant transformation: a proto-oncogene can be deregulated or activated to transmit increasing signals for cellular proliferation, or it may form a hybrid or chimera with the antigen receptor gene, leading to the translation of an abnormal protein with protein kinase activity.

REFERENCES

1. Le Beau MM: Chromosomal abnormalities in non-Hodgkin's lymphomas. *Semin Oncol* 17:20–29, 1990.
2. Griesser H, Tkachuk D, Reis MD, et al: Gene rearrangements and translocations in lymphoproliferative diseases. *Blood* 73:1402–1415, 1989.
3. Dewald GW, Noel P, Dahl RJ, et al: Chromosome abnormalities in malignant hematologic disorders. *Mayo Clin Proc* 60:675–689, 1985.
4. Nowell P, Finan J, Glover D, et al: Cytogenetic evidence for the clonal nature of Richter's syndrome. *Blood* 58:183–186, 1981.
5. Medeiros LJ, Bagg A, Cossman J: Molecular genetics in the diagnosis and classification of lymphoid neoplasms. In Jaffe ES (ed): *Surgical Pathology of the Lymph Node and Related Organs*, ed 2. Philadelphia, WB Saunders, 1995, pp 58–97.
6. Showe LC, Croce CM: Chromosome translocations in B and T cell neoplasias. *Semin Hematol* 23:237–244, 1986.
7. Gaidano G, Dalla-Favera R: protooncogenes and tumor suppressor genes. In Knowles DM (ed): *Neoplastic Hematopathology*. Baltimore, Williams & Wilkins, 1992, pp 245–261.
8. Slamon DJ: Proto-oncogenes and human cancers. *N Engl J Med* 317:955–957, 1987.
9. Friend SH, Dryja TP, Weinberg RA: Oncogenes and tumor-suppressing genes. *N Engl J Med* 318:618–622, 1988.
10. McKeithan TW: Molecular biology of non-Hodgkin's lymphomas. *Semin Oncol* 17:30–42, 1990.
11. Croce CM, Erikson J, Ar-Ruchdi A, et al: Translocated c-myc oncogene of Burkitt's lymphoma is transcribed in plasma cells and repressed in lymphoblastoid cells. *Proc Natl Acad Sci USA* 81:3170–3174, 1984.
12. Gale R, Canaani E: An 8-kilobase abl RNA transcript in chronic myelogenous leukemia. *Proc Natl Acad Sci USA* 81:5648–5652, 1984.

13. Kanopka JB, Watanabe SM, Witte ON: An alteration of the human *c-abl* protein in K562 leukemia cells unmasks associated tyrosine kinase acivity. *Cell* 37:1035–1038, 1984.
14. Kurzrock R, Shtalrid M, Remero P, et al: A novel *c-abl* protein product in Philadelphia-positive acute lymphoblastic leukemia. *Nature* 325:631–635, 1987.
15. Eisenberg A, Silver R, Soper L, et al: The location of breakpoints within the breakpoint cluster region (*bcr*) of chromosome 22 in chronic myeloid leukemia. *Leukemia* 2:642–647, 1988.
16. Mills KI, MacKenzie ED, Birnie GD: The site of the breakpoint within the *bcr* is a prognostic factor in Philadelphia-positive CML patients. *Blood* 72:1237–1241, 1988.
17. Morris SW, Daniel R, Ahmed CMI, et al: Relationship of *bcr* breakpoint to chronic phase duration, survival, and blast crisis lineage in chronic myelogenous leukemia patients presenting in early chronic phase. *Blood* 75:2035–2041, 1990.
18. Bakhkshi A, Jensen JP, Goldman P, et al: Cloning the chromosomal breakpoint of t(14;18) human lymphomas: Clustering around J on chromosome 14 and near a transcriptional unit on 18. *Cell* 41:899–906, 1985.
19. Cleary ML, Smith SD, Sklar J: Cloning and structural analysis of cDNA's for *bcl-2* and a hybrid *bcl-2*/immunoglobulin transcript resulting from the t(14;18) translocation. *Cell* 47:19–28, 1986.
20. Nowell PC, Shankey TV, Finan J, et al: Proliferation, differentiation, and cytogenetics of chronic leukemic B lymphocytes cultured with mitomycin-treated normal cells. *Blood* 57:444–451, 1981.
21. Tsujimoto Y, Yunis J, Onorato-Showe L, et al: Molecular cloning of the chromosomal breakpoint of B-cell lymphomas and leukemias with the (11;14) translocation. *Science* 226:1097–1099, 1984.
22. van den Berghe H, Vermaeleu K, Louwagie A, et al: High incidence of chromosome abnormalities in IgG3 myeloma. *Cancer Cytogenet* 11:381–387, 1984.
23. Croce CM: Chromosome translocations and human cancer. *Cancer Res* 46:6019–6023, 1986.
24. Tsujimoto Y, Gorham J, Cossman J, et al: The t(14;18) chromosome translocations involved in B-cell neoplasms result from mistakes in VDJ joining. *Science* 229:1390–1393, 1984.
25. Hockenberry D, Nunez G, Milliman C, et al: Bcl-2 is an inner-mitochondrial membrane protein that blocks programmed cell death. *Nature* 348:334–336, 1990.
26. Rosenberg CL, Wong E, Petty E, et al: PRAD1, a candidate *bcl-1* oncogene: Mapping and expression in centrocytic lymphoma. *Proc Natl Acad Sci USA* 88:9638–9642, 1991.
27. Rimokh R, Berger F, Delso G, et al: Detection of the chromosomal translocation t(11;14) by polymerase chain reaction in mantle cell lymphomas. *Blood* 83:1871–1875, 1994.
28. Shima EA, Le Beau MM, McKeitnon TW, et al: T-cell receptor α-chain gene moves immediately downstream of *c-myc* in a chromosomal 8;14 translocation in a cell line from a human T-cell leukemia. *Proc Natl Acad Sci USA* 83:3439–3443, 1986.
29. Erickson J, Finger L, Sun L, et al: *c-myc* deregulation by translocation of the alpha-locus of the T-cell receptor in T-cell leukemia. *Science* 232:884–887, 1986.
30. Erickson J, Williams DL, Finan J, et al: Locus of the α chain of T-cell receptor is split by chromosome translocation in T-cell leukemia. *Science* 229:784–787, 1985.
31. Denny CT, Hollis GF, Hecht F, et al: Common mechanism of chromosome inversion in B- and T-cell tumors: Relevance to lymphoid development. *Science* 234:197–200, 1986.
32. Russo G, Isobe M, Pegovaro L, et al: Molecular analysis of a t(7;14) (q35;q32) chromosome translocation in a T-cell leukemia of a patient with ataxia telangiectasia. *Cell* 53:137–144, 1988.
33. First International Workshop on Chromosome in Leukemia: Chromosomes in Ph'-positive granulocytic leukemia. *Br J Haematol* 39:305–309, 1978.
34. Fourth International Workshop on Chromosomes in Leukemia 1982: A prospective study of acute nonlymphocytic leukemia. *Cancer Genet Cytogenet* 11:249–360, 1984.
35. Second MIC Cooperative Study Group: Morphologic, immunologic and cytogenetic (MIC) working classification of the acute myeloid leukemias. *Br J Haematol* 68:487–494, 1988.
36. Bennett JM, Catovsky D, Daniel MT, et al: A variant form of hypergranular promyelocytic leukemia (M3). *Br J Haematol* 44:169–170, 1980.
37. Sun T, Weiss R: Hand-mirror variant of microgranular acute promyelocytic leukemia. *Leukemia* 5:266–269, 1991.
38. Washio S, Ido M, Azuma E, et al: Acute megakaryoblastic leukemia with translocation t(1;22)(p13;q13) in a 10-week-old infant. *Am J Hematol* 39:56–60, 1992.
39. Horiike S, Taniwaki M, Misawa S, et al: Chromosome abnormalities and karyotypic evolution in 83 patients with myelodysplastic syndrome and predictive value for prognosis. *Cancer* 62:1129–1138, 1988.
40. Yunis JJ, Lobell M, Arnesen MA, et al: Refined chromosome study helps define prognostic subgroups in most patients with primary myelodysplastic syndrome and acute myelogenous leukemia. *Br J Haematol* 68:189–194, 1988.
41. Kere J, Ruutu T, Chapelle ADL: Monosomy 7 in granulocytes and monocytes in myelodysplastic syndrome. *N Engl J Med* 316:499–503, 1987.
42. Nimer SD, Golde DW: The 5q- abnormality. *Blood* 70:1705–1712, 1987.
43. Pui CH, Crist WM, Look AT: Biology and clinical significance of cytogenetic abnormalities in childhood acute lymphoblastic leukemia. *Blood* 76:1449–1463, 1990.
44. Schouten HC, Sanger WG, Weisenburger DD, et al: Chromosomal abnormalities in untreated patients with non-Hodgkin's lymphoma: Associations with histology, clinical characteristics and treatment outcome. *Blood* 75:1841–1847, 1990.
45. Kristoffersson U, Heim S, Mandahl N, et al: Prognostic implications of cytogenetic findings in 106 patients with non-Hodgkin's lymphoma. *Cancer Genet Cytogenet* 25:55–64, 1987.
46. Kaneko Y, Rowley J, Variakojis D, et al: Prognostic implications of karyotype and morphology in patients with non-Hodgkin's lymphoma. *Int J Cancer* 32:683–692, 1983.

Chapter 9
CLINICAL APPLICATIONS

Accurate diagnosis of hematologic neoplasms is the basis for proper clinical management. Integration and recognition of the clinical and histopathologic features are required for proper classification and diagnosis of these diseases. This is obviously a complicated and difficult task because these diseases have diverse clinical, hematologic, and histologic manifestations. The sites of involvement in these diseases may not be the same, and the tissues available for study may vary. At the same time, many diagnostic techniques are available for accurate cell identification, which aids in the classification of these diseases.

Some techniques were developed many years ago; their sensitivity and specificity for diagnosis and cell identification, as well as their limitations, have been well recognized. The newly developed techniques, on the other hand, require further testing. The physician taking care of patients with hematologic diseases faces the significant challenge of remaining current with respect to both diagnostic and therapeutic modalities in providing optimal care.

The physician obtaining tissue for diagnosis must also be familiar with the diagnostic modalities because the new techniques require a variety of tissue fixatives and preservatives. Tissue improperly obtained or preserved may not be usable for diagnostic purposes. Sometimes this problem requires that new biopsy material be obtained; at other times, new material is not obtainable and the diagnosis must be made with what is at hand. It is not surprising that at times the plethora of diagnostic and clinical information becomes overwhelming and results in confusion. The tendency to perform a complete battery of special tests nonselectively for diagnostic purposes, although highly desirable in research environments, is cost prohibitive in clinical practice.

Three steps are involved in the diagnosis of hematologic neoplasms: (1) establishment of an accurate diagnosis, (2) proper classification of subtypes, and (3) evaluation of the extent of involvement. In general, the diagnosis of hematologic neoplasms is often established on the basis of clinical features of the disease and morphologic examination of the involved tissues. Proper classification and evaluation of the extent of the disease, however, are invariably based on accurate recognition of the cell type involved. Adequate identification of the cell type also demands recognition of the stage of maturation and, particularly in the lymphoid neoplasms, the clonality of the cells. Therefore, our diagnostic approach for hematologic neoplasms is to use morphologic studies as an initial step for diagnosis and to rely on special studies for accurate classification and evaluation of the extent of the disease.

This chapter deals with both the technical aspects of the tests and their practical application to aid in the diagnosis of hematologic neoplasms.

TECHNICAL CONSIDERATIONS

The technical details of the special diagnostic techniques are described in Part 2 of this text. The fine points concerning proper interpretation and some of the technical problems have been discussed in Chapters 2 to 8. Proper preparation of tissues is a prerequisite for a successful study. Tissues that are used for study may be prepared as fresh cell suspensions, smears and imprints, fresh frozen sections, paraffin-embedded tissue sections, and tissue embedded in plastics such as methacrylate. The merits and limitations of each of these preparations have been discussed in Chapters 3 and 4 and are summarized in Tables 9-1 and 9-2.

The choice of technique for clinical diagnosis is often determined by the type of specimen available for study, and the type of specimen available is often determined by the type of disease involved. In leukemias, for example, smears or cell suspensions prepared from blood and marrow specimens are often available for study; in lymphomas, imprints and tissue sections prepared from solid tissue masses (usually lymph node biopsy specimens) are used for diagnostic purposes. Morphologic examinations are usually done by light microscopy either on smears and imprints stained with Wright-Giemsa stain or on tissue sections stained with hematoxylin and eosin or Giemsa. The results

TABLE 9-1. Applicability of Cytochemical and Immunochemical Markers to Different Types of Specimens

Markers	Fresh Cell Suspensions	Smears, Imprints	Frozen Sections	Paraffin-Embedded Sections	Plastic-Embedded Sections
Cytochemical and Histochemical Markers					
Peroxidase	+	+	+	−	±
Cyanide-resistant peroxidase	+	+	+	±	±
Pseudoperoxidase	+	+	+	+	+
Sudan black B	±	+	±	±	±
Chloroacetate esterase	+	+	+	+	+
Nonspecific esterase	+	+	+	−	±
Fluoride-resistant esterase	+	+	+	−	±
Acid α-naphthyl acetate esterase	+	+	+	−	±
Aminocaproate esterase	+	+	+	−	+
Alkaline phosphatase	+	+	+	−	+
Acid phosphatase	+	+	+	−	+
Tartrate-resistant acid phosphatase	+	+	+	−	+
Toluidine blue O	±	+	+	+	+
Immunochemical Markers					
Cytoplasmic immunoglobulins	−	±	+	+	+
Terminal deoxynucleotidyl transferase	+	+	+	±	NT
Lysozyme	−	±	+	+	NT
Myeloperoxidase	+	+	+	+	NT
Factor VIII antigen	NT	±	+	+	NT
Hemoglobin	±	±	±	+	NT
Tryptase	−	+	+	+	NT
Surface Markers					
Surface immunoglobulin	+	−	+	−	−
Fc receptor	+	−	−	−	−
Complement receptor	+	−	−	−	−
Mouse erythrocyte receptor	+	−	−	−	−
Epstein-Barr virus receptor	+	−	−	−	−
Sheep erythrocyte receptor	+	−	−	−	−
Monoclonal Antibodies					
HLA	+	+	+	−	−
Myeloid antigens	+	+	+	−	−
T antigens	+	+	+	±	−
B antigens	+	+	+	±	−
Common ALL antigen	+	+	+	−	−

HLA-DR = IA-like antigen; ALL = acute lymphoblastic leukemia; NT = not tested.
Note: + means that the marker is applicable; − means that the marker is not applicable; ± means that the marker is not ideal.

of this morphologic examination serve as guides for further studies.

The general indications for special studies include (1) confirmation of an unusual diagnosis, such as hairy cell leukemia or systemic mast cell disease; (2) confirmation of a diagnosis in a patient with an unusual clinical setting, such as CLL in a person younger than 40 years; (3) difficult differential diagnosis between atypical reactive hyperplasia and neoplastic diseases; and (4) subclassification of neoplastic diseases in which the morphologic distinction is difficult, such as acute leukemias, CLLs, and non-Hodgkin's lymphomas, especially the diffuse, large-cell lymphomas.

When dealing with leukemias, morphologic studies are

TABLE 9-2. Cytochemical, Histochemical, Immunologic, and Immunochemical Markers for Identification of Blood Cells in Different Types of Specimens

Cell Types	Fresh Cell Specimens	Smears, Imprints	Frozen Sections	Paraffin-Embedded Sections	Plastic-Embedded Sections
Myeloblasts neutrophils	Peroxidase, Sudan black B, chloroacetate esterase, myeloid antigens (CD13, CD33), myeloperoxidase	Peroxidase, Sudan black B, chloroacetate esterase, myeloid antigens (CD13, CD33), myeloperoxidase	Peroxidase, chloroacetate esterase, lysozyme, myeloid antigens (CD13, CD33), myeloperoxidase	Chloroacetate esterase, lysozyme, myeloperoxidase	Chloroacetate esterase, lysozyme, peroxidase
Eosinophils	Cyanide-resistant peroxidase, chlorazol fast pink	Cyanide-resistant peroxidase, chlorazol fast pink	Cyanide-resistant peroxidase, chlorazol fast pink	Giemsa, chlorazol fast pink	Giemsa, cyanide-resistant peroxidase, chlorazol fast pink
Basophils	Toluidine blue O	Toluidine blue O	Toluidine blue O	Toluidine blue O	Toluidine blue O
Monocytes (blood)	Nonspecific esterase, myeloid antigens (CD13, CD14, CD33)	Nonspecific esterase, myeloid antigens (CD13, CD14, CD33)	Nonspecific esterase, lysozyme, myeloid antigens (CD13, CD14, CD33)	Lysozyme, CD68	Lysozyme, CD68
Histiocytes (tissue)	Fluoride-resistant esterase, CD68	Fluoride-resistant esterase, CD68	Fluoride-resistant esterase, CD68	Lysozyme, CD68	Lysozyme, CD68
Erythroblasts	Red cell antigen (RC82-4), glycophorin	Red cell antigen (RC82-4), glycophorin, hemoglobin antigen, pseudoperoxidase, Giemsa	Red cell antigen (RC82-4), glycophorin, hemoglobin antigen, pseudoperoxidase	Hemoglobin antigen, pseudoperoxidase, Giemsa	Giemsa
Megakaryocytes	Factor VIII antigen, CD41	Factor VIII antigen, CD41	Factor VIII antigen, CD41	Factor VIII antigen	NT
Plasma cells	CIg	CIg, Giemsa	CIg	CIg, Giemsa, methyl green-pyronine	CIg, Giemsa, methyl green-pyronine
Lymphocytes					
T cells	E-rosette, T antigens (CD2, CD3, CD5, CD7)	T antigens (CD2, CD3, CD5, CD7)	T antigens (CD2, CD3, CD5, CD7)	CD45RO, CD3	CD45RO
T_h	Focal ANAE, IgM receptor, CD4	Focal ANAE, CD4	Focal ANAE, CD4	NT	NT
T_s	IgG receptor, CD8	Wright-Giemsa (azurophilic granules), CD8	CD8	NT	NT
B cells	SIg, CIg, CD19, CD20, HLA-DR	SIg, CIg, CD19, CD20, HLA-DR	SIg, CIg, CD19, CD20, HLA-DR	CIg, CD20, CD74	CIg, CD20, CD74
Transformed Lymphocytes	HLA-DR, CD45	HLA-DR, CD45	HLA-DR, CD45	CD45	
T cells	Focal acid phosphatase, T antigens (CD2, CD3, CD5, CD7)	Focal acid phosphatase, T antigens (CD2, CD3, CD5, CD7)	Focal acid phosphatase, T antigens (CD2, CD3, CD5, CD7)	CD45RO, CD3	Focal acid phosphatase
B cells	SIg, CIg, CD20	SIg, CIg, CD20	SIg, CIg, CD20	CIg, CD20, CDw75	
Lymphoblasts (also see Table 9-4)					
T cells	TdT, focal acid phosphatase, T antigens (CD2, CD5, CD7), E-rosette	TdT, focal acid phosphatase, T antigens (CD2, CD5, CD7)	TdT, focal acid phosphatase, T antigens (CD2, CD5, CD7)	TdT	Focal acid phosphatase
B cells	SIg, CIg, B antigens (CD19, CD20)	SIg, CIg, B antigens (CD19, CD20)	SIg, CIg, B antigens (CD19, CD20)	CIg, CD20	CIg, CD20
Null cells (B-precursors)	TdT, CD19, CD10	TdT, CD19, CD10	TdT, CD19, CD10	TdT	TdT
Hairy cells	TRAP, CD22, CD11C	TRAP, CD22, CD11C	TRAP, CD22, CD11C	CD20	TRAP
Mast cells	Aminocaproate esterase, chloroacetate esterase, toluidine blue O, antiheparin, tryptase	Aminocaproate esterase, chloroacetate esterase, toluidine blue O, Giemsa, antiheparin, tryptase	Aminocaproate esterase, chloroacetate esterase, toluidine blue O, Giemsa, tryptase	Chloroacetate esterase, toluidine blue O, Giemsa, antiheparin, tryptase	Aminocaproate esterase, chloroacetate esterase, toluidine blue O, Giemsa, tryptase

ANAE = acid α-naphthyl acetate esterase; CIg = cytoplasmic immunoglobulin; NT = not tested; SIg = surface immunoglobulin; TRAP = tartrate-resistant acid phosphatase; TdT = terminal deoxynucleotidyl transferase; T_h = helper T cell; T_s = suppressor T cell.

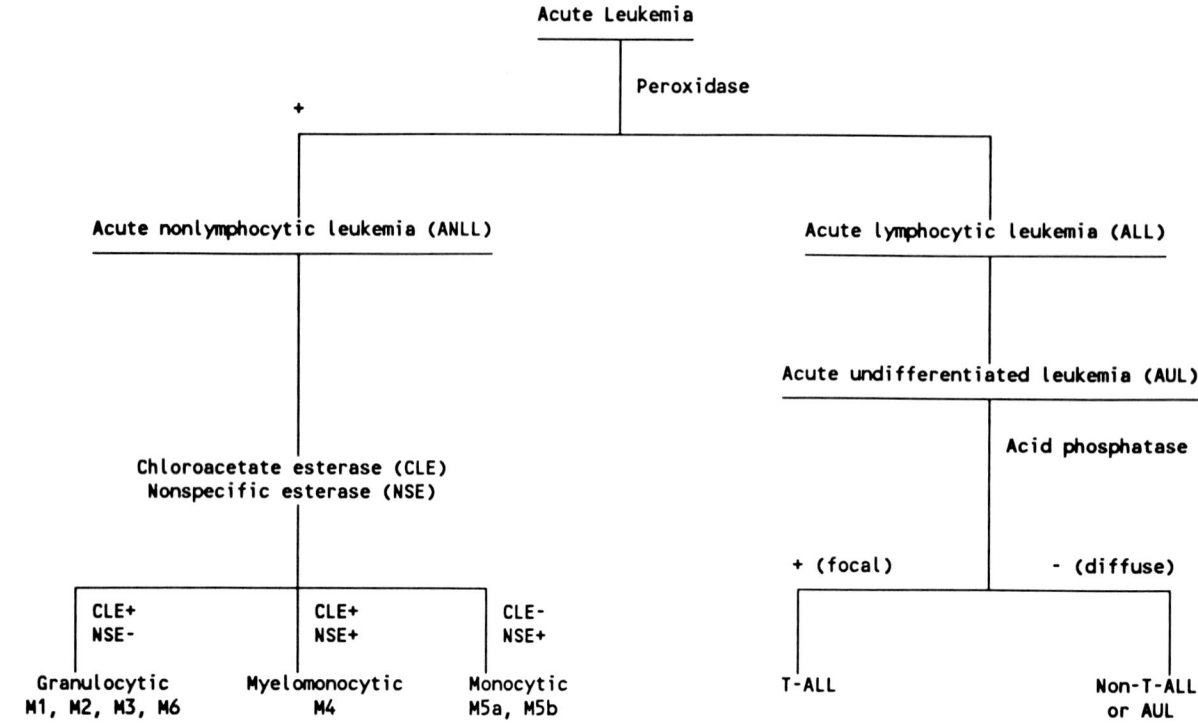

FIGURE 9-1. Classification of acute leukemia using cytochemical stains.

used initially to establish the diagnosis. If the type of leukemic cells can be identified with confidence by morphologic examination alone, special techniques will be used as indicated to confirm the initial diagnosis. If the leukemic cells cannot be identified with confidence by morphologic examination alone, special techniques will be used.

Because the cytochemical procedures are easy to perform, they are the method of choice when applicable, especially in dealing with nonlymphatic leukemias. For those cells not recognizable by both morphology and cytochemistry, the immunocytochemical method using monoclonal antibodies is another practical technique for subtyping leukemic cells. This technique can be applied to air-dried smears or cell suspensions tested by flow cytometry and is most useful in the study of lymphatic leukemias. The choice of additional special diagnostic studies for those situations in which the leukemic cells continue to escape recognition is guided by both the clinical features of the disease and the morphologic appearance of the leukemic cells. The diagnosis of undifferentiated or unclassified leukemia is made only when all efforts have failed to achieve positive identification of the leukemic cells.

In malignant lymphomas and lymphoma-like disorders, morphologic examination is made initially to ascertain neoplasia. For patients with benign or reactive features, no further studies are necessary unless clinically indicated. For patients in whom neoplastic changes cannot be recognized with certainty, special studies for cell types, maturation, and clonality will be needed (see Table 5-6 on page 44). Those cases showing monoclonal proliferation will be considered as neoplastic and will require further study. Cases with neoplastic changes will be examined and classified by morphologic studies, special studies, or both. The nodular (follicular) lymphomas usually can be satisfactorily diagnosed and classified by morphologic studies. For diffuse lymphomas, especially those of the large-cell type, morphologic studies may not be sufficient, and usually special histochemical or immunohistochemical studies are needed to accurately identify the neoplastic cells. If the neoplastic cells continue to defy proper recognition, the possibility of nonhematopoietic neoplasms should be considered. These general guides are flexible and should be modified as indicated by the symptoms of the patient and the impressions of the physicians concerning the diagnosis and management of such conditions. Some of the special considerations related to the diagnosis of various hematologic neoplasms are discussed in the remainder of this chapter. The cases referred to are those illustrated in Part 3.

CLASSIFICATION OF ACUTE LEUKEMIAS

Acute leukemias are classified according to the type of cell involved and the degree of differentiation. Morphologic examination of blood and marrow establishes the diagnosis of acute leukemia but is insufficient to identify the cell types for accurate classification of the disease without the assistance of special diagnostic tests (Case 1). In general, the cytochemical markers are most useful for myeloid leukemias,[1] whereas the immunologic markers are more helpful for lymphoblastic leukemias.[2] Additionally, monoclonal antibodies have greatly facilitated the identification of cell lineage in all leukemias. A practical approach to the classification of acute leukemia is outlined in Figure 9-1 and 9-2 and the characteristics of the leukemic cells in various subtypes of acute leukemia are summarized in Tables 9-3 and 9-4.

Lymphatic vs. Nonlymphatic

Myeloperoxidase or Sudan black staining remains the simplest and most sensitive method for positive identification of myeloid (nonlymphatic) leukemia[1,3,4] (Case 2). The aggregation of blocks for PAS-positive material was once considered a characteristic feature of the abnormal lymphoid cells of ALL. However, the same staining features have also been noted in approximately 10% to 20% of cases with acute monocytic leukemia and acute granulocytic leukemia.[3] Terminal deoxynucleotidyl transferase (TdT) has been recognized as a specific marker for lymphoblasts, although it was found in the blasts in rare cases of acute myeloid leukemia.[6,7] TdT positivity in acute myeloid leukemia may denote a poor prognosis.[8,9] Myeloid antigens have been reported to be present in the myeloid but not the lymphoid cells.[10-12] Lymphoid antigens may be occasionally seen in acute myeloid leukemias and may indicate a poor prognosis.[13] Expression of myeloid antigens in ALL, on the other hand, also identified a high-risk group among patients with ALL.[14]

Subclassification of Nonlymphatic Leukemias

The subclassification of nonlymphatic leukemias is achieved mainly by morphologic and cytochemical studies[15,16] (Figures 9-1 and Table 9-3). Myeloblasts predominate in both M1 and M2, although the cells in M1 can be firmly identified only by the combined use of morphology

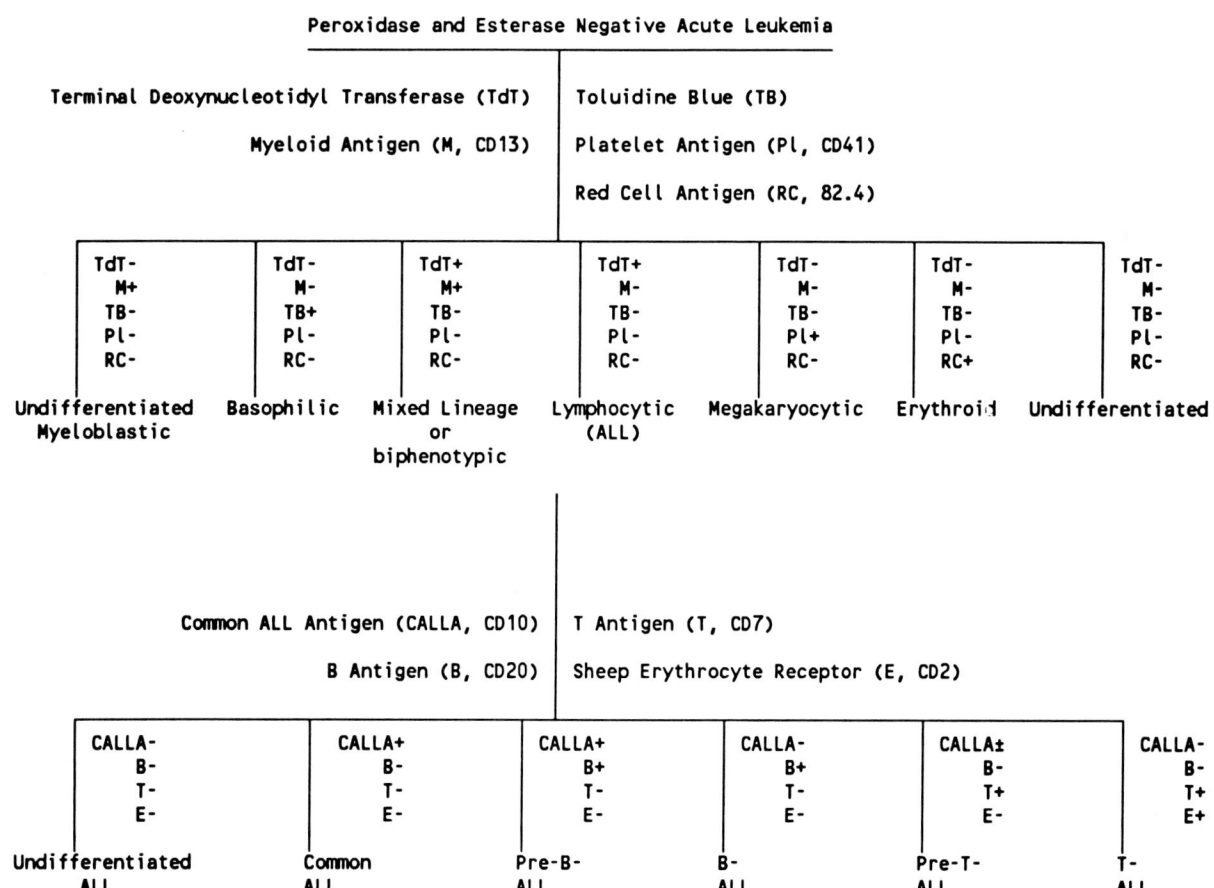

FIGURE 9-2. Classification of peroxidase- and esterase-negative acute leukemia using immunocytochemical methods.

TABLE 9-3. Markers Useful for Subclassification of Acute Myeloid Leukemias (Myeloid antigens[+], Peroxidase[+], Sudan Black[+], TdT[-], PAS[±])

Markers	M1	M2	M3	M4	M5	M6	M7	AEoL	ABaL
Myeloid antigens	+	+	+	+	+	+	+	−	NT
Peroxidase	+	+	+	+	±	+	−	+	−
Cyanide-resistant peroxidase	−	−	−	−	−	−	−	+	−
Sudan black B	+	+	+	+	±	+	−	+	−
Chloroacetate esterase	±	+	+	+	−	+	−	−	−
Nonspecific esterase	−	−	±	+	+	±	−	−	−
Toluidine blue O	−	−	−	−	−	−	−	−	+
RC82-4	−	−	−	−	−	+	−	−	−
Glycophorin	−	−	−	−	−	+	−	−	−
Hemoglobin	−	−	−	−	−	+	−	−	−
CD41	−	−	−	−	−	−	+	−	−

ABaL = acute basophilic leukemia; AEoL = acute eosinophilic leukemia; M1 to M7 refer to the FAB classification of acute leukemias; NT = not tested.
Note: Acute myeloid leukemias are characterized by reactions to the markers indicated in the title. + indicates a positive reaction; − indicates a negative reaction; ± indicates that in some cases the reaction is positive, and in other cases the reaction is negative.

and cytochemistry (Case 2). In M3, the leukemic myeloid cells can be recognized by their characteristic morphologic features[15] (Case 3). In M4, both myeloblasts and monocytes are increased in number and can be best recognized by the combined nonspecific esterase and chloroacetate esterase stain[1] (Cases 4 and 5). In M5, the nonspecific esterase stain is most helpful in confirming the monocytic nature of the leukemic cells[17-19] (Case 6).

M6 is characterized by the presence of many myeloblasts and erythroblasts; the morphologic features of these cells are often abnormal (Case 7). The myeloblasts can be recognized by peroxidase, Sudan black, and chloroacetate esterase; the erythroblasts, by pseudoperoxidase and immunochemical study for red cell antigen (RC82-4), glycophorin, and hemoglobin[20-23] (Case 7). A positive PAS reaction in the erythroblasts and the presence of many ringed sideroblasts would further reinforce the diagnosis.[24]

The latest addition to this classification is acute megakaryoblastic leukemia (M7)[25-29] (Case 10). Morphologically, the blasts usually show characteristic cytoplasmic budding (blebs) and signs of platelet formation. The blebs and newly formed platelets are PAS positive. Monoclonal antibodies specific for glycoprotein IIb/IIIa are helpful in identifying the blasts. Factor VIII antigen staining of megakaryoblasts is variable. The ultrastructural demonstration of platelet peroxidase is the earliest marker of megakaryocyte development and can be used to supplement immunologic methods. Most cases also have myelofibrosis.

The rare acute eosinophilic leukemia can usually be detected by morphologic identification of the early eosino-

TABLE 9-4. Markers Useful for Subclassification of ALLs (TdT[+], PAS[±], Myeloid antigen[−], Sudan Black[−], Peroxidase[−])

Markers	uALL	CALL	Pre-T-ALL	T-ALL	Pre-B-ALL	B-ALL
Sheep erythrocyte receptors (CD2)	−	−	−	+	−	−
SIg	−	−	−	−	−	+
CIg	−	−	−	−	+	+
TdT	+	+	+	+	+	−
HLA-DR	+	+	−	−	+	+
Common ALL antigen (CD10)	−	+	±	−	±	−
T antigen (CD7)	−	−	+	+	−	−
B antigen (CD19)	±	+	−	−	+	+
B antigen (CD20)	−	±	−	−	+	+
Focal acid phosphatase	−	−	+	+	−	−
Acid α-naphthyl acetate esterase	−	−	−	±	−	−
Morphology	L1/L2	L1/L2	L1/L2	L1/L2	L1/L2	L3

ALL = acute lymphoblastic leukemia; CALL = common ALL; HLA-DR = Ia-like antigen; L1 to L3 refer to the FAB classification of acute leukemias; uALL = unclassified or undifferentiated ALL (precursor B-ALL).
Note: ALLs are characterized by the reactions to markers indicated in the title. + indicates a positive reaction; − indicates a negative reaction; ± indicates that in some cases the reaction is positive, and in other cases the reaction is negative.

phils. In some cases in which the immature granules are not fully developed and are not eosinophilic, these abnormal eosinophils can be recognized by the cyanide-resistant peroxidase reaction or chlorazol fast pink[30-32] (Case 9).

Rarely, acute basophilic leukemia may cause confusion because of the presence of unusual peroxidase-negative cytoplasmic granules[23] (Case 8). Toluidine blue stain is helpful in demonstrating the metachromatic characteristic of basophilic granules and establishing the diagnosis of acute nonlymphatic leukemia with basophilic differentiation.

Subclassification of Lymphoblastic Leukemias

ALL can be separated by immunologic methods into six distinct subclassifications[2] (Figure 9-2 and Table 9-4): (1) "null" (unclassified) ALL, characterized by the absence of T antigens, SIg, and common ALL antigens; (2) common ALL, characterized by the presence of common ALL antigen on the surface of leukemic cells; (3) pre-T-ALL, characterized by the presence of T-cell antigen and absence of sheep erythrocyte receptor; (4) T-ALL, characterized by the presence of both T-cell antigen and sheep erythrocyte receptor; (5) pre-B-ALL, characterized by the presence of cytoplasmic immunoglobulin and the absence of SIg; and (6) B-ALL, characterized by the presence of SIg and B-cell antigen.

Morphologic and cytochemical studies are of less value in subclassifying the ALLs. The characteristic vacuolated, intensely basophilic cytoplasm of leukemic blasts (L3 subtype in the French-American-British classification) is helpful in recognizing the rare B-ALL[15] (Case 14). The demonstration of intense focal acid phosphatase activity in the Golgi region of T lymphoblasts by cytochemical methods is a relatively simple way of differentiating T-ALL from non-T-ALL,[34,35] although erythroblasts and early myeloblasts may also show similar focal acid phosphatase staining features. Since the 1980s, the immunocytochemical methods have been used for identification of common ALL, B-cell, and T-cell antigens. These methods are applicable to regular air-dried blood, marrow smears, or cell suspensions and have become most practical for subtyping the acute lymphoblastic leukemias[36-38] (Cases 12 and 13).

Erythroleukemia (M6) vs. Myelodysplastic Syndrome

The wide range of morphologic changes occurring both in erythroleukemia and in myelodysplastic syndrome makes morphologic distinction between these two types of disease difficult. Identification of Auer rods or peroxidase-positive abnormal granules (phi bodies)[39] in some of the myeloblasts is helpful in establishing the diagnosis of erythroleukemia or refractory anemia with excess blasts in transformation. The presence of large blocks of PAS-positive material in the cytoplasm of erythroid precursor cells is another characteristic of erythroleukemia.[24]

CLASSIFICATION OF CHRONIC LYMPHOCYTIC LEUKEMIAS

CLL represents a range of disorders of the mature lymphocytes (Figure 9-3 and Table 9-5). Most CLLs represent B-cell disease, as indicated by the presence of SIg and HLA-DR antigen and the absence of sheep erythrocyte receptors and most T-cell antigens[40,41] (Case 31). CD5 is the only T-cell antigen present; it is characteristic of CLL and mantle cell leukemia.[42] CD23 is usually present in CLL and absent in mantle cell leukemia. The SIg in B-CLL is characterized by its low density and the absence of capping, in contrast to the high-density SIg, with capping seen in B-cell prolymphocytic leukemia and in the leukemic phase of B-cell lymphomas, including mantle cell lymphoma and follicular center cell lymphomas[43-46] (Case 33). Another useful surface characteristic of B-CLL is the presence of mouse erythrocyte receptor (MER), which is not present in other B-cell lymphomas.[47-49]

T-CLL is uncommon, accounting for 2% to 5% of all cases of CLL. Because of the relatively aggressive nature of the helper T-CLL in comparison with the suppressor T-CLL or B-CLL, subtyping of the CLL is of clinical importance.[50-55] The morphologic appearance of the leukemic cells in T-CLL is more variable than that of B-CLL. In some cases, the leukemic cells may have abundant cytoplasm that contains azurophilic granules, as in normal suppressor T cells (T_s)[51-53] (Case 24). In other cases, the leukemic cells are variable in size and have indented or lobulated nuclei. Acid α-naphthyl acetate esterase (ANAE) stain may show dot-like cytoplasmic staining as in normal helper T cell (T_h)[54,55] (Case 23). The immunocytochemical methods using monoclonal antibodies for identification of various T-cell antigens and HLA-DR antigen are more useful than other methods in subtyping CLLs[36,37,56,57] (Cases 19, 23, and 24). A tentative subclassification of CLL according to the characteristics of leukemic cells is summarized in Figure 9-3 and Table 9-5.

Tγ Lymphoproliferative Disorder

Tγ lymphoproliferative disorder (TGLD) was originally called *T-cell chronic lymphocytic leukemia (CLL)* of the suppressor type or suppressor cell leukemia.[58] It is still so called in European literature,[59] but most American hema-

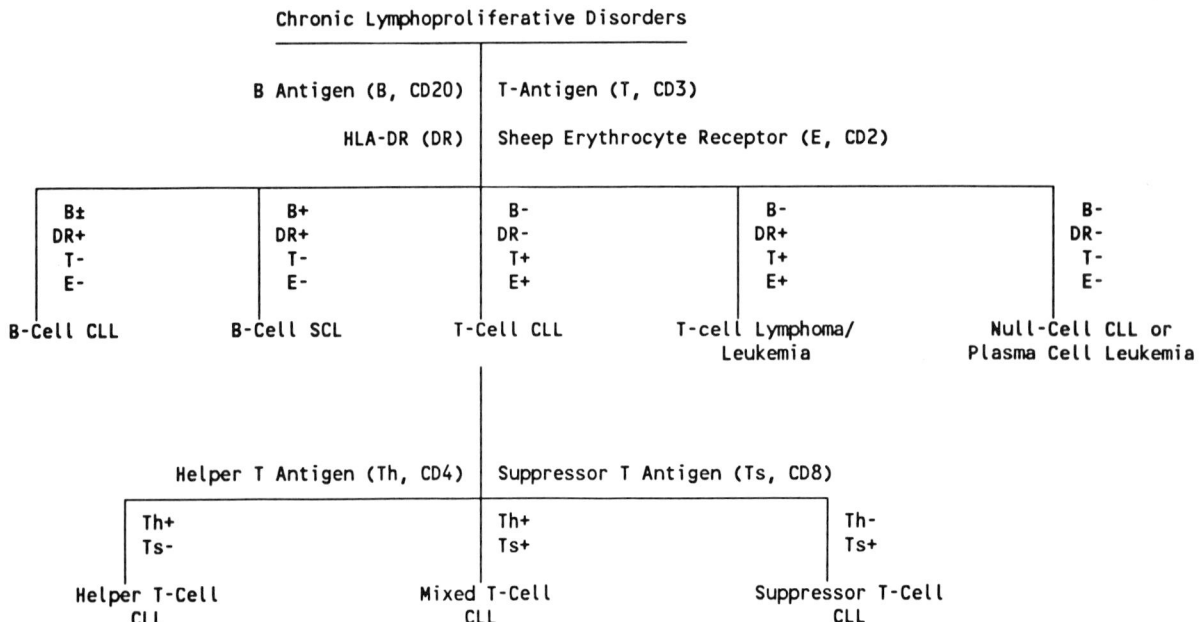

FIGURE 9-3. Classification of chronic lymphoproliferative disorders using immunocytochemical methods. CLL = chronic lymphocytic leukemia; SCL = small, cleaved, follicular center cell lymphoma/leukemia.

tologists consider it an entity separate from CLL. TGLD is probably composed of a heterogeneous group of diseases because its clinical manifestations cover a wide spectrum from a chronic stable to an acute fulminating course.[60,61]

Neutropenia, recurrent infections, splenomegaly, and rheumatoid arthritis are the salient features of this disease. The tumor cells are large granular lymphocytes; therefore, it was also called *large granular lymphocyte leukemia*.[62]

TABLE 9-5. Markers Useful for Subclassification of Chronic Lymphoid Leukemias

Markers	B-CLL	B-PLL	FCCL	MZL	SLVL	MBCL	HCL	PCL	T_h-CLL	T_m-CLL	T_s-CLL	T-LL
Surface (cytoplasmic) Ig	weak	strong	strong	moderate	strong	strong	strong	(strong)	−	−	−	−
CD2	−	−	−	−	−	−	−	−	+	+	+	+
CD3	−	−	−	−	−	−	−	−	+	+	+	+
CD4	−	−	−	−	−	−	−	−	+	+	−	±
CD8	−	−	−	−	−	−	−	−	−	+	+	±
CD5	+	±	−	+	−	−	−	−	+	+	±	+
HLA-DR	+	+	+	+	+	+	+	−	−	−	−	+
CD19	+	+	+	+	+	+	+	−	−	−	−	−
CD20	weak	strong	strong	moderate	strong	strong	strong	−	−	−	−	−
CD10	−	−	weak	±	−	−	−	−	−	−	−	−
CD23	+	−	±	−	−	−	−	−	−	−	−	−
CD25	−	−	−	−	−	−	+	−	−	−	−	+
CD38	−	−	±	−	±	−	±	+	−	−	−	−
FANAE	−	−	−	−	−	−	−	−	+	+	−	±
FAcP	−	−	−	−	−	−	−	−	±	±	−	+
TRAP	−	±	−	−	±	−	+	−	−	−	−	−
Morphology												
Nuclei	Round	Round	Cleaved	Variable	Round	Variable	Oval	Round	Convoluted	Convoluted	Round	Convoluted
Nucleolus	Absent	Prominent	Small	Absent	Absent	Absent	Absent	Small	Absent	Absent	Absent	Small
N/C ratio	High	Low	High	Variable	Variable	Low	Low	Low	High	High	Low	Low
Azurophilic granules	−	−	−	−	−	−	−	−	−	−	+	−

CLL = chronic lymphocytic leukemia; PLL = prolymphocytic leukemia; FCCL = follicular center cell lymphoma/leukemia; MZL = mantle zone lymphoma/leukemia; SLVL = splenic lymphoma with villous lymphocytes; MBCL = monocytoid B-cell lymphoma/leukemia; HCL = hairy cell leukemia; PCL = plasma cell leukemia; T_h = helper T cell; T_m = T cell with mixed-cell characteristics (i.e., both helper and suppressor T-cell characteristics); T_s = suppressor T cell; LL = lymphoma/leukemia; FANAE = focal α-naphthyl acetate esterase; FAcP = focal acid phosphatase; TRAP = tartrate-resistant acid phosphatase.

Since large granular lymphocytes represent either natural killer (NK) cells or NK-like T cells, markers for this cell type, such as CD16 (Leu-11), CD56 (Leu-19, NKH-1), or CD57 (Leu-7, HNK-1), are frequently demonstrated.[63] The phenotypes in most cases are suppressor/cytotoxic T cells, but phenotypes of helper/inducer T cells or coexistence of both helper and suppressor cells have also been reported.[64] A newly reported phenotype is CD3+, CD4−, CD8−, TGLD, in which the TCR γ/δ chain gene is rearranged.[65,66] The distinction between NK cells and NK-like T cells was controversial, but their identity has gradually been established.[67,68] The current definition of NK cells is CD3 negative, CD56 positive, and TCR negative, with no TCR gene rearrangement, while that of NK-like T cells is CD3 positive, CD16/CD57 positive, and TCR positive, with TCR gene rearrangement. Clinically, TGLD can be divided into chronic lymphocytic leukemia, acute lymphocytic leukemia, lymphoma, and lymphoblastic crisis (in chronic myelogenous leukemia) subtypes.[69,70]

DIAGNOSIS OF HAIRY CELL LEUKEMIA

Accurate diagnosis of hairy cell leukemia rests on the identification of the hairy cells in blood, marrow, spleen, or liver.[71,72] However, the characteristic cytoplasmic filamentous projections of the hairy cells may be inconspicuous in the regular Wright-stained smear or touch imprint preparation. Cytochemical demonstration of intense tartrate-resistant acid phosphatase (TRAP) activity in the neoplastic cells is most helpful in identifying small numbers of hairy cells in peripheral blood or buffy coat smears[72-75] (Case 28). The morphologic observation of tissue sections stained with hematoxylin and eosin usually shows diffuse round cell infiltration, with the clear cell pattern in bone marrow and red cell lakes in the spleen that are typical of hairy cell leukemia (Case 29). The combination of cytochemical study and morphologic observation should be sufficient for establishing the diagnosis of hairy cell leukemia.

In most cases, the predominant markers belong to the B-cell phenotype, including SIg, Fc receptor, B-cell antigens, and HLA-DR.[76,77] The complement receptor is, however, absent in hairy cell leukemia.[78] The results from mouse E-rosette studies have been disputed.[47,76,79] The SIg can be monoclonal or polyclonal, expressing one heavy chain determinant or several determinants.[78] Fc receptors, including IgG-Fc and IgM-Fc, have been demonstrated in hairy cell leukemia.[76,78] Cytoplasmic immunoglobulin (CIg) is expressed in a few cases, and monoclonal or biclonal paraproteins are occasionally found in the sera of patients with hairy cell leukemia.

In terms of monoclonal antibodies, some cases of hairy cell leukemia react with CD11b, FMC7, CD24, and BA-2.[51,80,81] The relatively specific monoclonal antibodies for hairy cell leukemia are CD11c and CD22. When a group of cells present both the monocyte (CD11c) and B-cell (CD22) markers simultaneously on their surface, hairy cell leukemia should be considered.[82] If these cells also carry CD25 (IL-2 or Tac antigen),[83] together with positivity of CD11c and CD22, the diagnosis is almost definite. A monoclonal antibody against TRAP has been developed. It is now possible to use this antibody, 9C5, to identify hairy cells in paraffin-embedded tissue sections.[84] Phagocytosis, a function of the monocyte-histiocyte, is also demonstrated in hairy cell leukemia.[76,85-87] A few cases of T-cell hairy cell leukemia have been identified by the reaction of the hairy cells with sheep erythrocytes and anti-T antiserum.[76,88-90] We have found that the hairy cells are positive for HLA-DR, SIg, and CD11b (OKM1).[91] At present, the diagnostic significance of these immunologic findings is uncertain.

Two new entities may mimic hairy cell leukemia: splenic lymphoma with villous lymphocytes (SLVL) and monocytoid B-cell lymphoma (MBCL).[92-98] The cells of these two lymphomas may show cytoplasmic projections (rare in MBCL) and a monoclonal B-cell pattern with coexistence of the monocyte marker CD11c.[93] TRAP has also been demonstrated occasionally in SLVL.[93] The presence of the CD25 marker on hairy cells may help to distinguish hairy cell leukemia from the other two entities.[83] Microscopic examination of the spleen tissue may show the typical red pulp infiltrations forming pseudosinus or red cell lakes in hairy cell leukemia; the other two entities involve mainly the white pulp of the spleen. In addition, extranodal lesions are seldom seen in MBCL. Occasionally, prolymphocytic leukemia also may mimic hairy cell leukemia.[99]

DIAGNOSIS OF MAST CELL DISEASE

Accurate diagnosis of mast cell disease rests on the proper recognition of the mast cell lesions either in smears or in tissue sections.[100,101] (Cases 30 and 31). Mast cells are not easily recognized with conventional hematoxylin and eosin stains and can be confused with a variety of other cells (e.g., fibroblasts, histiocytes, plasma cells, hairy cells, and immature granulocytes). Special stains are necessary for conclusive identification of the mast cell diseases. Wright-Giemsa stain is helpful in demonstrating the basophilic granules of mast cells and the accompanying eosinophilic reaction.[101,102] Toluidine blue stain is useful in confirming the metachromatic property of mast cell granules. However, the metachromasia of mast cell granules is diminished or totally abolished by conventional tissue processing, particularly decalcification with acidified solutions. Mast cells are rich in chloroacetate esterase, which can be easily demonstrated in paraffin sections, but this enzyme is also present in neutrophilic myelocytes. Aminocaproate esterase is a more specific enzyme marker for mast cells. However, this enzyme is less stable and requires a special procedure for tissue preparation (i.e., fixation in cold formalin and, in the case of bone marrow biopsy specimens, decalcification with ethylenediaminetetraacetic acid [EDTA] followed by cryostat sectioning or plastic embedding without decalcification).[103,104] Recently, a monoclonal antibody (AA1) specific for human mast cell tryptase became available. It can be used on routinely processed paraffin sections for identification of mast cells and aids in the practical diagnosis of mast cell diseases.[105]

DIAGNOSIS OF GRANULOCYTIC DISORDERS

Chronic Myeloid Leukemia and Unclassified Myeloproliferative Disorders

The leukocyte alkaline phosphatase score has been helpful in differentiating between chronic myeloid leukemia (low score) and the granulocytic leukemoid reaction (high score)[106] (Case 25). The leukocyte alkaline phosphatase score is, however, high in rare neutrophilic leukemia.[107] The demonstration of TdT in leukemic blasts has also been shown to be useful in differentiating between lymphoblastic and myeloblastic transformation of CML.[108] The peroxidase stain may help distinguish a myeloproliferative disorder with only subtle morphologic abnormality from a secondary granulocytic hyperplasia such as infection.[109,110] The former may show acquired partial myeloperoxidase deficiency, but the latter does not.[109,110] The butyrate esterase stain is helpful in identifying the monocytic component of chronic myelomonocytic leukemia in order to distinguish it from chronic myeloid leukemia[111] (Case 26).

Granulocytic Sarcoma

Granulocytic sarcoma is a localized tumor composed of granulocytic precursor cells. It is an uncommon tumor and may occur in a variety of clinical settings.[112] Granulocytic sarcoma is commonly misdiagnosed as diffuse large-cell lymphoma because in conventional hematoxylin and eosin-stained sections it is morphologically similar to lymphoma. Both histochemical stains for chloroacetate esterase and immunoperoxidase stains for lysozyme are useful in revealing the granulocytic identity of the tumor cells (Case 49). An unusual case of chronic myeloid leukemia with extramedullary T-lymphoblastic transformation has been reported recently.[113]

CLASSIFICATION OF MALIGNANT LYMPHOMAS (NON-HODGKIN'S LYMPHOMAS)

The follicular non-Hodgkin's lymphomas have distinctive pathologic features.[114] Although they are traditionally subclassified as poorly differentiated lymphocytic, mixed, and histiocytic types, they are all considered to be B-cell neoplasms in different stages of transformation.[115,116] The diffuse non-Hodgkin's lymphomas, however, are heterogeneous in cell origin. Most are recognized as neoplasms corresponding to various subtypes of lymphocytes at certain developmental stages, and few are of true histiocytic origin.[117] Identification of cell type by immunologic or histochemical characteristics has proved helpful in objective subclassification of lymphomas when morphologic distinction is difficult.

Lymphoblastic vs. Small Noncleaved Follicular Center Cell Lymphoma (Undifferentiated Lymphoma)

Both lymphoblastic and undifferentiated lymphomas (Burkitt's or non-Burkitt's) are high-grade lymphomas of intermediate cell size with some morphologic similarity, such as high mitotic rate and the "starry sky" appearance.[118-120] Morphologic distinction may be difficult, particularly with suboptimally prepared tissue. Because lymphoblastic lymphoma is recognized as a pre-T-cell or T-cell neoplasm[121] and the undifferentiated lymphoma as a B-cell neoplasm (small, noncleaved follicular center cell),[122] special stains for identification of cell type are helpful in differentiating these neoplasms. Demonstration of focal acid phosphatase activity in the Golgi region by cytochemical stains[121] (Case 33) or demonstration of nuclear TdT activity by immunocytochemical stain[7] is helpful in establishing the diagnosis of lymphoblastic lymphoma. On the other hand, demonstration of the presence of monoclonal SIg and CIg or B-cell antigen (CD20) by immunoperoxidase staining is helpful in confirming the diagnosis of Burkitt's or non-Burkitt's undifferentiated lymphoma (CY Li, unpublished data) (Case 34). Flow cytometric study may demonstrate a monoclonal SIg pattern and B-cell antigens in Burkitt's lymphoma.

Subclassification of Diffuse Large-Cell Lymphomas

Diffuse large-cell lymphomas was formerly called *reticulum cell sarcoma* or *histiocytic lymphoma*. The latter is a misnomer because most cases are not composed of true histiocytes. Diffuse large-cell lymphoma includes a group of disorders of diverse cell lineage that can be subclassified by morphologic, cytochemical, and immunologic studies.[117,120,123–126] These disorders include large follicular center cell lymphoma (cleaved and noncleaved, B cell), B-immunoblastic lymphoma, large T-cell lymphoma (including T-immunoblastic lymphoma), and true histiocytic lymphoma. Most large-cell lymphomas are of B-cell origin (60%); 25% are of null cell origin; and 15% are of T-cell origin.[127–129] In addition, some undifferentiated carcinomas (Case 48) and granulocytic sarcomas (Cases 1 and 49) may mimic large-cell lymphomas morphologically.

Several enzyme histochemical and immunohistochemical markers are useful in differentiating histiocytes, activated T lymphocytes and activated B lymphocytes, and granulocytes (Table 9-6). With these methods, granulocytic sarcomas can be identified easily (Case 49); occasional cases of B-cell lymphoma with morphologic features of undifferentiated epithelial neoplasm can be recognized,[130] and the diffuse large-cell lymphomas can be subclassified more objectively into B-cell, T-cell, and true histiocytic types.[117] The B-cell type is characterized by the presence of B-cell antigens, monoclonal SIg or CIg, and negative or weakly positive diffuse acid phosphatase activity (Cases 35, 36, 40, and 52). The T-cell type is characterized by intense focal acid phosphatase activity in the Golgi region or T-cell antigens (Cases 37, 38, and 51) and is frequently associated with a convoluted or multilobulated nuclear appearance and a history of preceding skin manifestations. The histiocytic type is characterized by strong, nonspecific esterase activity and diffuse acid phosphatase activity, as well as the presence of lysozyme and CD68 or phagocytic activity, or both (Case 39).

Recently, anaplastic large-cell (CD30-positive) lymphoma (ALCL) has been recognized as a distinct clinicopathologic entity.[131–133] The tumor usually shows sheets of uniformly CD30-positive large, pleomorphic lymphoid cells with abundant cytoplasm and often preferentially involves the lymph node sinuses as well as extranodal sites, such as soft tissue, bone, and skin. It also appears to be correlated with the presence of a unique chromosomal abnormality, t(2;5)(p23;q35).[134,135] The majority of tumors express one or more T-cell-associated antigens, some express neither T- nor B-cell-associated antigens, and rare cases express B-cell antigens. The tumor also frequently expresses epithelial membrane antigen (EMA), especially nodal ALCL,[136] and may not show reactivity for the leukocyte common antigen (CD45) in paraffin sections.[137] It is important to be aware of the existence of CD30-positive/CD45-negative ALCLs, as they can mimic the poorly differentiated, nonhematopoietic tumors both morphologically (the sinusoidal growth pattern) and phenotypically (the expression of EMA).

Extranodal Lymphocytic Lymphoma vs. Pseudolymphoma

The histologic distinction between a reactive pseudolymphoma and a lymphocytic lymphoma in an extranodal site is not always possible.[138,139] The presence of germinal centers within the lymphocytic infiltrate was emphasized previously as a cardinal feature of pseudolymphoma[140]; however, apparent germinal centers may also be occasionally found within lymphomas[139] (Case 53). Because malignant lymphomas are thought to be monoclonal proliferative processes,[141] in contrast to the polyclonal reactive process of pseudolymphoma, the immunoperoxidase stain for κ and λ light chains has been helpful in determining the clonality of these lymphoproliferative processes and thereby differentiating between them[139,142,143] (Case 53). The relatively rare extranodal T-cell lymphoma requires

TABLE 9-6. Markers Useful for Subclassification of Diffuse Large-Cell Lymphomas

Markers	FCC	B-IBL	T-IBL	T Cell	Histiocytic	Granulocytic	Metastatic Tumors
Acid phosphatase	0-2 + D	0-2 + D	2-3 + F	2-3 + F	4 + D	2 + D	Variable
Nonspecific esterase	0	0	0	0-1 + F	4 + D	0	Variable
Chloroacetate esterase	0	0	0	0	0	4+	0
Myeloperoxidase	0	0	0	0	0	4+	0
Lysozyme	0	0	0	0	1-3+	4+	Variable
Monocytic antigen (CD68)	0	0	0	0	1-4+	0	0
CIg	0-2 + M	1-3 + M	0	0	0-1 + P	0-1 + P	0-1 + P
SIg	2-3 + M	±M	0	0	±P	±P	0
B antigen (CD20)	+	+	−	−	−	−	−
T antigen (CD3)	−	−	+	+	−	−	−

D = diffuse cytoplasmic staining; F = focal staining confined to the Golgi area; FCC = follicular center cell type; IBL = immunoblastic lymphoma; M = monoclonal; P = polyclonal.
Note: The intensity of reaction is graded on a scale from 0 to 4+, with 0 indicating no reaction and 4+ indicating the strongest reaction.

monoclonal antibodies and, sometimes, genotyping for identification.[144,145]

Lymphoepithelioid Cell Lymphoma (Lennert's Lymphoma)

Lymphoepithelioid cell lymphoma was originally considered a variant of Hodgkin's disease but is actually a heterogeneous group of lymphomas characterized by abundant epithelioid histiocytes.[146,147] The epithelioid histiocytes are reactive histiocytes containing lysozyme and the Ia antigen (HLA-DR surface antigen).[148] The malignant lymphocytes in most cases are T cells that are positive for E-rosette formation[148] or reactive with the monoclonal antibodies CD3[149] and CD4.[150]

However, lymphoplasmacytic immunocytoma with a high content of epithelioid cells has also been reported.[151] Immunohistochemical demonstration of monotypic Ig in the cytoplasm of those plasmacytoid cells is helpful in establishing the diagnosis (Case 54) and distinguishing it from the typical lymphoepithelioid cell lymphoma of the helper T-cell type.[152]

Sézary Syndrome and Mycosis Fungoides

Mycosis fungoides is a T-cell neoplasm that is confined to the skin (Case 51). When the neoplastic cells spread into the circulation, with involvement of lymph nodes and the spleen, the condition is called *Sézary syndrome*.[153–155] The tumor cells in both conditions are identical, showing characteristic cerebriform nuclei and scanty cytoplasm. The tumor cells are positive for E-rosettes, human T-lymphocyte antigen, acid phosphatase, and β-glucuronidase.[149–154] Most neoplastic cells are helper/inducer cells, as defined on the basis of functional tests in culture, the presence of IgM-Fc receptor, and reactions to monoclonal antibodies (positive for CD3, CD4, and CD5).[51,155,156] Other types of lymphomas, including B cell (Case 52) and histiocytic, may also involve the skin. Histochemical and immunohistochemical characterizations of the tumor cells in skin lesions are helpful in the differential diagnosis of various cutaneous lymphomas.[157,158]

DIAGNOSIS AND CLASSIFICATION OF HODGKIN'S DISEASE

Hodgkin's disease is defined as a malignant process in which diagnostic Reed-Sternberg cells are found in the background of one of the various histologic types described.[159] Although the cell of origin of the Hodgkin's cell (Reed-Sternberg cells and their variants) is still controversial, some unusual immunohistochemical characteristics have been recognized that may be useful in differential diagnosis of Hodgkin's disease and non-Hodgkin's lymphoma, as well as other diseases with the presence of Reed-Sternberg-like cells. In the nodular sclerosing, mixed cellularity, and lymphocyte-depletion types of Hodgkin's disease, the Reed-Sternberg cells are characteristically positive for Leu-M1 (CD15), Ber-H2 (CD30), LN-2 (CD74), peanut agglutinin lectin (PNA), HLA-DR antigen, and Lewis X antigen but negative for LCA (CD45).[160–166] The Reed-Sternberg cells often contain a polyclonal cytoplasmic immunoglobulin as well.[167–172] Among these immunohistochemical markers, CD15 and CD45 are most commonly used for clinical diagnosis. The demonstration of CD15-positive and CD45-negative large cells in the lesion supports the diagnosis of Hodgkin's disease (Case 32). Conversely, the demonstration of strongly CD45-positive large cells in the lesion supports the diagnosis of non-Hodgkin's lymphoma.

Another interesting phenomenon is the in vivo attachment of lymphocytes to the surface of Hodgkin's cells (Figure 9-4). These lymphocytes are predominantly T lymphocytes.[173,174] Although the significance of this phenomenon is uncertain, a similar close interaction with T cells has been noted in interdigitating reticulum cells.[175,176] Further studies comparing the Reed-Sternberg cell and interdigitating reticulum cells may be helpful in understanding the nature of Hodgkin's cells.[175,177]

The lymphocyte-predominance type of Hodgkin's disease has been recently recognized as a distinct entity with different immunohistochemical characteristics suggestive of B-cell origin. The large, atypical cells (L and H variants of Reed-Sternberg cells) seen in this subtype are characteristically negative for CD15 and positive for CD45, L26 (CD20), and J chain.[178,181]

Recently, several studies have demonstrated the pres-

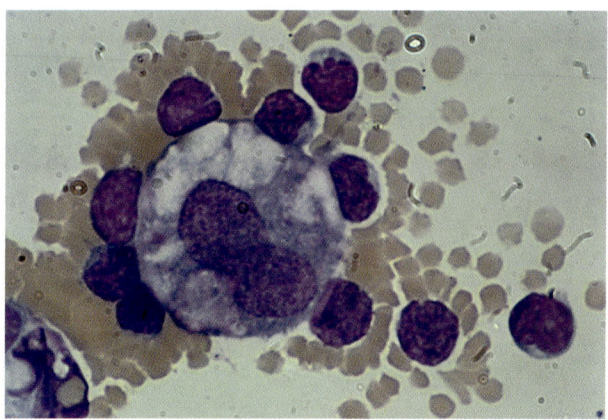

FIGURE 9-4. Reed-Sternberg cell. A cytocentrifuge preparation showing a Reed-Sternberg cell in the center surrounded by a circle of T lymphocytes, identified by simultaneous sheep erythrocyte rosette formation. (Wright-Giemsa, ×1,000)

ence of Epstein-Barr virus (EBV)-encoded small nuclear RNA (EBER) and latent membrane protein (LMP) in Hodgkin's and Reed-Sternberg cells by using sensitive, nonisotopic in situ hybridization and immunohistochemical techniques on routinely processed, paraffin-embedded tissues.[182-185] The prevalence of EBV varied among different subtypes of Hodgkin's disease. EBV-positive tumor cells were most frequently found in the mixed-cellularity type and least frequently in the lymphocyte-predominant type, with the nodular sclerosing type in between. A study with morphologic correlation further indicated that EBV is present in virtually all tumor cells in cases with an EBV-infected tumor cell population. In all cases with EBV-infected tumor cells, LMP was demonstrable on these cells. These findings strongly suggest that EBV is significantly involved in the pathogenesis of a large portion of Hodgkin's disease cases.

Bone Marrow Staging for Lymphoma

Examination of the bone marrow biopsy specimen is essential for lymphoma staging. Morphologic identification of early lymphomatous involvement and distinction of small lymphocytic lymphoma from normal benign lymphocytic aggregates are often difficult. The immunohistochemical stain of leukocyte common antigen (CD45) is helpful in highlighting the lymphoid cells in the bone marrow specimen. More specifically, the CD20 immunostain is helpful for identifying B-cell lymphoma with early interstitial or paratrabecular marrow involvement, except for small lymphocytic lymphomas, which are generally weak or negative for CD20 but positive for CD74 (Cases 40 and 41). Although CD74 is known to be less specific as a B-cell marker, it is helpful for identifying excess numbers of small B cells in small lymphocytic lymphoma (Case 43). This is in contrast to the benign lymphoid aggregates that usually consist of an equal mixture of T cells identified by UCHL-1 (CD45RO) predominantly in the periphery of aggregates and B cells identified by CD20 and CD74 predominantly in the center of the aggregates, including the follicular center. The lesions of T-cell lymphomas usually show conspicuous absence of B cells, and the CD45RO and CD3 immunostains are helpful in identifying small T cells and occasionally large cells in these lesions[186-188] (Cases 44, 46, and 47).

DIAGNOSIS OF PLASMAPROLIFERATIVE DISORDERS

Neoplastic vs. Reactive

The morphologic diagnosis of B-cell neoplasms involving the bone marrow is possible in most cases of advanced disease. However, difficulties arise in differentiating early multiple myeloma or monoclonal gammopathy of undetermined significance from reactive plasmacytosis or lymphoma from lymphocytosis. Immunoperoxidase or immunofluorescent staining of κ and λ light chains is helpful in differentiating the monoclonal neoplastic plasmaproliferative diseases, in which positive staining is present for one light chain only (Case 56), from polyclonal reactive plasmacytosis, in which plasma cells positive for κ and λ light chains are present in normal proportions.[189]

Multiple Myeloma and Waldenström's Macroglobulinemia

Multiple myeloma and Waldenström's macroglobulinemia may represent neoplasms that consist of medullary cord B cells that are in a more mature form than the B cells of other B-cell tumors.[128] Typical multiple myeloma cells are positive for CIg, CD38, PC-1, and PCA-1 but negative for SIg, HLA-DR, and surface B antigens—characteristics that distinguish multiple myeloma from other B-cell tumors[79,189-192] (Case 21). Waldenström's macroglobulinemia cells are similar to CLL cells, which are positive for SIg, HLA-DR, and surface B antigens.[191] Unlike CLL cells, both multiple myeloma and Waldenström's macroglobulinemia are negative for mouse E-rosette.[47,79] Under most circumstances, however, the laboratory diagnosis of multiple myeloma and Waldenström's macroglobulinemia is based mainly on the presence of a monoclonal gammopathy in serum rather than on the phenotypes of tumor cells.

Myeloma With Unusual Morphology

The morphology of myeloma cells varies widely. This variation may sometimes cause myeloma to be confused with other neoplastic diseases. The unusual morphology of neoplastic plasma cells includes signet-ring cells simulating metastatic adenocarcinoma (Case 57); large, foamy, histiocyte-like cells resembling lipid storage cells; mononuclear cells with abundant clear cytoplasm simulating hairy cells; and large, anaplastic cells simulating proerythroblasts, large-cell lymphoma, undifferentiated carcinoma, or acute leukemia (Case 58). Demonstration of intense monoclonal CIg in the tumor cells by immunohistochemical stain is helpful in establishing the diagnosis of myelomas with unusual morphology.[189]

Heavy Chain Diseases

Heavy chain diseases are uncommon and have diverse clinical and histopathologic features. The diagnosis of these diseases is usually established by identifying the abnormal fragments of heavy chains in serum or urine, or both.[193]

The morphologic differential diagnosis includes atypical hyperplasia, undetermined lymphoplasmaproliferative processes, plasmacytoma, and malignant lymphoma of various subclassifications.[194-197] Immunohistochemical staining of various components of immunoglobulin in cells or tissue sections is helpful in correlating the histopathologic findings with the serologic findings in these diseases (Case 50).

Amyloidosis

Amyloidosis is characterized by extracellular deposition of an insoluble fibrillar protein (i.e., amyloid) in a variety of tissues and organs. Although the amyloid fibroid proteins have common morphologic and staining properties, such as congophilia with characteristic apple-green birefringence in polarized light, recent advances in protein purification and sequence determination techniques have led to the disclosure of different amyloid proteins in different clinicopathologic forms of amyloidosis.[198] Isolation of the amyloid proteins and determination of their precise chemical nature have also led to the development of specific antibodies. Immunohistochemical methods using antibodies against different types of amyloid-related proteins (amyloid-related light chain [AL], amyloid A [AA], prealbumin, and β_2-microglobulin) are helpful in distinguishing primary, secondary, senile, familial, and dialysis-associated amyloidosis (Table 9-7)[199-201] (Cases 59–61).

AL amyloid usually consists of all or part of the variable region of immunoglobulin light chain in protein deposits and is associated with primary amyloidosis, with or without plasma cell dyscrasia.

DIAGNOSIS OF MALIGNANT HISTIOCYTOSIS

Malignant histiocytosis is generally considered to be a true histiocytic disorder characterized by a systemic, progressive, invasive proliferation of morphologically atypical histiocytes.[114,202] It is considered to be synonymous with histiocytic medullary reticulosis.[203] The diagnosis is established based on the morphologic recognition of the characteristic infiltration pattern (predominantly involving the red pulp of the spleen and sinuses of the lymph node) and the identification of cytologically atypical, pleomorphic, phagocytic, neoplastic cells. However, the histopathologic changes of this disease are heterogeneous, and no pathognomonic feature is recognized. Erythrophagocytosis or leukophagocytosis in cytologically atypical neoplastic cells may not be evident in sections stained with hematoxylin and eosin. Based on morphologic features alone, it may be difficult to differentiate this disease from other large-cell malignancies, such as undifferentiated carcinoma or large-cell lymphoma with sinusoidal involvement (Case 62). Extranodal T-cell lymphoma[144,145] or Ki-1 anaplastic large-cell lymphoma[204] may also masquerade as malignant histiocytosis. Demonstration of strong diffuse acid phosphatase and nonspecific esterase activity in the cytoplasm of neoplastic cells by histochemical methods is helpful in establishing the histiocytic nature of the tumor cells.[205] Demonstration of cytoplasmic lysozyme or CD68 by the immunoperoxidase method is also helpful in confirming the histiocytic nature of the neoplastic cells, particularly when only paraffin-embedded tissue is available for study.[125,126,158,205-207]

Diagnosis of Round Cell Tumors

The group of round cell tumors that commonly involve the marrow or lymph nodes (including malignant lymphoma, small-cell carcinoma of the lung, neuroblastoma, rhabdomyosarcoma, and Ewing's sarcoma) can cause difficulty in morphologic differential diagnosis. Among the many immunohistochemical markers now available, the most useful include CD45 for identification of malignant lymphoma, epithelial membrane antigen (EMA) and keratin for small-cell carcinoma, chromogranin and synaptophysin for neuroblastoma, and muscle actin and desmin for rhabdomyosarcoma.[208-214] The simple PAS stain for demonstration of abundant glycogen in tumor cells of Ewing's sarcoma or rhabdomyosarcoma is also helpful.[215,216] Although some of these markers are not unique to a specific cell type, their combined use as a panel provides a practical approach to

TABLE 9-7. Markers Useful for Subclassification of Amyloidosis

Protein Type	Related Protein	Clinicopathologic Form
AL	Immunoglobulin light chain (κ or λ)	Primary and myeloma associated
AA	Amyloid A protein	Secondary, familial Mediterranean fever
AS	Prealbumin (transthyretin)	Senile
AF	Prealbumin (transthyretin)	Heredofamilial
AP	Amyloid P component	All amyloid

TABLE 9-8. Markers Useful for Characterization of Round Cell Tumors

	LCA	Keratin	EMA	Chromogranin	Muscle Actin	Desmin	Vimentin	PAS
Lymphoma	+	−	−	−	−	−	−	−
Small cell carcinoma	−	+	+	+	−	−	−	−
Neuroblastoma	−	−	−	+	−	−	−	−
Rhabdomyosarcoma	−	−	−	±	+	+	+	+
Ewing's sarcoma	−	−	−	−	−	−	+	+

LCA = leukocyte common antigen (CD45); EMA = epithelial membrane antigen.

the differential diagnosis of round cell tumors on routinely processed biopsy specimens (Table 9-8) (Cases 16–18).

REFERENCES

1. Yam LT, Li CY, Crosby WH: Cytochemical identification of monocytes and granulocytes. *Am J Clin Pathol* 55:283–290, 1971.
2. Greaves MF, Janossy G, Petro J, et al: Immunologically defined subclasses of acute lymphoblastic leukemia in children: Their relationship to presentation features and prognosis. *Br J Haematol* 48:179–197, 1981.
3. Bennett JM, Reed CJR: Acute leukemia cytochemical profile: Diagnostic and clinical implications. *Blood Cells* 1:101–108, 1975.
4. Hayhoe FGJ, Quaglino D: *Haematological Cytochemistry*. New York, Churchill Livingstone, 1980.
5. Bennett JM, Dutcher TF: The cytochemistry of acute leukemia: Observations on glycogen and neutral fat in bone marrow aspirates. *Blood* 33:341–347, 1969.
6. Bollum FJ: Terminal deoxynucleotidyl transferase as a hematopoietic cell marker. *Blood* 54:1203–1215, 1979.
7. Hecht T, Forman SJ, Winkler US, et al: Histochemical demonstration of terminal deoxynucleotidyl transferase in leukemia. *Blood* 58:856–858, 1981.
8. Jani PW, Verbi MF, Greaves MF, et al: Terminal deoxynucleotidyl transferase in acute myeloid leukemia. *Leuk Res* 7:17–29, 1983.
9. Coco FL, Lopez M, Pasqualetti D, et al: Terminal transferase positive acute myeloid leukemia: Immunophenotypic characterization and response to induction therapy. *Hematol Oncol* 7:167–174, 1989.
10. Foon KA, Fitchen JH, Billing RJ, et al: An antigen expressed by cells of the myelomonocytic lineage. *Am J Hematol* 10:259–267, 1981.
11. Roberts M, Greaves MF: Maturation-linked expression of a myeloid cell surface antigen. *Br J Haematol* 38:439–452, 1978.
12. Beard J, Reinherz EL, Kung PC, et al: A monoclonal antibody reactive with human peripheral blood monocytes. *J Immunol* 124:1943–1968, 1980.
13. Cross AH, Goorha RM, Nuss R, et al: Acute myeloid leukemia with T-lymphoid features: A distinct biologic and clinical entity. *Blood* 72:579–587, 1988.
14. Sobol RE, Mick R, Royston I, et al: Clinical importance of myeloid antigen expression in adult acute lymphoblastic leukemia. *N Engl J Med* 316:1111–1117, 1987.
15. Bennett JM, Catovsky D, Daniel MT, et al: Proposals for the classification of the acute leukemias. *Br J Haematol* 33:451–458, 1976.
16. Shibata A, Bennet J, Castoldi GL, et al: Recommended methods for cytological procedures in hematology. *Clin Lab Hematol* 7:55–74, 1985.
17. Li CY, Lam KW, Yam LT: Esterases in human leukocytes. *J Histochem Cytochem* 21:1–12, 1973.
18. McKenna RW, Bloomfield CD, Dick F, et al: Acute monoblastic leukemia: Diagnosis and treatment of ten cases. *Blood* 46:481–494, 1975.
19. Shaw MT: The distinctive features of acute monocytic leukemia. *Am J Hematol* 4:97–103, 1978.
20. Li CY, Yam LT, Crosby WH: Histochemical characterization of cellular and structural elements of the human spleen. *J Histochem Cytochem* 20:1049–1058, 1972.
21. Solberg LA, Oles KJ, Kimlinger TK, et al: A new murine monoclonal antibody for the diagnosis of erythroleukemia. *Am J Clin Pathol* 93:387–390, 1990.
22. Second MIC Cooperative Group: Morphologic, immunologic and cytogenetic (MIC) working classification of the acute myeloid leukemias. *Cancer Genet Cytogenet* 30:1–16, 1988.
23. Neiman RS: Erythroblastic transformation in myeloproliferative disorders: Confirmation by an immunohistologic technique. *Cancer* 46:1636–1640, 1980.
24. Hayhoe FGJ, Quaglino D: Refractory sideroblastic anaemia and erythaemic myelosis: Possible relationship and cytochemical observations. *Br J Haematol* 6:381–387, 1960.
25. Huang MJ, Li CY, Nichols WLZ, et al: Acute leukemia with megakaryocytic differentiation: A study of 12 cases identified immunocytochemically. *Blood* 64:427–439, 1984.
26. Bennett JM, Catovsky D, Daniel M-T, et al: Criteria for the diagnosis of acute leukemia of megakaryocyte lineage (M7): A report of the French-American-British Cooperative Group. *Ann Intern Med* 103:460–462, 1985.
27. San Miguel JF, Gonzalez M, Canizo MC, et al: Leukemia with megakaryoblastic involvement: Clinical, hematologic, and immunologic characteristics. *Blood* 72:402–407, 1988.
28. Windebank KP, Tefferi A, Smithson A, et al: Acute megakaryocytic leukemia (M7) in children. *Mayo Clin Proc* 64:1339–1351, 1989.

29. de Oliveira MSP, Gregory C, Matutes E, et al: Cytochemical profile of megakaryoblastic leukemia: A study with cytochemical methods, monoclonal antibodies, and ultrastructural cytochemistry. J Clin Pathol 40:663–669, 1987.
30. Maeda R, Kanazawa K, Nakano E, et al: Studies on the specificity of the chlorazol fast pink staining method. Acta Histochem Cytochem 3:65–73, 1970.
31. Yam LT, Li CY, Necheles TF, et al: Pseudoeosinophilia, eosinophilic endocarditis and eosinophilic leukemia. Am J Med 53:193–202, 1972.
32. Gabbas AG, Li CY: Acute nonlymphocytic leukemia with eosinophilic differentiation. Am J Hematol 21:29–38, 1986.
33. Wick MR, Li CY, Pierre RV: Acute nonlymphocytic leukemia with basophilic differentiation. Blood 60:38–45, 1982.
34. Catovsky D, Greaves MF, Pain C, et al: Acid phosphatase reaction in acute lymphoblastic leukemia. Lancet 1:749–751, 1978.
35. Smithson WA, Li CY, Pierre RV, et al: Acute lymphoblastic leukemia in children: Immunologic, cytochemical, morphologic, and cytogenetic studies in relation to pretreatment risk factors. Med Pediatr Oncol 7:83–93, 1979.
36. Li CY, Ziesmer SC, Yam LT, et al: Practical immunocytochemical identification of human blood cells. Am J Clin Pathol 81:204–212, 1984.
37. Li CY: Immunocytochemical techniques for identifying leukemias. Mayo Clin Proc 59:185–188, 1984.
38. Li CY, Ziesmer SC, Lazcano-Villareal O: Use of azide and hydrogen peroxide as an inhibitor for endogenous peroxidase in the immunoperoxidase method. J Histochem Cytochem 35:1457–1460, 1987.
39. Hanker JS, Laszlo J, Moore JO: The light microscopic demonstration of hydroperoxidase-positive Phi bodies and rods in leukocytes in acute myeloid leukemia. Histochemistry 58:241–252, 1978.
40. Aisenberg AC, Wilkes BM, Long TC, et al: Cell surface phenotype in lymphoproliferative diseases. Am J Med 68:206–213, 1980.
41. Aisenberg AC: Cell surface markers in lymphoproliferative disease. N Engl J Med 304:331–336, 1981.
42. Coumsell L, Coppin H, Pham D, et al: An antigen shared by a human T-cell subset and B-cell chronic lymphocytic cells. J Exp Med 152:229–234, 1980.
43. Aisenberg AC, Wilkes B: Lymphosarcoma cell leukemia: The contribution of cell surface study to diagnosis. Blood 48:707–715, 1976.
44. Cohen HJ: B-cell lymphosarcoma cell leukemia: Dynamics of surface membrane immunoglobulin. Value of differentiation from chronic lymphocytic leukemia. Ann Intern Med 88:317–322, 1978.
45. Liebes L, Duagliata F, Silber R: The anomalous capping behavior of chronic lymphocytic leukemia lymphocytes: Studies with an antilymphocyte antiserum. Clin Immunol Immunopathol 10:222–232, 1978.
46. Bennett JM, Catovsky D, Daniel M-T, et al: Proposals for the classification of chronic (mature) B and T lymphoid leukemias. J Clin Pathol 42:567–584, 1989.
47. Burns GF, Cawley JC: Spontaneous mouse erythrocyte-rosette formation: Correlation with surface immunoglobulin phenotype in hairy-cell leukemia. Clin Exp Immunol 39:83–89, 1980.
48. Kosinos B, Filipa D, Mortelsmann R, et al: Characterization of malignant lymphomas in leukemic phase by multiple differentiation markers of mononuclear cells: Correlation with clinical features and conventional morphology. Am J Med 63:556–567, 1977.
49. Stathopoulos A, Elliott EV: Formation of mouse or sheep red blood cell rosettes by lymphocytes from normal and leukemic individuals. Lancet 1:600–602, 1974.
50. Brouet JC, Flandarin G, Sasportes M, et al: Chronic lymphocytic leukemia of T-cell origin: Immunological and clinical evaluation in eleven patients. Lancet 2:890–893, 1975.
51. Foon KA, Schroff RW, Gale RP: Surface markers on leukemia and lymphoma cells: Recent advances. Blood 60:1–19, 1982.
52. McKenna RW, Paskin J, Kersey JH, et al: Chronic lymphoproliferative disorder with unusual clinical, morphologic, ultrastructural and membrane surface marker characteristics. Am J Med 62:588–596, 1977.
53. Phyliky RL, Li CY, Yam LT: T-cell chronic lymphocytic leukemia with morphologic and immunologic characteristics of cytotoxic/suppressor phenotype. Mayo Clin Proc 58:709–720, 1983.
54. Grossi CE, Webb SR, Zicca A, et al: Morphological and histochemical analysis of two human T-cell subpopulations bearing receptors for IgM or IgG. J Exp Med 147:1405–1417, 1978.
55. Witzig TE, Phyliky RL, Li CY, et al: T-cell chronic lymphocytic leukemia with a helper/inducer membrane phenotype: A distinct clinicopathologic subtype with a poor prognosis. Am J Hematol 21:139–155, 1986.
56. Aisenberg AC, Wilkes BM, Harris NL, et al: T-cell chronic lymphocytic leukemia: Report of a case studied with monoclonal antibody. Am J Med 72:695–699, 1982.
57. Schroff RW, Foon KA, Billing RJ, et al: Immunologic classification of lymphocytic leukemias based on monoclonal antibody–defined cell surface antigens. Blood 59:207–215, 1982.
58. Broder S, Poplack D, Whang-Peng J, et al: Characterization of a suppressor-cell leukemia. N Engl J Med 298:66–72, 1978.
59. Foa R, Matutes E, Britobabapulle V, et al: T-cell chronic lymphocytic leukemia: A proliferation of large granular lymphocytes. Immunological, clinical, ultrastructural and molecular studies. In Polliack A, Catavsky D (eds): Chronic Lymphocytic Leukemia. Chur, Switzerland, Harwood Academic, 1988, pp 369–381.
60. McKenna RW, Arthur DC, Gajl-Peczalska KJ, et al: Granulated T-cell lymphocytosis with neutropenia: Malignant or benign chronic lymphoproliferative disorder? Blood 66:259–266, 1985.
61. Dhodapkar MV, Li CY, Lust JA, et al: Clinical spectrum of clonal proliferations of T-large granular lymphocytes: A T-cell clonopathy of undetermined significance? Blood 84:1620–1627, 1994.

62. Loughran TP, Starkebaum G: Large granular lymphocyte leukemia. *Medicine* 66:397–405, 1987.
63. Ritz J, Schmidt RE, Michon J, et al: Characterization of functional surface structures on human natural killer cells. *Adv Immunol* 42:181–211, 1988.
64. Berliner N: T gamma lymphocytosis and T-cell chronic leukemia. *Hematol Oncol Clin North Am* 4:473–487, 1990.
65. Vie H, Chevalier S, Garand R, et al: Clonal expansion of lymphocytes bearing the γδ T-cell receptor in a patient with large granular lymphocyte disorder. *Blood* 74:285–290, 1989.
66. Sun T, Cohen NS, Marino J, et al: CD3+, CD4−, CD8− large granular T-cell lymphoproliferative disorder. *Am J Hematol* 37:173–178, 1991.
67. Robertson MJ, Ritz J: Biology and clinical relevance of human natural killer cells. *Blood* 76:2421–2438, 1990.
68. Loughran TP Jr: Clonal diseases of large granular lymphocytes. *Blood* 82:1–14, 1993.
69. Sun T, Schulman P, Kolitz J, et al: A study of lymphoma of large granular lymphocytes with modern modalities: Report of two cases and review of the literature. *Am J Hematol* 40:135–145, 1992.
70. Sun T, Brody J, Koduru P, et al: Study of the major phenotype of large granular T-cell lymphoproliferative disorder. *Am J Clin Pathol* 98:516–521, 1992.
71. Bouroncle BA: Leukeic reticuloendotheliosis (hairy cell leukemia). *Blood* 53:412–436, 1979.
72. Li CY: Lymphoma-like disorders. In Fairbanks VF (ed): *Current Hematology*, vol 1., New York, Wiley Medical, 1981, pp 451–469.
73. Janckila AJ, Li CY, Lam KW, et al: The cytochemistry of tartrate-resistant acid phosphatase: Technical considerations. *Am J Clin Pathol* 70:45–55, 1978.
74. Yam LT, Li CY, Finkel HE: Leukemic reticuloendotheliosis: The role of tartrate-resistant acid phosphatase in diagnosis and splenectomy in treatment. *Arch Intern Med* 130:248–256, 1972.
75. Yam LT, Janckila AJ, Li CY, et al: Cytochemistry of tartrate-resistant acid phosphatase: 15 years' experience. *Leukemia* 1:285–288, 1987.
76. Gupta S, Good RA: Markers of human lymphocyte subpopulations in primary immunodeficiency and lymphoproliferative disorders. *Semin Hematol* 17:1–29, 1980.
77. Jansen J, Schuit HRE, van Zwet TL, et al: Hairy-cell leukaemia: A B-lymphocytic disorder. *Br J Haematol* 42:21–33, 1979.
78. Jansen J, Schuit HRE, Meijer CJLM et al: Cell markers in hairy cell leukemia studied in cells from 51 patients. *Blood* 59:52–60, 1982.
79. Kozimer B, Kempin S, Pass S, et al: Characterization of B-cell leukemias: A tentative immunomorphological scheme. *Blood* 56:815–823, 1980.
80. Brooks DA, Beckman GR, Bradley J, et al: Human lymphocyte markers defined by antibody derived from somatic cell hybrids, IV: A monoclonal antibody reacting specifically with a subpopulation of human B lymphocytes. *J Immunol* 126:1373–1377, 1981.
81. Jansen J, LeBien TW, Kersey JH: The phenotype of the neoplastic cells of hairy cell leukemia studies with monoclonal antibodies. *Blood* 59:609–614, 1982.
82. Schwarting R, Stein H, Wang CY: The monoclonal antibodies S-HCL1 (α Leu-14) and S-HCL3 (α Leu-M5) allow the diagnosis of hairy cell leukemia. *Blood* 65:974–983, 1985.
83. Korsmeyer J, Green WC, Cossman J, et al: Rearrangement and expression of immunoglobulin genes and expression of Tac antigens in hairy cell leukemia. *Proc Natl Acad Sci USA* 80:4452–4526, 1983.
84. Janckila AJ, Cardwell EM, Yam LT, et al: Hairy cell identification by immunohistochemistry of tartrate-resistant acid phosphatase. *Blood* 85:2839–2844, 1995.
85. Fu SM, Winchester RJ, Rai KR, et al: Hairy cell leukemia: Proliferation of a cell with phagocytic and B-lymphocyte properties. *Scand J Immunol* 3:847–851, 1974.
86. Palutke M, Weise RW, Tabaczka P, et al: Hairy cells and macrophages: A comparative study. *Lab Invest* 39:267–280, 1978.
87. Utsinger PD, Yount WJ, Fuller CR, et al: Hairy cell leukemia: B lymphocyte and phagocytic properties. *Blood* 49:19–27, 1977.
88. Cawley JC, Burns GF, Nash AA, et al: Hairy-cell leukemia with T-cell features. *Blood* 51:61–69, 1978.
89. Hernandez D, Cruz C, Carnot J, et al: Hairy-cell leukemia of T-cell origin. *Br J Haematol* 40:504–506, 1978.
90. Saxon A, Stevens RH, Golde DW: T-lymphocyte variant of hairy-cell leukemia. *Ann Intern Med* 88:323–326, 1978.
91. Janckila AJ, Stelzer GT, Wallace JH, et al: Phenotype of the hairy cells of leukemic reticuloendotheliosis defined by monoclonal antibodies. *Am J Clin Pathol* 79:431–437, 1983.
92. Melo JV, Robinson DSF, Gregory C, et al: Splenic B-cell lymphoma with villous lymphocytes in peripheral blood: A disorder distinct from hairy cell leukemia. *Leukemia* 1:294–299, 1987.
93. Melo JV, Hedge U, Parreira A, et al: Splenic B-cell lymphoma with circulating villous lymphocytes: Differential diagnosis of B-cell leukemia with large spleens. *J Clin Pathol* 40:642–651, 1987.
94. Vardiman JW, Gilenski TA, Ratain MJ, et al: Evaluation of Leu-M5 (CD11c) in hairy cell leukemia by the alkaline phosphatase antialkaline phosphatase technique. *Am J Clin Pathol* 90:250–256, 1988.
95. Sheibani K, Burke JS, Swartz WG, et al: Monocytoid B-cell lymphoma: Clinicopathologic study of 21 cases of a unique type of low-grade lymphoma. *Cancer* 62:1531–1538, 1988.
96. Carbone A, Gloghini A, Pinto A, et al: Monocytoid B-cell lymphoma with bone marrow and peripheral blood involvement at presentation. *Am J Clin Pathol* 92:228–236, 1989.
97. Traweek ST, Sheibani K, Winberg CD, et al: Monocytoid B-cell lymphoma: Its evolution and relationship to other low-grade B-cell neoplasms. *Blood* 73:573–578, 1989.
98. Sun T, Susin M, Shevde N, et al: Hybrid form of hairy cell leukemia and chronic lymphocytic leukemia. *Hematol Oncol Clin North Am* 8:283–294, 1990.
99. Yam LT, Phyliky RL, Li CY: Benign and neoplastic disorders

99. simulating hairy cell leukemia. *Semin Oncol* 11:353–361, 1984.
100. Sagher F, Even-Paz Z: *Mastocytosis and the Mast Cell.* Chicago, Year Book Medical, 1967.
101. Webb TA, Li CY, Yam LT: Systemic mast cell disease: A clinical and hematopathologic study of 26 cases. *Cancer* 49:927–938, 1982.
102. Yam LT, Yam CF, Li CY: Eosinophilia in systemic mastocytosis. *Am J Clin Pathol* 73:48–54, 1980.
103. Li CY, Travis WD, Van Hale PC, et al: Useful cytochemical stains for the diagnosis of systemic mast cell disease (SMCD). *J Histochem Cytochem* 34:1355, 1986.
104. Travis WD, Li CY, Bergstrath EJ, et al: Systemic mast cell disease: Analysis of 58 cases and literature review. *Medicine* 67:345–368, 1988.
105. Walls AF, Jones DB, Williams JH, et al: Immunohistochemical identification of mast cells in formaldehyde-fixed tissue using monoclonal antibodies specific for tryptase. *J Pathol* 162:119–126, 1990.
106. Kaplow LS: Leukocyte alkaline phosphatase cytochemistry: Applications and methods. *Ann NY Acad Sci* 155:911–947, 1968.
107. Yam LT: Neutrophilic leukemia. *South Med J* 75:870–872, 1982.
108. Janossy G, Woodruff RK, Pippard MJ, et al: Relation of "lymphoid" phenotype and response to chemotherapy incorporating vincristine-prednisolone in the acute phase of Ph^1 positive leukemia. *Cancer* 43:426–434, 1979.
109. Breton-Gorins J, Houssay D, Dreyfus B: Partial myeloperoxidase deficiency in a case of preleukemia, I: Studies of fine structure and peroxidase synthesis of promyelocytes. *Br J Haematol* 30:273–278, 1975.
110. Cech P, Schneider P, Bachmann F: Partial myeloperoxidase deficiency. *Acta Haematol* 67:180–184, 1982.
111. Seo IS, Li CY, Yam LT: Myelodysplastic syndrome: Diagnostic implication of cytochemical and immunocytochemical studies. *Mayo Clin Proc* 68:47–53, 1993.
112. Neiman RS, Barcos M, Berard CW, et al: Granulocytic sarcoma: A clinicopathologic study of 61 biopsied cases. *Cancer* 48:1426–1437, 1981.
113. Sun T, Susin M, Koduru P, et al: Extramedullary blast crisis in chronic myelogenous leukemia: Demonstration of T-cell lineage and Philadelphia chromosome in a paraspinal tumor. *Cancer* 68:605–610, 1991.
114. Rappaport H: Tumors of the hematopoietic system. In *Atlas of Tumor Pathology*, Section 3, Fascicle 8. Washington DC, Armed Forces Institute of Pathology, 1966, pp 49–63.
115. Jaffe ES, Shevach EM, Frank MM, et al: Nodular lymphoma: Evidence for origin from follicular B lymphocytes. *N Engl J Med* 290:813–819, 1974.
116. Warnke R, Levy R: Immunology of follicular lymphomas: A model of B-lymphocyte homing. *N Engl J Med* 298:481–486, 1978.
117. Li CY, Harrison EG: Histochemical and immunohistochemical study of diffuse large-cell lymphomas. *Am J Clin Pathol* 70:721–732, 1978.
118. Berard CW, O'Conor GT, Thomas LB, et al: Histopathological definition of Burkitt's tumour. *Bull WHO* 40:601–607, 1969.
119. Nathwani BM, Kim H, Rappaport H: Malignant lymphoma, lymphoblastic. *Cancer* 38:964–983, 1976.
120. National Cancer Institute-sponsored study of classification of non-Hodgkin's lymphomas. In Rosenberg SA, Berard CW, Brown BW Jr, et al (eds): Summary and description of a working formulation for clinical usage. *Cancer* 49:2112–2135, 1982.
121. Stein H, Petersen N, Gaedicke G, et al: Lymphoblastic lymphoma of convoluted or acid phosphatase type: A tumor of T precursor cells. *Int J Cancer* 17:292–295, 1976.
122. Mann RB, Jaffe ES, Braylan RC, et al: Non-endemic Burkitt's lymphoma: A B-cell tumor related to germinal centers. *N Engl J Med* 295:685–691, 1976.
123. Strauchen JA, Young RC, DeVita VT Jr, et al: Clinical relevance of the histopathological subclassification of diffuse "histiocyte" lymphoma. *N Engl J Med* 299:1382–1387, 1978.
124. Whitcomb CC, Cousar JB, Flint A, et al: Subcategories of histiocytic lymphoma: Associations with survival and reproducibility of classification. The Southeastern Cancer Study Group experience. *Cancer* 48:2464–2474, 1981.
125. Pulford KAF, Rigney EM, Micklem KJ, et al: KP1: A new monoclonal antibody that detects a monocyte/macrophage associated antigen in routinely processed tissue sections. *J Clin Pathol* 42:414–421, 1989.
126. Warnke RA, Plford KAF, Pallesen G, et al: Diagnosis of myelomonocytic and macrophage neoplasms in routinely processed tissue biopsies with monoclonal antibody KP1. *Am J Pathol* 135:1089–1095, 1989.
127. Brouet JC, Preud'homme JL, Flandrin G, et al: Membrane markers in "histiocytic" lymphomas (reticulum cell sarcomas). *J Natl Can Inst* 46:631–633, 1976.
128. Jaffe ES: Non-Hodgkin's lymphomas as neoplasms of the immune system. In Berard CW (moderator): A multidisciplinary approach to non-Hodgkin's lymphoma. *Ann Intern Med* 94:218–235, 1980.
129. Warnke R, Miller R, Grogan T, et al: Immunologic phenotype in 30 patients with diffuse large-cell lymphoma. *N Engl J Med* 303:293–300, 1980.
130. Li CY, Banks PM: Immunoperoxidase stain in the diagnosis of B-cell lymphoma with morphological features of undifferentiated epithelial neoplasm. *J Histochem Cytochem* 26:211, 1978.
131. Agnarsson BA, Kadin ME: Ki-1 positive large cell lymphoma: A morphologic and immunologic study of 19 cases. *Am J Surg Pathol* 12:264–274, 1988.
132. Chott A, Kaserer K, Augustin I, et al: Ki-1-positive large cell lymphoma: A clinicopathologic study of 41 cases. *Am J Surg Pathol* 14:439–448, 1990.
133. Nakamura S, Takagi N, Kojima M, et al: Clinicopathologic study of large cell anaplastic lymphoma (Ki-1-positive large cell lymphoma) among the Japanese. *Cancer* 68:118–129, 1991.
134. Mason DY, Bastard C, Rimokh R, et al: CD30-positive large cell lymphomas ("Ki-1 lymphoma") are associated with a

chromosomal translocation involving 5q35. *Br J Haematol* 74:161–168, 1990.
135. Bitter MA, Franklin WA, Larson RA, et al: Morphology in Ki-1 (CD30)-positive non-Hodgkin's lymphoma is correlated with clinical features and the presence of a unique chromosomal abnormality, t(2;5)(p23;q35). *Am J Surg Pathol* 14:305–316, 1990.
136. DeBruin PC, Beljaards RC, Van Heerde P, et al: Differences in clinical behaviour and immunophenotype between primary cutaneous and primary nodal anaplastic large cell lymphoma of T-cell or null-cell phenotype. *Histopathology* 23:127–135, 1993.
137. Falini B, Pileri S, Stein H, et al: Variable expression of leucocyte-common (CD45) antigen in CD30 (Ki-1)-positive anaplastic large-cell lymphoma: Implications for the differential diagnosis between lymphoid and nonlymphoid malignancies. *Hum Pathol* 21:624–629, 1990.
138. Greenberg SD, Heisler JG, Gyorkey F, et al: Pulmonary lymphoma versus pseudolymphoma: A perplexing problem. *South Med J* 65:775–784, 1972.
139. Julsrud PR, Brown LR, Li CY, et al: Pulmonary processes of mature-appearing lymphocytes: Pseudolymphoma, well-differentiated lymphocytic lymphoma, and lymphocytic interstitial pneumonitis. *Radiology* 127:289–296, 1978.
140. Saltzstein SL: Pulmonary malignant lymphomas and pseudolymphomas: Classification, therapy, and prognosis. *Cancer* 16:928–955, 1963.
141. Levy R, Warnke R, Dorfman RF, et al: The monoclonality of human B-cell lymphomas. *J Exp Med* 145:1014–1028, 1977.
142. Humphrey DM, Cortez EA, Spira DA: Immunohistologic studies of cytoplasmic immunoglobulins in rheumatic diseases including two patients with monoclonal patterns and subsequent lymphoma. *Cancer* 49:2049–2069, 1982.
143. Knowles CM II, Halper JP, Jakobiec FA: The immunologic characterization of 40 extranodal lymphoid infiltrates: Usefulness in distinguishing between benign pseudolymphoma and malignant lymphoma. *Cancer* 49:2321–2335, 1982.
144. Sun T, Brody J, Susin M, et al: Extranodal T-cell lymphoma mimicking malignant histiocytosis. *Am J Hematol* 35:269–274, 1990.
145. Farcet J-P, Garland P, Marolleau J-P, et al: Hepatosplenic T-cell lymphoma: Sinusal/sinusoidal localiation of malignant cells expressing the T-cell receptor. *Blood* 75:2213–2219, 1990.
146. Lennert K, Mohri N, Stein H, et al: The histopathology of malignant lymphoma. *Br J Haematol* 31(Suppl):193–203, 1975.
147. Burke JS, Butler JJ: Malignant lymphoma with a high content of epithelioid histiocytes (Lennert's lymphoma). *Am J Clin Pathol* 66:1–9, 1976.
148. Knowles DM: Non-Hodgkin's lymphomas, II: Current immunologic concepts. *Prog Surg Pathol* 2:107–143, 1980.
149. Knowles DM, Halper JP: Human T-cell malignancies: Correlative clinical, histopathologic, immunologic, and cytochemical analysis of 23 cases. *Am J Pathol* 106:187–203, 1982.
150. Feller AC, Griesser GH, Mak TW, et al: Lymphoepithelioid lymphoma (Lennert's lymphoma) is a monoclonal proliferation of helper/inducer T cells. *Blood* 68:663–667, 1986.
151. Patsouris E, Noël H, Lennert K: Lymphoplasmacytic/lymphoplasmacytoid immunocytoma with a high content of epithelioid cells: Histologic and immunohistochemical findings. *Am J Surg Pathol* 14:660–670, 1990.
152. Patsouris E, Noël H, Lennert K: Histological and immunohistological findings in lymphoepithelioid cell lymphoma (Lennert's lymphoma). *Am J Surg Pathol* 12:341–350, 1988.
153. Miller RA, Coleman CN, Fawcett HD, et al: Sézary syndrome: A model for migration of T lymphocytes to skin. *N Engl J Med* 303:89–92, 1980.
154. Haynes BF, Metzbar RS, Minna JK, et al: Phenotype characterization of cutaneous T-cell lymphoma: Use of monoclonal antibodies to compare with other malignant T cells. *N Engl J Med* 304:1319–1323, 1981.
155. Flandrin G, Brouet JC: The Sézary cell: Cytologic, cytochemical and immunologic studies. *Mayo Clin Proc* 49:575–583, 1974.
156. Broder S, Edelson RL, Lutzner MA, et al: The Sézary syndrome: A malignant proliferation of helper T cells. *J Clin Invest* 58:1287–1306, 1976.
157. Krishnan J, Li CY, Su WPD: Cuatneous lymphomas: Correlation of histochemical and immunohistochemical characteristics and clinicopathologic features. *Am J Clin Pathol* 79:157–165, 1983.
158. Arai E, Su WPD, Roche PC, et al: Cutaneous histiocytic malignancy. Immunohistochemical reexamination of cases previously diagnosed as cutaneous "histiocytic lymphoma" and "malignant histiocytosis." *J Cutan Pathol* 20:115–120, 1993.
159. Lukes RJ, Craver LF, Hall TC, et al: Report of the nomenclature committee. *Cancer Res* 26:1311, 1966.
160. Chittal SM, Caveriviere P, Schwarting R, et al: Monoclonal antibodies in the diagnosis of Hodgkin's disease: Search for a rational panel. *Am J Surg Pathol* 12:9–21, 1988.
161. Pinkus GS, Thomas P, Said JW: Leu M1: A marker for Reed-Sternberg cells in Hodgkin's disease. An immunoperoxidase study of paraffin-embedded tissue. *Am J Pathol* 119:244–252, 1985.
162. Dorfman RF, Gatter KC, Pulford KAF, et al: An evaluation of the utility of antigranulocyte and antileukocyte monoclonal antibodies in the diagnosis of Hodgkin's disease. *Am J Pathol* 123:508–519, 1986.
163. Fellbaum C, Hansmann ML, Parwaresch MR, et al: Monoclonal antibodies Ki-B3 and Leu-M1 discriminate giant cells of infectious mononucleosis and of Hodgkin's disease. *Hum Pathol* 19:1168–1173, 1988.
164. Ree HJ, Neiman RS, Martin AW, et al: Paraffin section markers for Reed-Sternberg cells: A comparative study of peanut agglutinin, Leu-M1, LN-2, and Ber-H2. *Cancer* 63:2030–2036, 1989.
165. Agnarsson BA, Kadin ME: The immunophenotype of Reed-Sternberg cells: A study of 50 cases of Hodgkin's disease using fixed frozen tissues. *Cancer* 63:2083–2087, 1989.

166. Ree HJ, Teplitz C, Khan A: The Lewis X antigen: A new paraffin section marker for Reed-Sternberg cells. *Cancer* 67:1338–1346, 1991.
167. Kadin ME, Stites DP, Levy R, et al: Exogenous immunoglobulin and the macrophage origin of Reed-Sternberg cells in Hodgkin's disease. *N Engl J Med* 299:1208–1214, 1978.
168. Landaas TO, Godal T, Halvorsen TB: Characterization of immunoglobulins in Hodgkin cells. *Int J Cancer* 20:717–722, 1977.
169. Papadimitriou CS, Stein H, Lennert K: The complexity of immunohistochemical staining pattern of Hodgkin and Reed-Sternberg cells: Demonstration of immunoglobulin, albumin, α_1-antichymotrypsin and lysozyme. *Int J Cancer* 21:531–541, 1978.
170. Poppema S, Elema JD, Halie MR: The significance of intracytoplasmic proteins in Reed-Sternberg cells. *Cancer* 42:1793–1803, 1978.
171. Taylor CR: An immunohistological study of follicular lymphoma, reticulum cell sarcoma and Hodgkin's disease. *Eur J Cancer* 12:61–75, 1976.
172. Mir R, Kahn LB: Immunohistochemistry of Hodgkin's disease: A study of 20 cases. *Cancer* 52:2064–2071, 1983.
173. Kadin ME, Newcom SR, Gold SB, et al: Origin of Hodgkin's cell. *Lancet* 2:167–168, 1974.
174. Stuart AE, Williams DRW, Habershaw JA: Rosetting and other reactions of the Reed-Sternberg cell. *J Pathol* 122:81–90, 1977.
175. Kadin ME: A reappraisal of the Reed-Sternberg cell: A commentary. *Blood Cells* 6:525–532, 1980.
176. Kaiserling E, Lennert K: Die interdigitierende reticulumzelle im menschlichen lymphknoten: Eine spezifische zelle der thymusabhängigen region. *Virchows Arch (Cell Pathol)* 16:51–61, 1974.
177. Hansmann ML, Kaiserling E: The lacunar cell and its relationship to interdigitating reticulum cells. *Virchows Arch (Cell Pathol)* 39:323–332, 1982.
178. Pinkus GS, Said JW: Hodgkin's disease, lymphocyte predominance type, nodular: A distinct entity? Using staining profile for L and H variants of Reed-Sternberg cells defined by monoclonal antibodies to leukocyte common antigen, granulocyte-specific antigen, and B-cell specific antigen. *Am J Pathol* 118:1–6, 1985.
179. Pinkus GS, Said JW: Hodgkin's disease, lymphocyte predominance type, nodular: Further evidence for a B cell deviation. L and H variants of Reed-Sternberg cells express L26, a pair B cell marker. *Am J Pathol* 133:211–217, 1988.
180. Chittal SM, Alard C, Rossi JF, et al: Further phenotypic evidence that nodular, lymphocyte-predominant Hodgkin's disease is a large B-cell lymphoma in evolution. *Am J Surg Pathol* 14:1024–1035, 1990.
181. Bishop PW, Harris M, Smith AP, et al: Immunophenotypic study of lymphocyte predominance Hodgkin's disease. *Histopathology* 18:19–24, 1991.
182. Hummel M, Anagnostopoulos I, Dallenbach F, et al: EBV infection patterns in Hodgkin's disease and normal lymphoid tissue: Expression and cellular localization of EBV gene products. *Br J Haematol* 82:689–694, 1992.
183. Khan G, Norton AJ, Slavin G: Epstein-Barr virus in Hodgkin's disease: Relation to age and subtype. *Cancer* 71:3124–3129, 1993.
184. Armstrong AA, Alexander FE, Pinto Paes R, et al: Association of Epstein-Barr virus with pediatric Hodgkin's disease. *Am J Pathol* 142:1683–1688, 1993.
185. Weiss LM, Movahed AM, Warnke RA, et al: Detection of Epstein-Barr virus genomes in Reed-Sternberg cells of Hodgkin's disease. *N Engl J Med* 320:502–506, 1989.
186. Li CY, Chan YJ: Useful immunohistochemical markers for distinguishing lymphoid lesions in paraffin sections of bone marrow biopsies. International Congress of 25 years of immunoenzymatic techniques. In *Abstract Book*. Athens, Triaena Congress, p 165, 1991.
187. Van der Valk P, Mullink H, Huijgins PC, et al: Immunohistochemistry in bone marrow diagnosis: Value of a panel of monoclonal antibodies on routinely processed bone marrow biopsies. *Am J Surg Pathol* 13:97–106, 1989.
188. Kubic VL, Brunning RD: Immunohistochemical evaluation of neoplasms in bone marrow biopsies using monoclonal antibodies reactive in paraffin-embedded tissue. *Mod Pathol* 2:618–629, 1989.
189. Hitzman JL, Li CY, Kyle RA: Immunoperoxidase staining of bone marrow sections. *Cancer* 48:2438–2446, 1981.
190. Halper J, Fu SM, Wang CY, et al: Patterns of expression of human "Ia-like" antigens during the terminal stages of B-cell development. *J Immunol* 120:1480–1484, 1978.
191. Nadler LM, Stashenko P, Hardy R, et al: Characterization of human B-cell specific antigen (B2) distinct from B1. *J Immunol* 126:1941–1947, 1981.
192. Deegan MJ: Membrane antigen analysis in the diagnosis of lymphoid leukemias and lymphomas. *Arch Pathol Lab Med* 113:606–618, 1989.
193. Kyle RA, Greipp PR, Banks PM: The diverse picture of gamma heavy-chain disease: Report of seven cases and review of literature. *Mayo Clin Proc* 56:439–451, 1981.
194. Galian A, Lecestre MJ, Scotto J, et al: Pathological study of alpha chain disease, with special emphasis on evolution. *Cancer* 39:2081–2101, 1977.
195. Lewin KJ, Kahn LB, Novis BH: Primary intestinal lymphoma of "western" and "mediterranean" type, alpha chain disease and massive plasma cell infiltration: A comparative study of 37 cases. *Cancer* 38:2511–2528, 1976.
196. Chang CS, Lin SF, Chen TP, et al: Leukemic manifestation in a case of alpha-chain disease with multiple polypoid intestinal lymphocytic lymphoma. *Am J Hematol* 41:209–214, 1992.
197. Wester SM, Banks PM, Li CY: The histopathology of γ heavy-chain disease. *Am J Clin Pathol* 78:427–436, 1982.
198. Kisilevsky R: Amyloidosis: A familial problem in the light of current pathogenetic developments. *Lab Invest* 49:381–390, 1983.
199. Shirahama T, Cohen AS, Skinner M: Immunohistochemis-

try of amyloid. In De Lellis RA (ed): *Advances in Immunohistochemistry*. New York, Masson, 1984, pp 277–302.
200. Fujihara S, Balow JE, Costa JC, et al: Identification and classification of amyloid in formalin-fixed, paraffin-embedded tissue sections by the unlabeled immunoperoxidase method. *Lab Invest* 43:358–365, 1980.
201. Shirahama T, Skinner M, Cohen AS: Histochemical and immunohistochemical characterization of amyloid associated with chronic hemodialysis as β_2 microglobulin. *Lab Invest* 53:705–709, 1985.
202. Warnke RA, Kim H, Dorfman DF: Malignant histiocytosis (histiocytic medullary reticulosis), I: Clinicopathologic study of 29 cases. *Cancer* 35:215–230, 1975.
203. Scott RB, Robb-Smith AHT: Histiocytic medullary reticulosis. *Lancet* 2:194–198, 1939.
204. Pallesen G: The diagnostic significance of the CD30 (Ki-1) antigen. *Histopathology* 16:409–413, 1990.
205. Carbone A, Michaeau C, Caillaud JM, et al: A cytochemical and immunohistochemical approach to malignant histiocytosis. *Cancer* 47:2862–2871, 1981.
206. Mendelsohn G, Eggleston JC, Mann RB: Relationship of lysozyme (muramidase) to histiocytic differentiation in malignant histiocytosis: An immunohistochemical study. *Cancer* 45:273–279, 1980.
207. Falini B, Flarghi L, Pileri S, et al: PG-M1: A new monoclonal antibody directed against a fixative-resistant epitope on the macrophage-restricted form of the CD68 molecule. *Am J Pathol* 142:1359–1372, 1993.
208. Chang TK, Li CY, Smithson WA: Immunocytochemical study of small round tumors in routinely processed specimens. *Arch Pathol Lab Med* 113:1343–1348, 1989.
209. Kurtin PJ, Pinkus GS: Leukocyte common antigen: A diagnostic discriminant between hematopoietic and nonhematopoietic neoplasms in paraffin sections using monoclonal antibodies. Correlation with immunologic studies and ultrastructural localization. *Hum Pathol* 16:353–365, 1985.
210. Hachitanda Y, Tsuneyoshi M, Enjoji M: An ultrastructural and immunohistochemical evaluation of cytodifferentiation in neuroblastic tumors. *Mod Pathol* 2:13–19, 1989.
211. Gould VE, Lee I, Wiedenmann B, et al: Synaptophysin: A novel marker for neurons, certain neuroendocrine cells and their neoplasms. *Hum Pathol* 17:979–983, 1986.
212. Schmidt RA, Cone R, Haas JE, et al: Diagnosis of rhabdomyosarcomas with HHF35, a monoclonal antibody directed against muscle actins. *Am J Pathol* 131:19–28, 1988.
213. Azumi N, Ben-Ezra J, Buttifora H: Immunophenotypic diagnosis of leiomyosarcomas and rhabdomyosarcomas with monoclonal antibodies to muscle-specific actin and desmin in formalin-fixed tissue. *Mod Pathol* 1:469–474, 1988.
214. Cho KR, Olson JL, Epstein JI: Primitive rhabdomyosarcoma presenting with diffuse bone marrow involvement: An immunohistochemical and ultrastructural study. *Mod Pathol* 1:23–28, 1988.
215. Fitzmaurice RJ, Johnson PRE, Liu Yin JA, et al: Rhabdomyosarcoma presenting as "acute leukemia." *Histopathology* 18:173–175, 1991.
216. Schajowicz F: Ewing's sarcoma and reticulum-cell sarcoma of bone, with special reference to the histochemical demonstration of glycogen as an aid to differential diagnosis. *J Bone Joint Surg* 41A:349–356, 1959.

Part Two
PROCEDURES

All clinical laboratories, including hematopathology laboratories, must operate under standards and guidelines set forth by the Occupational Safety and Health Administration (OSHA) of the U.S. government. Of particular relevance to the hematology laboratory is the Bloodborne Pathogens Standard, which defines potentially infectious materials, contaminated waste, personal protective equipment, universal precautions, and work practice controls. The U.S. Department of Health and Human Services (HHS) has published guidelines on how to contain potentially infectious materials, how to discard contaminated waste, and how to use personal protective equipment. When practiced, these guidelines minimize the risk of exposure of health care and laboratory workers to infectious agents that may unknowingly be present in blood, body fluids, and tissue specimens. HHS has also listed criteria for four laboratory biosafety levels, Biosafety Levels (BSLs) 1–4, depending on the pathogenicity of the specimens and the risk level of activities in the lab. Most hematopathology labs would be classified as BSL-2. This level of risk dictates the use of standard and special laboratory practices, universal precautions, and personal protective equipment when handling specimens in the laboratory. Access to the lab should be limited, and a hazard warning sign should be posted on the lab door. Use of sharps should be minimized and should be discarded in a labeled, puncture-proof, spill-proof container ("sharps box"). Contaminated waste should be discarded in a labeled, leak-proof container ("red bag"). Generation of aerosols should be avoided when manipulating and processing specimens. If this cannot be avoided, the procedure should be done in a regularly inspected, approved laminar flow hood. Centrifuges should be equipped with tube holders and buckets specifically designed to contain the specimen in the event of a catastrophic tube failure.

Many of the procedures that follow involve the handling of potentially infectious materials. We advise the use of appropriate precautions and protective equipment when performing these procedures and tests.

Section 1
BUFFER SOLUTIONS

1.1 PHOSPHATE BUFFERS

Purpose

This series of phosphate buffers is commonly used in cytochemical and histochemical stains, especially for nonspecific esterase, naphthol AS acetate esterase, chloroacetate esterase, and aminocaproate esterase. Buffers with a variety of pH values can easily be obtained from two stock solutions.

Method

1. Solution A. Dissolve 9.47 g sodium phosphate (Na_2HPO_4) in 1.0 L distilled water (0.067 M).
2. Solution B. Dissolve 9.07 g potassium phosphate (KH_2PO_4) in 1.0 L distilled water (0.067 M).
3. With constant stirring, slowly add solution B to any volume of solution A until the desired pH is obtained.
4. These buffers are stable at room temperature for at least 3 months.

The pH of Common Phosphate Buffers

1. For nonspecific esterase in monocytes and for fluoride-resistant esterases: pH 6.3.
2. As a diluent for both Wright's and Giemsa stains: pH 6.6.
3. For naphthol AS acetate esterase in sinus lining cells: pH 7.0.
4. For chloroacetate esterase in neutrophilic granules and mast cells and for aminocaproate esterase in mast cells: pH 7.4.

1.2 TRIS BUFFERS

Purpose

A series of Tris buffers is often used in cytochemical and histochemical stains. The method of preparation is similar to that for the phosphate buffers.

Method

1. Solution A. Dissolve 6.06 g Trizma base in 1.0 L distilled water (0.05 M).
2. Solution B. Dissolve 7.88 g Trizma hydrochloride in 1.0 L distilled water (0.05 M).
3. With constant stirring, slowly add solution B to any volume of solution A until the desired pH is reached.
4. Tris buffers are stable at room temperature for at least 3 months.

The pH of Common Tris Buffers

1. For the demonstration of peroxidases and immunoalkaline phosphatase stains: pH 7.6.
2. For alkaline phosphatase of the blood vessels in tissue specimens (frozen): pH 8.0.
3. For leukocyte alkaline phosphatase in cytologic preparations: pH 9.1.

1.3 ACETATE BUFFER, 0.1 M, pH 5.2

Purpose

Acetate buffer is recommended for demonstrating leukocyte acid phosphatase and for demonstrating horseradish peroxidase activity in the immunoperoxidase method.

Method

1. Solution A. Dissolve 13.6 g sodium acetate in 1.0 L distilled water (0.1 M).
2. Solution B. Dilute 6.0 mL glacial acetic acid to 1.0 L with distilled water (0.1 M).
3. With constant stirring, add solution B to any volume of solution A until the solution reaches pH 5.2.

1.4 ACETATE-TARTRATE BUFFER, 0.1 M, pH 5.2

Purpose

Acetate-tartrate buffer is recommended for demonstrating TRAP.

Method

1. Dissolve 3.75 g l(+)-tartaric acid in 500.0 mL 0.1 M acetate buffer (Section 1.3).
2. Adjust the pH to 5.2 by adding 10.0 N sodium hydroxide in drops.

1.5 PROPANEDIOL BUFFER, 0.05 M, pH 9.8

Purpose

Propanediol buffer is recommended for demonstrating leukocyte alkaline phosphatase.

Method

1. Propanediol stock solution, 2.0 M
   a. Combine 35.64 g 2-amino-2-methyl-1,3-propanediol (previously liquefied by warming), 75.0 mL distilled water, and 32.0 mL 6.0 N hydrochloric acid.
   b. Add 4.0 mL 0.01 M magnesium chloride.
   c. Mix well and let stand overnight.
   d. Adjust pH to 9.8 with concentrated hydrochloric or sodium hydroxide and bring volume to 200.0 mL with distilled water.
2. Working propanediol buffer, 0.05 M, pH 9.8
   a. Dilute 1.0 mL stock propanediol buffer to 40.0 mL with distilled water.
   b. This buffer is stable at room temperature for at least 1 year.

SUGGESTED READING

Johnson B Jr: A new fluorometric method for the estimation or detection of total and fractionated alkaline phosphatase. *Clin Chem* 15:108–123, 1969.

1.6 CACODYLATE BUFFER, 0.1 M, pH 7.0 AND 7.4

Purpose

Cacodylate buffer is used to wash tissue specimens after fixation but before plastic embedding.

Method

1. Dissolve 13.8 g cacodylic acid in 900.0 mL distilled water.
2. Adjust pH to 7.0 or 7.4 with 10.0 N sodium hydroxide.
3. Bring volume to 1.0 L with distilled water.
4. Stored refrigerated, this buffer is stable for at least 6 months.

1.7 VERONAL BUFFER, 0.04 M, pH 7.6 AND 8.0

Purpose

Veronal buffer at pH 7.6 is for calf intestinal alkaline phosphatase, which is used as a positive control in the immunoalkaline phosphatase method. Veronal buffer at pH 8.0 is good for demonstrating alkaline phosphatase in vascular endothelial cells and in intestinal epithelium.

Method

1. Dissolve 3.89 g sodium acetate trihydrate and 5.32 g sodium barbiturate in 280.0 mL distilled water.
2. Add 160.0 mL of 0.1 N hydrochloric acid.
3. Adjust pH to 7.6 or 8.0 with concentrated sodium hydroxide and bring volume to 1.0 L with distilled water.
4. Stored refrigerated, this buffer is stable for at least 3 months.

1.8 PHOSPHATE-BUFFERED SALINE (PBS)

Purpose

The use of PBS is similar to that of the phosphate buffers (see Section 1.1) in cytochemical and histochemical stains.

Method

1. Dissolve 165.12 g sodium phosphate (Na_2HPO_4), 59.52 g potassium phosphate (KH_2PO_4), and 204.0 g sodium chloride in 2.0 L distilled water with stirring rod and heating.
2. Bring volume to 24.0 L with distilled water.
3. Stored at room temperature, this solution is stable for at least 3 months.

Section 2
FIXATIVES

2.1 BUFFERED FORMOL-ACETONE

Purpose

Buffered formol-acetone is a good general fixative for cytochemistry. It can be used with the esterases, peroxidase, β-glucuronidase, and Sudan black B stains.

Method

1. Dissolve 20.0 mg sodium phosphate (Na_2HPO_4) and 100.0 mg potassium phosphate (KH_2PO_4) in 30.0 mL distilled water.
2. Add 45.0 mL acetone and 25.0 mL of 37% formaldehyde solution.
3. Mix well before use. This solution has a final pH of approximately 6.6.
4. Stored at 4°C to 10°C, this solution will remain stable for 2 months.

2.2 BUFFERED METHANOL-ACETONE

Purpose

Buffered methanol-acetone is the preferred fixative for cytochemical demonstration of the acid phosphatases.

Method

1. Dissolve 0.63 g citric acid in 30.0 mL distilled water.
2. Add 60.0 mL acetone and 10.0 mL methanol.
3. Adjust pH to 5.4 with sodium hydroxide or hydrochloric acid.
4. Stored at 4°C to 10°C, this solution will remain stable for 2 months.

2.3 BUFFERED 60% ACETONE IN CITRATE

Purpose

Buffered 60% acetone in citrate is a suitable fixative for peroxidases and for acid and alkaline phosphatases.

Method

1. Dissolve 0.63 g citric acid in 40.0 mL distilled water.
2. Add 60.0 mL acetone.
3. Adjust pH to 5.0 with sodium hydroxide or hydrochloric acid.
4. Stored at 4°C to 10°C, this solution will remain stable for 2 months.

2.4 FORMOL-METHANOL

Purpose

Formol-methanol is a fixative used for leukocyte alkaline phosphatase.

Method

1. Add 10.0 mL of 37% formaldehyde solution to 90.0 mL absolute methanol.
2. Chill before use.
3. Stored at 4°C to 10°C, this solution will remain stable for 2 months.

2.5 FORMOL-ETHANOL

Purpose

Formol-ethanol is a satisfactory fixative for peroxidases and for demonstration of Epstein-Barr virus with in situ hybridization.

Method

1. Add 10.0 mL of 37% formaldehyde solution to 90.0 mL absolute ethanol.
2. Chill before use.
3. Stored at 4°C to 10°C, this solution will remain stable for 2 months.

2.6 MOTA'S FIXATIVE

Purpose

Mota's fixative is excellent for preservation of the metachromatic granules of mast cells and basophils.

Method

1. Add 1.0 g lead subacetate [$Pb_2O\ (CH_3COO)_2$)], 50.0 mL ethanol, and 0.5 mL glacial acetic acid to 40.0 mL distilled water.
2. Mix well.
3. Stored at room temperature, this fixative is stable for at least 1 month.

2.7 NEUTRAL BUFFERED FORMALDEHYDE

Purpose

Neutral buffered formaldehyde is a good general fixative for preservation of histologic specimens.

Method

1. Dissolve 7.572 g sodium phosphate (Na_2HPO_4) and 1.814 g potassium phosphate (KH_2PO_4) in 900.0 mL distilled water.
2. Add 100.0 mL of 37% formaldehyde solution.
3. Adjust to pH 7.4 with sodium hydroxide or hydrochloric acid.
4. Stored at room temperature, this fixative is stable for at least several months.

2.8 BAKER'S FORMOL-CALCIUM SOLUTION

Purpose

Baker's formol-calcium solution is used for preservation of enzyme activity in tissue specimens either before or after frozen sectioning.

Method

1. Dissolve 10.0 g calcium chloride in 900.0 mL distilled water.
2. Add 100.0 mL of 37% formaldehyde solution.
3. Add a handful of marble chips.
4. Stored at 4°C to 10°C, this solution will remain stable for 2 months.
5. Mix vigorously before use.

2.9 FORMOL-CALCIUM IN CACODYLATE BUFFER, pH 7.4

Purpose

Formol-calcium in cacodylate buffer is generally good for enzyme histochemistry in plastic-embedded sections. It is especially useful for preserving alkaline phosphatase and naphthol AS esterase in the sinusoidal cells of the spleen.

Method

1. Dissolve 10.0 g calcium chloride in 900.0 mL of 0.1 M cacodylate buffer at pH 7.4 (Section 1.6).
2. Add 100.0 mL of 37% formaldehyde solution.
3. Mix well.
4. Adjust pH to 7.4 with concentrated sodium hydroxide.
5. Stored refrigerated, this solution will remain stable for 2 months.

2.10 PARAFORMALDEHYDE-GLUTARALDEHYDE-ACROLEIN BUFFER

Purpose

Paraformaldehyde-glutaraldehyde-acrolein buffer (PGA) has been recommended as a fixative for enzyme histochemistry in plastic sections.

Method

1. Dissolve 9.0 g paraformaldehyde in 142.0 mL distilled water at 60°C.
2. To this solution add 150.0 mL of 0.2 M phosphate buffer [27.8 g sodium biphosphate (NaH_2PO_4) and 28.4 g sodium phosphate (Na_2HPO_4) in 1.0 L], 2.4 mL of 25% glutaraldehyde (electron microscopy grade), and 6.0 mL of 10% acrolein (electron microscopy grade).
3. Mix well and cool to room temperature.

4. Titrate final pH to 7.4 with concentrated sodium hydroxide.
5. Store in a dark bottle at 4°C to 10°C.
6. Shake well before use.
7. Prepare fixative fresh weekly.

SUGGESTED READING

Beckstead JH, Halverson PS, Ries CA, et al: Enzyme histochemistry and immunohistochemistry on biopsy specimens of pathologic human bone marrow. *Blood* 57:1088–1098, 1981.

2.11 B-5 FIXATIVE

Purpose

B-5 fixative is used for paraffin embedding of bone marrow biopsy specimens. It also preserves well the antigenicity of lysozyme, prostatic acid phosphatase, and immunoglobulin.

Method

1. Dissolve 13.3 g mercury chloride and 2.8 g sodium acetate (anhydrous) in 200.0 mL hot distilled water with stirring.
2. Allow the mixture to cool at room temperature for 24 hr and then filter into a brown jug for storage. Stored at room temperature, this solution is stable for 2 months.
3. Add 2.0 mL of 37% formaldehyde to a 20.0 mL aliquot of this mercury chloride solution for each biopsy specimen immediately before use.

Section 3
COUNTERSTAINS

3.1 BUFFERED 1% METHYL GREEN SOLUTION

Purpose

A buffered 1% methyl green solution is a suitable counterstain for chloroacetate esterase, nonspecific esterase, alkaline phosphatase, peroxidase, naphthol AS acetate esterase, and acid phosphatase.

Method

1. Dissolve 1.0 g methyl green (CI 42585) in 100.0 mL of 0.1 N acetate buffer at pH 5.2 (Section 1.3).
2. Mix well.
3. Titrate the pH of this solution to 4.2 to 4.5 with dilute hydrochloric acid or sodium hydroxide.
4. Place this solution in a separating funnel and extract it several times with chloroform until the chloroform layer is free of violet color. The supernatant is the pure buffered methyl green solution, which is used as a counterstain.
5. Stored refrigerated, this solution is stable for at least 2 months.

3.2 BUFFERED 0.5% NEUTRAL RED SOLUTION

Purpose

Buffered 0.5% neutral red solution is used as a counterstain for naphthol AS acetate esterase, peroxidase, and iron stains.

Method

1. Dissolve 1.0 g neutral red (CI 50040) in 200.0 mL warm 0.1 N acetate buffer at pH 5.2 (Section 1.3).
2. Mix well.
3. Filter and add a small amoun of sodium azide as a preservative.
4. Stored at room temperature, this solution is stable for at least 2 months.

3.3 GIEMSA STAIN

Purpose

Giemsa stain is used as a counterstain for the peroxidase stain and the Sudan black B stain.

Method

1. Filter commercially available Giemsa stain into a plasic bottle.
2. Cover bottle tightly to prevent evaporation of stain.
3. Store according to manufacturer's instructions.

3.4 MAYER'S HEMATOXYLIN

Purpose

Hematoxylin is a good counterstain for the PAS stain and for the TRAP stain.

Method

1. Dissolve 1.0 g hematoxylin, 50.0 g ammonium alum, and 50.0 g chloral hydrate in 1.0 L distilled water.
2. Add 0.2 g sodium iodate as the ripening agent.
3. Store at room temperature and allow 3 to 7 days for ripening before use. This solution is stable for at least 2 months.

Section 4
MISCELLANEOUS SOLUTIONS

4.1 HOLT'S GUM SUCROSE SOLUTION

Purpose

Holt's gum sucrose solution preserves most hydrolytic enzymes well, except naphthol AS acetate esterase and alkaline phosphatase.

Method

1. Add 60.0 g sucrose and 2.0 g gum arabic to 200.0 mL distilled water.
2. Mix well.
3. Add one small crystal of thymol as a preservative.
4. This solution has a final pH of approximately 4.8 to 5.2, which may drop to 4.0 on storage.
5. Stored at 4°C to 10°C, this solution will remain stable for at least 2 months. Discard when the solution appears turbid or contains fungal balls.

4.2 BUFFERED GUM SUCROSE SOLUTION

Purpose

Buffered gum sucrose solutions preserve many tissue hydrolytic enzymes, including alkaline phosphatase and naphthol AS acetate esterase.

Method

1. Add 60.0 g sucrose and 2.0 g gum arabic to 4.28 g sodium cacodylate in 100.0 mL distilled water.
2. Mix well.
3. Titrate to pH 6.6 with concentrated hydrochloric acid and bring volume to 200.0 mL with distilled water.
4. Add one small crystal of thymol as a preservative.
5. Stored at 4°C to 10°C, this solution is stable for at least 1 month.

4.3 PARAROSANILINE SOLUTION, 4%

Purpose

Pararosaniline, a coupling agent, is used for cytochemical and histochemical studies of chloroacetate esterase, acid phosphatase, nonspecific esterase, α-naphthyl acetate esterase, and β-glucuronidase.

Method

1. Dissolve 1.0 g pararosaniline (CI42500) in 25.0 mL hot 2.0 N hydrochloric acid.
2. Filter this mixture when it is cool.
3. Kept at room temperature away from direct sunlight, this solution is stable for at least 2 to 3 months.

4.4 NEW FUCHSIN SOLUTION, 4%

Purpose

New fuchsin, a coupling agent, is used for cytochemical and histochemical studies of chloroacetate esterase, aminocaproate esterase, and alkaline phosphatase.

Method

1. Dissolve 1.0 g new fuchsin (CI 42520) in 25.0 mL hot 2.0 N hydrochloric acid.
2. Filter this mixture when it is cool.
3. Kept at room temperature away from direct sunlight, this solution is stable for at least 2 to 3 months.

4.5 MOUNTING MEDIA

Media for Stains Not Soluble in Organic Solvents

1. Permount (Fisher Scientific): xylene-based synthetic medium.
2. Diatex (American Scientific Products): xylene-based synthetic medium.

Medium for Stains Soluble in Organic Solvents

1. Glycerin jelly
   a. Mix 10.0 g gelatin and 60.0 mL distilled water.
   b. Heat until gelatin is dissolved.
   c. Add 70.0 mL glycerin and 1.0 mL phenol.
   d. Mix well.
   e. Stored at room temperature, this solution is stable for at least 3 months.

4.6 AMINOALKYLSILANE-TREATED (SILANIZED) GLASS SLIDES

Purpose

To prepare glass slides to provide increased adhesiveness for tissue sections.

Method

1. Fill slide racks with glass microscope slides and soak in absolute ethanol to remove dirt and grease for two changes, 10 dips on each change. Prepare 500–600 slides at a time.
2. Drain slides and air-dry or dry in oven at 60°C.
3. Soak slides for 2 min in ethanol containing 490.0 mL of absolute ethanol and 10.0 mL of 3-amino-propyl-triethoxysilane (Sigma, St. Louis).
4. Rinse well in three changes of distilled water.
5. Drain and place slides in oven at 60°C for 30 min or until dry.
6. Store slides in a dust-free box, as everything will stick to them.

Comment

This method of coating slides is particularly useful, if not absolutely essential, when tissue sections are to be pepsinized for immunohistochemical staining. It can also be used for coating slides for routine staining. The greatest difficulty is that the section must be mounted in the desired place on the slide the first time the tissue is attached. The adhesive is so effective that the tissue is fastened to the slide, never to be removed.

SUGGESTED READING

Rentrop M, Knapp B, Winter H, et al: Amino-alkylsilane-treated glass slides as support for *in situ* hybridization of keratin cDNAs to frozen tissue sections under varying fixation and pretreatment conditions. *Histochem J* 18:271–276, 1986.

Section 5
CYTOLOGY AND CYTOCHEMISTRY

5.1 PREPARATION OF PERIPHERAL BLOOD SMEARS

Coverslip Method

1. Add one small drop of blood about 2.0 mm in diameter to the center of a coverslip (22 × 22 mm). Hold two corners of this coverslip between the tip of the index finger and thumb.
2. Place a second coverslip over the first so that an eight-pointed star is formed by the two coverslips.
3. Allow the blood to spread between the coverslips.
4. Grasp one of the corners of the second coverslip with the tip of the thumb and the index finger of the other hand.
5. Pull the coverslips horizontally away from each other.
6. Air-dry smears before staining.

Slide Method

1. Place one drop of blood about 3.0 to 4.0 mm in diameter on a microscope slide (75 × 25 mm) in an area about 10.0 mm from one end. Hold the slide in a horizontal position.
2. Place the end of a second slide on the first at an angle of 45°. The second slide should touch the first one between the end closest to the drop of blood and the drop of blood.
3. Move the second slide (still at a 45° angle) toward the blood until its edge touches the blood. Allow the blood to spread evenly between the point of contact between the two slides.
4. Push the second slide forward smoothly.
5. Air-dry smears quickly before staining.

5.2 PREPARATION OF SMEARS OF MARROW ASPIRATE

Coverslip Method

1. Place one drop of marrow aspirate with adequate marrow particles on a coverslip (22 × 22 mm). Remove excess blood with a Pasteur pipette.
2. Prepare smears in a manner identical to that for peripheral blood (Section 5.1). If the marrow blood with marrow particles does not spread evenly between the two coverslips, press or tap on the second coverslip gently to facilitate spreading.
3. Air-dry smears quickly before staining.

Slide Method

1. Place one large drop of marrow aspirate with adequate marrow particles on a microscope slide (75 × 25 mm). Remove excess blood with a pipette.
2. Place a second slide over the first. The longitudinal axis of the second slide is parallel to the longitudinal axis of the first.
3. Allow the marrow blood to spread evenly between the two slides.
4. Pull the two slides horizontally away from each other.
5. Air-dry smears quickly before staining.

5.3 PREPARATION OF TISSUE IMPRINTS

Method

1. Obtain fresh unfixed tissue and slice it with a sharp scalpel or razor blade. If necessary, trim the tissue into a small block (about 1 × 2 × 2 cm).
2. Pick up the tissue block gently with forceps. Blot the

freshly cut surface gently with blotting paper or gauze several times to remove excess blood or tissue fluids.
3. Imprint tissue on a clean slide gently two to four times. Allow enough room for labeling. Do not use a cut surface to make more than 10 to 12 impressions (three or four slides). For marrow biopsies, prepare imprints by rolling the biopsy specimen between two slides.
4. Air-dry imprints.
5. Stain with Wright-Giemsa stain (Section 5.7).
6. Rinse in water, dry, and mount in synthetic mounting medium (Section 4.5).

5.4 CAPILLARY METHOD FOR LEUKOCYTE CONCENTRATE (BUFFY COAT)

Method

1. Collect blood or marrow in four or more heparinized capillary tubes (1.5 × 75 mm, the kind used in microhematocrit determinations). Fill each tube at least three-fourths full.
2. Seal one end of each tube with clay, Critoseal (Sherwood Medical), or Critocaps (Sherwood Medical).
3. Centrifuge in an International hematocrit centrifuge (Damon/IEC) at 8000 g for 1 min.
4. Attach smallpox vaccination bulb to the end of the tube with the plasma layer (the open end). Break tubes about 2.0 mm below the buffy coat level with the aid of an ampule file.
5. Squeeze the bulb to deliver the leukocyte concentrate (buffy coat) layer to a glass slide or coverslip.
6. Prepare smears by placing another slide or coverslip over that with the leukocyte concentrates, compressing gently and pulling the slides or coverslips away from each other (Section 5.1).
7. Air-dry smears, stains, and mount in synthetic mounting medium (Section 4.5).

Comments

The capillary method is used to prepare buffy coat smears with a small amount of blood. It is most useful in blood with marked leukopenia and in "dry" marrow with few or no marrow spicules.

Note: Human blood and body fluids are potentially infectious materials. Breaking the capillary tubes may cause spraying of small glass fragments, and of blood and body fluids. Use universal precautions and appropriate personal protective devices when preparing smears.

Caution: Centrifugation can cause aerosols; exercise care when centrifuging blood or body fluids.

SUGGESTED READINGS

Mudrick P, Lee CL, Davidsohn I: Capillary test for "L.E." cells. *Am J Clin Pathol* 35:516–519, 1961.

Yam LT: Cytology of leukocyte concentrates. *Am J Clin Pathol* 62:679–684, 1974.

5.5 PREPARATION OF EFFUSIONS FOR CYTODIAGNOSIS

Method

1. Place 5.0 to 10.0 mL of effusion in a clean test tube containing a small amount of ethylenediaminetetraacetate (EDTA) or heparin. Mix well.
2. Centrifuge at 500 g for 5 min; discard supernatant. Remove excess fluid with gauze.
3. Mix sediment well, either with an applicator stick or with a siliconized Pasteur pipette.
4. Place one small drop of sediment on a clean slide. Place a second slide at right angles to the first slide. Slowly lower the second slide onto the specimen on the first slide. Apply gentle pressure to the second slide to facilitate spreading of the drop. The smear is made by pulling the second slide horizontally along the first slide.
5. Air-dry smears.
6. Stain with Wright-Giemsa stain (Section 5.7) or Riu's stain (Section 5.8).
7. Rinse in water, dry, and mount in synthetic mounting medium (Section 4.5).

Comments

Care must be taken to avoid clot formation in the effusion. After a clot is formed, the true cytologic pattern of the effusion is altered, and many cells are trapped in the clot. Effusions can be kept at 4°C to 10°C for 48 hr without significant deterioration of cell morphology. For solid mass aspirates, the aspirate is expelled directly onto a clean slide from the aspirating needle and smears are made according to steps 4 through 7.

SUGGESTED READING

Yam LT: A rapid method of preparing smears of effusions and solid mass aspirates for cytologic diagnosis. *Am J Clin Pathol* 47:797–801, 1967.

5.6 PREPARATION OF CEREBROSPINAL FLUID FOR CYTODIAGNOSIS

Method

1. Place 1.0 mL or more of fresh cerebrospinal fluid in a plastic or siliconized glass conical test tube. Centrifuge at about 500 g for 5 min.
2. Decant one-half to two-thirds of the supernatant. Add one or two drops of the patient's own serum or egg albumin. Mix with a siliconized Pasteur pipette.
3. Place two drops of fluid in each centrifuge cup of a cytocentrifuge. Centrifuge at 700 rpm for 5 to 7 min.
4. Allow sediment to air-dry for 10 to 30 min.
5. Stain with Wright's stain or Wright-Giemsa stain (Section 5.7).
6. Wash gently with water, dry, and mount in synthetic mounting medium (Section 4.5).

5.7 WRIGHT-GIEMSA STAIN

Reagents

1. 0.067 M phosphate buffer, pH 6.6 (Section 1.1)
2. Synthetic mounting medium (Section 4.5)
3. Wright's stain
   a. Filter commercially available Wright's stain into a plastic bottle.
   b. Cover the bottle tightly to prevent evaporation of stain.
4. Giemsa stain
   a. Filter commercially available Giemsa stain into a plastic bottle.
   b. Cover the bottle tightly to prevent evaporation of stain.

Method

1. Cover smears with Wright's stain for 3 min.
2. Add an equal volume of distilled water to smears and mix well by gentle blowing. Allow to stain for 5 min.
3. Wash smears with water.
4. Stain with dilute buffered Giemsa solution (1.0 mL Giemsa in 19.0 mL phosphate buffer) for 10 to 15 min.
5. Rinse in water, dry, and mount in synthetic mounting medium.

Comments

Wright's stain alone (steps 1 through 3) is sufficient for peripheral blood smears. In cytologic materials, such as smears of marrow, lymph node, spleen, and serous effusion sediments, Wright-Giemsa stain will result in better staining.

5.8 RIU'S STAIN

Reagents

1. Eosin yellow (CI 45380)
2. Methylene blue (CI 52015)
3. Methanol
4. Azure I (methylene azure, CI 52010)
5. Potassium phosphate (KH_2PO_4)
6. Sodium phosphate ($Na_2HPO_4 \cdot 12\ H_2O$)
7. Synthetic mounting medium (Section 4.5)
8. Solution A
   a. Dissolve 0.18 g eosin yellow and 0.07 g methylene blue in 100.0 mL methanol.
   b. Filter before storage.
   c. Store in a dark-colored bottle.
   d. This solution is stable at room temperature for 6 months.
9. Solution B
   a. Dissolve 0.7 g methylene blue, 0.6 g azure I, 6.25 g potassium phosphate, and 2.6 g sodium phosphate in 500.0 mL distilled water.
   b. Mix well and allow to stand at room temperature for 24 hr.
   c. Titrate the pH of this mixture to 6.4 to 6.6 with sodium hydroxide or hydrochloric acid.
   d. Filter before storage.
   e. Stored at room temperature, this solution is stable for at least 6 months.

Method

1. Cover air-dried smear with Solution A for 30 sec.
2. Add Solution B to Solution A on slide; mix well by gentle blowing. The amount of Solution B used is approximately twice that of Solution A. Allow to stain for 90 sec to 2 min.
3. Rinse in distilled water, dry, and mount in synthetic medium.

Results

Riu's stain is comparable to Giemsa stain, except that it gives a slight blue tint. The red blood cells are stained red-yellow, but they are not as bright red as those stained with the Wright-Giemsa stain. Excessive amounts of heparin may interfere slightly with the staining quality. This stain is useful for cytologic materials from effusions and solid-mass aspirates.

Comments

The staining of the cells with Riu's stain is similar to that of the May-Grünwald-Giemsa stain or other Romanovsky stains.

SUGGESTED READING

Yam LT: A rapid method of preparing smears of effusions and solid mass aspirates for cytologic diagnosis. *Am J Clin Pathol* 47:797–801, 1967.

5.9 PEROXIDASE METHOD (MODIFIED AFTER GRAHAM & KARNOVSKY)

Reagents

1. Fixative: cold buffered formol acetone (Section 2.1)
2. 3,3,diaminobenzidine tetrahydrochloride (DAB)
3. 3% hydrogen peroxide
4. 0.05 M Tris buffer, pH 7.6 (Section 1.2)
5. Counterstains
   a. Mayer's hematoxylin (Section 3.4)
   b. Giemsa stain (Section 3.3)
6. Synthetic mounting medium (Section 4.5)
7. Incubation medium
   a. Dissolve 5.0 mg of DAB in 10.0 mL of 0.05 M Tris buffer.
   b. Add 0.05 mL (one drop) of 3% hydrogen peroxide
   c. Mix well and use immediately.

Method

1. Fix smears in a cold fixative for 30 sec, rinse with water, and air-dry.
2. Incubate smears for 15 min at room temperature in the incubation medium.
3. Wash in water.
4. Counterstain for 3 to 5 min in hematoxylin. Rinse well and soak in tap water for several minutes. If Giemsa stain is used as the counterstain, immerse smears in a 1:20 dilution of Giemsa made in phosphate buffer, pH 6.6, for 5 to 10 min. Wash smears in water and rinse (dip twice) in 0.1 N acetate buffer, pH 5.2 (Section 1.4). Wash again in water.
5. Air-dry and mount in synthetic mounting medium.

Results

Enzyme activity in the leukocytes is indicated as dark brown granules in the cytoplasm of the granulocytes and monocytes. It may appear brown-black when Giemsa stain is used as the counterstain.

Comments

1. Enzyme activity may be enhanced if 0.01 M imidazole buffer, pH 7.6, is used.
2. Myeloperoxidase is most active at pH 7.6. Its activity decreases as the pH declines. On the other hand, horseradish peroxidase continues to be active at pH as low as 5.2. With the immunoperoxidase procedure, we prefer to carry out the peroxidase reaction at pH 5.2 to minimize the endogenous myeloperoxidase activity in the leukocytes.

SUGGESTED READING

Graham RC, Karnovsky MJ: The early stages of absorption of injected horseradish peroxidase in the proximal tubules of mouse kidney: Ultrastructural cytochemistry by a new technique. *J Histochem Cytochem* 14:291–301, 1966.

5.10 PEROXIDASE METHOD (MODIFIED AFTER GRAHAM, ET AL)

Reagents

1. Fixative: cold buffered formol acetone (Section 2.1)
2. 3-amino-9-ethylcarbazole
3. N,N-dimethylformamide
4. 0.05 M Tris buffer, pH 7.6 (Section 1.2)
5. 3% hydrogen peroxide
6. Mayer's hematoxylin (Section 3.4)
7. Glycerine jelly (Section 4.5)
8. Incubating medium
   a. Dissolve 2.0 mg of 3-amino-9-ethylcarbazole in 0.5 mL N,N-dimethylformamide.
   b. Add 9.5 mL Tris buffer and 0.05 mL (one drop) hydrogen peroxide.
   c. Use immediately.

Method

1. Fix smears in cold buffered formol acetone for 60 sec, rinse with water, and air-dry.
2. Incubate smears for 15 min at room temperature in the incubating medium and rinse well.

3. Counterstain for 3 to 5 min in hematoxylin. Rinse well and soak in tap water for several minutes.
4. Mount in glycerin jelly.

Results

Enzyme activity is indicated by a bright red precipitate in the cytoplasm.

Comments

Enzyme activity in the leukocytes may be further enhanced when 0.01 M imidazole buffer, pH 7.6, is used.

SUGGESTED READINGS

Graham RC, Lundholm U, Karnovsky MJ: Cytochemical demonstration of peroxidase activity with 3-amino-9-ethylcarbazole. *J Histochem Cytochem* 13:150–152, 1965.

Straus W: Peroxidase procedures: Technical problems encountered during their application. *J Histochem Cytochem* 27:1349–1351, 1979.

5.11 PEROXIDASE METHOD (HANKER'S METHOD)

Reagents

1. Fixative: cold buffered formal acetone (Section 2.1)
2. *p*-phenylenediamine dihydrochloride
3. Pyrocatechol
4. 0.05 M Tris buffer, pH 7.6 (Section 1.2)
5. 1% hydrogen peroxide
6. Buffered 0.5% neutral red solution, pH 5.2 (Section 3.2)
7. Synthetic mounting medium (Section 4.5)
8. Incubating medium
   a. Dissolve 5.0 mg *p*-phenylenediamine dihydrochloride and 10.0 mg pyrocatechol in 10.0 mL Tris buffer.
   b. Add 10.0 mL Tris buffer and 0.1 mL hydrogen peroxide.
   c. Use immediately.

Method

1. Fix smears in cold buffered formol acetone for 30 sec, rinse with water, and air-dry.
2. Incubate smears or sections in the incubating medium for 10 to 30 min at room temperature.
3. Wash in water.
4. Counterstain with neutral red for 1 min.
5. Wash in water, dry, and mount in synthetic mounting medium.

Results

Enzyme activity appears as dark brown to black granules in the cytoplasm of the leukocytes.

SUGGESTED READING

Hanker JS, Yates PE, Metz CE, et al: A new, specific, sensitive and noncarcinogenic reagent for the demonstration of horseradish peroxidase. *Histochem J* 9:789–792, 1977.

5.12 PEROXIDASE METHOD FOR PHI BODIES (MODIFIED AFTER HANKER ET AL.)

Reagents

1. Fixative: cold buffered formol acetone (Section 2.1)
2. 3,3-diaminobenzidine tetrahydrochloride
3. 0.067 M phosphate buffer, pH 7.4 (Section 1.1)
4. 0.1% hydrogen peroxide
5. Giemsa stain (Section 5.7)
6. Synthetic mounting medium (Section 4.5)
8. Incubating medium
   a. Dissolve 30.0 mg of 3,3-diaminobenzidine tetrahydrochloride in 40.0 mL phosphate buffer.
   b. Add 0.4 mL of 0.1% hydrogen peroxide.
   c. Use immediately.

Method

1. Fix smears in cold buffered formol acetone for 30 sec, rinse with water, and air-dry.
2. Incubate smears for 15 min at room temperature in the incubating medium.
3. Wash gently in running water.
4. Counterstain with Giemsa stain for 40 min.
5. Rinse with water, dry, and mount in synthetic mounting medium.

Results

Enzyme activity appears as dark brown granules in the cytoplasm of granulocytes and monocytes. Red blood cells also stain dark brown owing to the pseudoperoxidase activity of hemoglobin. The abnormal fusiform or spindle-shaped particles (phi bodies) and rods with hydroperoxidase activity in leukemic cells of acute myelogenous leukemia may be easily identified by this method.

Comments

3,3-Diaminobenzidine tetrahydrochloride may be a carcinogen and should be used with caution.

SUGGESTED READING

Hanker JS, Lazlo J, Moore JO: The light microscopic demonstration of hydroperoxidase-positive phi bodies and rods in leukocytes in acute myeloid leukemia. *Histochemistry* 58:241–252, 1978.

5.13 CYANIDE-RESISTANT PEROXIDASE FOR EOSINOPHILS

Reagents

1. Fixative: cold buffered formol acetone (Section 2.1)
2. 3,3-Diaminobenzidine tetrahydrochloride
3. 0.05 M Tris buffer, pH 7.6 (Section 1.2)
4. 3% hydrogen peroxide
5. Sodium cyanide
6. 1 N hydrochloric acid
7. 1 N sodium hydroxide
8. Synthetic mounting medium (Section 4.5)
9. Counterstains
   a. Mayer's hematoxylin (Section 3.4)
   b. Giemsa stain (Section 3.3)
10. Incubating medium
    a. Dissolve 5.0 mg of 3,3-diaminobenzidine tetrahydrochloride in 10.0 mL 0.05 M Tris buffer.
    b. Add 0.05 mL (one drop) of 3% hydrogen peroxide.
    c. Add 5.0 mg of sodium cyanide and mix well.
    d. Adjust pH to 7.6 with hydrochloric acid solution or sodium hydroxide solution.
    e. Use immediately.

Method

1. Fix smears in cold buffered formol acetone for 30 sec, wash with tap water, and air-dry.
2. Stain smears with the cyanide-containing incubation medium for 15 min at room temperature.
3. Wash in water.
4. Counterstain with hematoxylin or Giemsa stain for 5 min.
5. Wash in water, dry, and mount in synthetic mounting medium.

Results

Eosinophils and their precursors stain dark brown. Monocytes and granulocytes other than eosinophils are negative for this stain.

SUGGESTED READINGS

Archer RK, Broome J: Studies on the peroxidase reaction of living eosinophils and other leukocytes. *Acta Haematol* 29:147–156, 1963.

Graham RC, Karnovsky MJ: The early stages of absorption of injected horseradish peroxidase in the proximal tubules of mouse kidney: Ultrastructural cytochemistry by a new technique. *J Histochem Cytochem* 14:291–301, 1966.

Yam LT, Li CY, Crosby WH: Cytochemical identification of monocytes and granulocytes. *Am J Clin Pathol* 55:283–290, 1971.

5.14 CHLOROACETATE ESTERASE (NEW FUCHSIN METHOD)

Reagents

1. Fixative: buffered formol acetone (Section 2.1)
2. 0.067 M phosphate buffer, pH 7.4 (Section 1.1)
3. 4% new fuchsin solution (Section 4.4)
4. Fresh 4% sodium nitrite solution
   a. Stored at 4°C to 10°C, this solution should remain for 1 week without negative effects when used with the cytochemical stain.
5. Naphthol AS-D chloroacetate
6. N,N-dimethylformamide
7. Buffered 1% methyl green solution (Section 3.1)
8. Synthetic mounting medium (Section 4.5)
9. Fresh hexazotized 4% new fuchsin solution
   a. Mix equal volumes of 4% new fuchsin solution and 4% sodium nitrite solution.
   b. Allow to react for 1 min before use.
   c. This solution is fairly unstable and should be freshly prepared each time.
10. Substrate solution
    a. Dissolve 10.0 mg naphthol AS-D chloroacetate in 5.0 mL N,N-dimethylformamide.
    b. Stored at 4°C to 10°C, this solution is stable for 1 month.
11. Incubating medium
    a. Mix together 9.5 mL phosphate buffer, 0.05 mL fresh hexazotized 4% new fuchsin, and 0.5 mL substrate solution.
    b. Do *not* Filter
    c. Use immediately.

Method

1. Fix smears in cold buffered formol acetone for 30 sec. Wash in distilled water and dry.
2. Incubate fixed smears at room temperature for 10 min in the incubating medium.
3. Wash with tap water.
4. Counterstain with methyl green solution for 2 min.
5. Rinse in tap water, dry, and mount in synthetic mounting medium.

Results

Enzyme activity appears as bright red granules in the cytoplasm of mast cells and neutrophilic granulocytes, including promyelocytes and many myeloblasts. An occasional histiocyte may also be weakly positive for this enzyme.

Comments

Fast garnet GBC and fast blue BB or RR can also be used as couplers.

SUGGESTED READINGS

Moloney WC, McPherson K, Fliegelman L: Esterase activity in leukocytes demonstrated by the use of napthol AS-D chloroacetate substrate. *J Histochem Cytochem* 8:200–207, 1960.

Yam LT, Li CY, Crosby WH: Cytochemical identification of monocytes and granulocytes. *Am J Clin Pathol* 55:283–290, 1971.

5.15 NONSPECIFIC ESTERASE

Reagents

1. Fixative: cold buffered formol acetone (Section 2.1)
2. 0.067 M phosphate buffer, pH 6.6 (Section 1.1)
3. 4% pararosaniline solution (Section 4.3)
4. Fresh 4% sodium nitrite solution
5. α-Naphthyl butyrate
6. Ethylene glycol monomethyl ether
7. a. Buffered 1% methyl green solution (Section 3.1)
   or
   b. Mayer's hematoxylin (Section 3.4)
8. Synthetic mounting medium (Section 4.5)
9. Fresh hexazotized 4% pararosaniline solution
   a. Mix equal volumes of 4% pararosaniline solution and 4% sodium nitrite solution.
   b. Allow solutions to react for 1 min before use.
10. Substrate solution
    a. Dissolve 100.0 mg α-naphthyl butyrate in 5.0 mL ethylene glycol monomethyl ether.
    b. Stored at 4°C to 10°C, this solution is stable for 2 months.
11. Incubating medium
    a. Mix 9.4 mL phosphate buffer, 0.1 mL fresh hexazotized pararosaniline solution, and 0.5 mL substrate solution.
    b. Filter before use.
    c. Use immediately.

Method

1. Fix smears in cold buffered formol acetone for 30 sec, wash with water, and air-dry.
2. Incubate smears in the filtered incubating medium at room temperature for 45 min.
3. Rinse in water.
4. Counterstain with methyl green or Mayer's hematoxylin for 1 to 5 min.
5. Rinse in water, dry, and mount with synthetic mounting medium.

Results

Enzyme activity appears as dark red granules in the cytoplasm of the blood cells. The pattern of enzyme activity in the monocytes and histiocytes is intense and diffuse, whereas that in the lymphocytes is focal and well demarcated.

Comments

α-Naphthyl acetate is also a suitable substrate for the incubating medium, although it will be hydrolyzed by some granulocytes and plasma cells to give a positive staining reaction.

When the incubation time is increased to 2 hr, the enzyme activity in the lymphocytes also can be demonstrated.

Fluoride-resistant esterase activity in the histiocytes may be demonstrated by adding sodium fluoride, 15.0 mg/10.0 mL, to the incubating medium.

SUGGESTED READINGS

Li CY, Lam KW, Yam LT: Esterase in human leukocytes. *J Histochem Cytochem* 21:1–12, 1973.

Yam LT, Li CY, Crosby WH: Cytochemical identification of the granulocytes and monocytes. *Am J Clin Pathol* 55:283–290, 1971.

5.16 COMBINED METHODS FOR NONSPECIFIC ESTERASE AND CHLOROACETATE ESTERASE

Reagents

1. Fixative: cold buffered formol acetone (Section 2.1)
2. Incubating medium for nonspecifc esterase (α-naphthyl butyrate-hexazotized pararosaniline, Section 5.15)
3. 0.067 M phosphate buffer, pH 7.4 (Section 1.1)
4. Fast blue BBN (CI 37175)
5. a. Buffered 1% methyl green solution (Section 3.1)
   or
   b. Mayer's hematoxylin (Section 3.4)
6. Synthetic mounting medium (Section 4.5)
7. Substrate solution
   a. Dissolve 10.0 mg naphthol AS-D chloroacetate in 5.0 mL N,N-dimethylformamide.
   b. Stored at 4°C to 10°C, this solution is stable for 1 month.
8. Incubating medium for chloroacetate esterase
   a. Mix 9.5 mL phosphate buffer, 0.5 mL substrate solution, and 5.0 mg fast blue BBN.
   b. Use immediately.

Method

1. Fix smears in cold buffered formol acetone solution for 30 sec, rinse in water, and air-dry.
2. Stain smears for nonspecific esterase with the incubating medium for nonspecific esterase (Section 5.15).
3. Rinse in water and dry.
4. Incubate smears in the freshly prepared incubating medium for chloroacetate esterase at room temperature for 10 min.
5. Rinse in water
6. Counterstain with methyl green or Mayer's hematoxylin for 1 to 5 min.
7. Wash, dry, and mount in synthetic mounting medium.

Results

Nonspecific esterase activity appears dark red in the cytoplasm of the monocytes, and chloroacetate esterase activity appears blue in the neutrophilic granulocytes.

Comments

The cytoplasmic chloroacetate esterase activity, as demonstrated by this method, may not be entirely specific. Interpretation of weak enzyme activity in the blood cells should be made with caution.

SUGGESTED READINGS

Li CY, Lam KW, Yam LT: Esterase in human leukocytes. *J Histochem Cytochem* 21:1–12, 1973.

Yam LT, Li CY, Crosby WH: Cytochemical identification of the granulocytes and monocytes. *Am J Clin Pathol* 55:283–290, 1971.

5.17 ACID α-NAPHTHYL ACETATE ESTERASE FOR T LYMPHOCYTES

Reagents

1. Fixatives: use either of the following
   a. Cold general cytochemical fixative (Section 2.1)
   or
   b. Cold formol calcium in cacodylate buffer (Section 2.9)
2. 0.067 M phosphate buffer, pH 6.3 (Section 1.1)
3. α-Naphthyl acetate
4. Acetone
5. Fresh hexazotized 4% pararosaniline solution (Section 5.15)
6. Concentrated sodium hydroxide
7. a. Buffered 1% methyl green solution (Section 3.1)
   or
   b. Mayer's hematoxylin (Section 3.4)
8. Synthetic mounting medium (Section 4.5)
9. Incubating medium
   a. Dissolve 10.0 mg α-naphthyl acetate in 0.4 mL acetone.
   b. Add 37.0 mL phosphate buffer and 2.4 mL fresh hexazotized pararosaniline solution.
   c. Mix well.
   d. Adjust to pH 5.8 with sodium hydroxide.
   e. Use immediately.

Method

1. Fix smears for 30 sec at 4°C to 10°C, wash with water, and air-dry.
2. Incubate smears in the incubating medium at 37°C for 3 hr.
3. Rinse briefly with water.
4. Counterstain with either methyl green or Mayer's hematoxylin for 1 to 5 min.
5. Rinse with water, air-dry, and mount in synthetic mounting medium.

Results

Enzyme activity appears dark red. It is discrete and dot-like in the lymphocytes and diffuse and intense in the monocytes and histiocytes.

SUGGESTED READINGS

Knowles DM II, Halper JP, Machin GA, et al: Acid α-Naphthyl acetate esterase activity in human neoplastic lymphoid cells. *Am J Pathol* 96:257–278, 1979.

Pinkus GS, Hargreaves HK, McLeoad TA, et al: α-Naphthyl acetate esterase activity: A cytochemical marker for T lymphocytes. *Am J Pathol* 97:17–42, 1979.

5.18 PERIODIC ACID-SCHIFF (PAS) REACTION

Reagents

1. Fixative: absolute methanol
2. Malt diastase
3. Periodic acid
4. Basic fuchsin (CI 42500)
5. 1 N hydrochloric acid
6. Anhydrous sodium bisulfite
7. Activated charcoal
8. Mayer's hematoxylin (Section 3.4)
9. Synthetic mounting medium (Section 4.5)
10. Diastase solution
    a. Dissolve 500.0 mg malt diastase in 50.0 mL saline.
    b. Use immediately.
11. 1% periodic acid solution
    a. Dissolve 1.0 g periodic acid in 100.0 mL distilled water.
    b. Stored in the dark and at room temperature, this solution is stable for several days.
12. Schiff's solution
    a. Dissolve 1.0 g basic fuchsin in 200.0 mL boiling distilled water.
    b. Mix and cool to 50°C.
    c. Filter and add 20.0 mL of 1 N hydrochloric acid to the filtrate.
    d. Cool further to 20°C to 30°C and add 1.0 g anhydrous sodium bisulfite with gentle mixing.
    e. Keep this solution in the dark for 1 to 3 days.
    f. Add 2.0 g activated charcoal and shake for 1 min.
    g. Filter and keep the filtrate in the dark at 4°C to 10°C.
    h. This solution keeps well for several months.

Method

1. Fix smears in methanol for 10 min at room temperature, decant methanol, and air-dry.
2. If diastase treatment is desirable, place smears in the diastase solution at 37°C for 1 hr. Rinse in distilled water and dry.
3. Add periodic acid solution to smears for 7 min at room temperature, rinse in distilled water, and dry.
4. Stain with Schiff's solution at room temperature in the dark for 30 min to 1 hr.
5. Wash with running water for 10 min, dry, and counterstain with Mayer's hematoxylin for 1 to 5 min.
6. Wash, dry, and mount in synthetic mounting medium.

Results

Positive PAS stain is indicated by a diffuse pink color in the cytoplasm of the granulocytes and a granular pink color in the megakaryocytes, lymphocytes, and erythroblasts.

SUGGESTED READING

Wislocki GB, Rheingold JJ, Dempsey EW: The occurrence of the periodic acid–Schiff reaction in various normal cells of blood and connective tissue. *Blood* 4:562–568, 1949.

5.19 SUDAN BLACK B STAIN

Reagents

1. Fixative: cold buffered formol acetone (Section 2.1)
2. Crystal phenol
3. Absolute ethanol
4. Sodium phosphate ($Na_2HPO_4 \cdot 12\ H_2O$)
5. Sudan black B (CI 26150)
6. 70% ethanol
7. Buffered 0.5% neutral red solution (Section 3.2)
8. Synthetic mounting medium (Section 4.5)
9. Alcoholic phenol phosphate buffer
    a. Dissolve 32.0 g crystal phenol in 60.0 mL absolute ethanol
    b. Add 0.6 g sodium phosphate; then add distilled water until the volume reaches 200.0 mL.
    c. Stored at room temperature, this solution is stable for 6 months.
10. Stock Sudan black B solution
    a. Dissolve 0.3 g Sudan black B in 100.0 mL ethanol.
    b. Add alcoholic phenol phosphate buffer to a final volume of 200.0 mL.

c. Mix well.
d. Stored at room temperature, this solution is stable for 3 months.
11. Working Sudan black B solution
    a. Add 60.0 mL stock Sudan black B solution to 40.0 mL alcoholic phenol phosphate buffer.
    b. Mix well and filter before use.
    c. Stored at room temperature, this solution is stable for 1 month.

Method

1. Fix smears in cold buffered formol acetone solution for 30 to 60 sec, wash with tap water, and dry.
2. Stain smears in working Sudan black B solution for 30 min to 1 hr at room temperature.
3. Wash with 70% ethanol for 2 min.
4. Wash with tap water for 2 min and air-dry.
5. Counterstain with buffered neutral red for 10 min.
6. Rinse with water, dry, and mount in synthetic mounting medium.

Results

Positive staining is dark brown to black in the cytoplasm of mature and immature granulocytes and many myeloblasts. Monocytes are also weakly positive.

Comment

Giemsa stain also may be used as the counterstain.

SUGGESTED READING

Sheehan HL, Storey GW: An improved method of staining leukocyte granules with Sudan black B. *J Pathol Bacteriol* 59:336–337, 1947.

5.20 ACID PHOSPHATASE

Reagents

1. Fixative: cold buffered methanol acetone (Section 2.2)
2. 0.1 M acetate buffer, pH 5.2 (Section 1.3)
3. Naphthol AS-BI phosphoric acid
4. N,N-dimethylformamide
5. Fast garnet GBC salt (CI 37210)
6. Mayer's hematoxylin (Section 3.4)
7. Glycerin jelly (Section 4.5)
8. Substrate solution
    a. Dissolve 20.0 mg naphthol AS-BI phosphoric acid in 0.5 mL N,N-dimethylformamide.
    b. Add enough 0.1 M acetate buffer to make 100.0 mL.
    c. Stored at 4°C to 10°C, this solution is stable for 2 months.
9. Incubating medium
    a. Dissolve 5.0 mg fast garnet GBC in 10.0 mL substrate solution.
    b. Filter.
    c. Use immediately.

Method

1. Fix smears with cold fixative for 30 sec. Rinse briefly with distilled water and air-dry.
2. Incubate in the incubating medium at 37°C for 45 min.
3. Rinse with water.
4. Counterstain with Mayer's hematoxylin for 1 to 5 min.
5. Wash with water, dry, and mount with glycerin jelly.

Results

Enzyme activity appears as discrete red granules in the cytoplasm of the blood cells.

SUGGESTED READINGS

Janckila AJ, Li CY, Lam KW, et al: The cytochemistry of tartrate-resistant acid phosphatase: I. Technical considerations. *Am J Clin Pathol* 70:45–55, 1978.

Li CY, Yam LT, Lam KW: Acid phosphatase isoenzyme in human leukocytes in normal and pathologic conditions. *J Histochem Cytochem* 18:473–481, 1970.

5.21 TARTRATE-RESISTANT ACID PHOSPHATASE

Reagents

1. Fixative: cold buffered methanol acetone (Section 2.2).
2. 0.1 M acetate buffer, pH 5.2 (Section 1.3)
3. Naphthol AS-BI phosphoric acid
4. N,N-dimethylformamide
5. l(+)-tartaric acid
6. Fast garnet GBC salt (CI 37210)
7. Mayer's hematoxylin (Section 3.4)
8. Glycerin jelly (Section 4.5)
9. Substrate solution
    a. Dissolve 20.0 mg naphthol AS-BI phosphoric acid in 0.5 mL N,N-dimethylformamide.

b. Add 100.0 mL 0.1 M acetate buffer and 750.0 mg l(+)-tartaric acid.
c. Mix well.
d. Titrate pH to 5.2 with concentrated sodium hydroxide.
e. Stored at 4°C to 10°C, this solution is stable for 2 months.
10. Incubating medium
   a. Dissolve 5.0 mg fast garnet GBC in 10.0 mL of substrate solution.
   b. Filter.
   c. Use immediately.

Method

1. Fix smears with cold buffered methanol acetone for 30 sec. Wash briefly with distilled water and air-dry.
2. Incubate smears in the incubating medium at 37°C for 45 min.
3. Wash with water.
4. Counterstain with Mayer's hematoxylin for 1 to 5 min.
5. Wash with water, dry, and mount with glycerin jelly.

Results

Acid phosphatase activity appears as discrete purple to dark red granules in the cytoplasm of the blood cells. The presence of tartrate in the incubating medium almost completely inhibits enzyme activity in all types of blood cells. The neoplastic reticulum cells of hairy cell leukemia and a rare histiocyte from spleen and lymph node imprints from patients with other diseases have tartrate-resistant acid phosphatase activity.

SUGGESTED READINGS

Janckila AJ, Li CY, Lam KW, et al: The cytochemistry of tartrate-resistant acid phosphatase: I. Technical considerations. *Am J Clin Pathol* 70:45–55, 1978.

Li CY, Yam LT, Lam KW: Studies of acid phosphatase isoenzymes in human leukocytes: Demonstration of isoenzyme cell specificity. *J Histochem Cytochem* 18:901–910, 1970.

5.22 LEUKOCYTE ALKALINE PHOSPHATASE (KAPLOW'S METHOD)

Reagents

1. Fixatives: Use either of the following (see "Comments")
   a. Cold buffered formol methanol (Section 2.4)
   b. Cold buffered 60% acetone in citrate (Section 2.3)
2. Working 0.05 M propanediol buffer, pH 9.8 (Section 1.5)
3. Naphthol AS-BI phosphoric acid
4. N,N-dimethylformamide
5. Fast violet B salt (CI 37165)
6. Mayer's hematoxylin (Section 3.4)
7. Incubating medium
   a. Dissolve 5.0 mg naphthol AS-BI phosphoric acid in 0.2 mL N,N-dimethylformamide.
   b. Add 60.0 mL propanediol buffer and 40.0 mg fast violet B salt.
   c. Mix well.
   d. Filter.
   e. Use immediately.

Method

1. Fix air-dried smears in buffered acetone in citrate for 30 sec at 4°C to 10°C. Wash with gently running water and air-dry.
2. Incubate smears in the incubating medium at room temperature for 15 min.
3. Wash in tap water.
4. Counterstain with Mayer's hematoxylin for 1 to 5 min.
5. Wash in tap water, air-dry, and examine.

Results

Enzyme activity appears as bright red granules in the cytoplasm of both segmented and stab forms of human neutrophils. A rare lymphocyte also may be weakly stained. All other types of cells in blood are negatively stained. In human marrow, the capillary endothelial cells and the osteoblasts are also strongly stained.

Scoring Procedure and Interpretations

One hundred segmented or stab forms of neutrophils are rated visually from 0 to 4+ on the basis of the intensity of the precipitating dye:

0 = no granules
1+ = very few red granules
2+ = few to moderate number of granules
3+ = moderate to numerous granules
4+ = cytoplasm of the neutrophils is filled with granules

The sum of ratings in these 100 neutrophils is the score for the test.

The leukocyte alkaline phosphatase score in normal

adults is approximately 60 (range, 15 to 130). Because the scoring of enzyme activity is influenced by technical bias and by the reagents used, the normal range should be determined in each laboratory.

Comments

Both the fast violet B and naphthol salts should be kept in the refrigerator, preferably in a desiccator. Other substrates, such as naphthol AS phosphate, and couplers, such as fast blue BBN, also give satisfactory results.

Tris buffer, 0.2 M, at pH 9.1 to 9.4 is a suitable substitute for the propanediol buffer.

The formol methanol mixture exerts a stronger inhibitory effect on the enzyme activity but preserves the morphology of the cells better than the buffered acetone in citrate fixative. Formal methanol is not suitable as a fixative to preserve smears that are to be kept for long periods of time and serve for quality control procedures. It is the fixative of choice for specimens with eosinophilia and basophilia, in which preservation of excellent cell morphology for accurate cell indentification is essential.

Scoring of enzyme activity should be made in areas of the slide with optimal cell morphology. Avoid the edges of the smear and areas with cell overlapping and shrinkage.

Positive controls (specimens with high enzyme scores) should be run with the test slides. The control slides may be obtained from blood of patients with polycythemia vera, from patients with infectious leukocytosis with prominent toxic granules in the neutrophils, or from women in the third trimester of pregnancy. Several slides from the blood of such patients can be prepared, fixed in buffered acetone in citrate, dried, wrapped in Parafilm, and stored at −70°C for as long as 1 year without significant loss of enzyme activity.

If a blue precipitate is desired, the method using naphthol AS phosphate and fast blue BBN may be used. In cytologic material or tissue sections that are intended to be mounted and kept permanently, the method using naphthol AS-BI phosphate and hexazotized new fuchsin is the most suitable.

When the leukocyte alkaline phosphatase stain is used for demonstration of enzyme activity on the surface of the lymphocytes, the staining time may have to be extended to 30 min or 1 hr.

SUGGESTED READINGS

Kaplow LS: Cytochemistry of leukocyte alkaline phosphatase: Use of a complex naphthol AS phosphate in azo dye coupling technique. *Am J Clin Pathol* 39:439–449, 1963.

Kaplow LS: Alkaline phosphatase activity in peripheral blood lymphocytes. *Arch Pathol* 88:69–72, 1969.

Nanba K, Jaffe ES, Braylan RC, et al: Alkaline phosphatase–positive malignant lymphoma: A subtype of B-cell lymphomas. *Am J Clin Pathol* 68:535–542, 1977.

5.23 LEUKOCYTE ALKALINE PHOSPHATASE (RUTENBERG'S METHOD)

Reagents

1. Fixative:
   a. Cold buffered formol methanol (Section 2.4)
   b. Cold buffered 60% acetone in citrate (Section 2.3)
2. 0.2 M Tris buffer, pH 9.1 (Section 1.2)
3. Naphthol AS phosphate
4. N,N-dimethylformamide
5. Fast blue BBN (CI 37175)
6. Buffered 0.5% neutral red solution (Section 3.2)
7. Synthetic mounting medium (Section 4.5)
8. Substrate solution
   a. Dissolve 30.0 mg naphthol AS phosphate in 0.5 mL N,N-dimethylformamide.
   b. Add enough 0.2 M Tris buffer to bring the volume to 100.0 mL.
   c. Stored at 4°C to 10°C, this solution is stable for 2 months.
9. Incubating medium
   a. Dissolve 10.0 mg fast blue BBN in 10.0 mL substrate solution.
   b. Filter.
   c. Use immediately.

Method

1. Fix smears with cold buffered formol methanol for 30 sec. Rinse with several changes of distilled water and air-dry.
2. Incubate smears in the incubating medium for 15 min at room temperature.
3. Rinse with several changes of water and air-dry.
4. Counterstain with neutral red for 1 min.
5. Wash, dry, and mount in synthetic mounting medium.

Results

Enzyme activity appears as discrete blue granules in the cytoplasm of the neutrophils. Nucleus stains red.

Scoring Procedure and Interpretations

One hundred consecutive neutrophils are rated visually from 0 to 4+ on the basis of the number of stained granules in each cell:

0 = no granules
1+ = very few blue granules
2+ = few to moderate number of granules
3+ = moderate to numerous granules
4+ = cytoplasm of the neutrophils is filled with granules

The sum of ratings in these 100 neutrophils is the score of the test.

Normal scores range from 40 to 100. In patients who have chronic granulocytic leukemia, the score is less than 40, and often below 10. In patients who have polycythemia vera and bacterial infections, the score is greater than 100, and frequently above 150.

SUGGESTED READING

Rutenberg AM, Rosales CL, Bennett JM: An improved histochemical method for the demonstration of leukocyte alkaline phosphate activity: Clinical application. *J Lab Clin Med* 65:698–705, 1965.

5.24 ALKALINE PHOSPHATASE METHOD (MODIFIED AFTER LEARY ET AL.)

Reagents

1. Fixatives:
   a. Cold buffered formol acetone (Section 2.1)
   b. Cold buffered formol methanol (Section 2.4)
   c. Cold buffered 60% acetone in citrate (Section 2.3)
2. 0.05 M Tris buffer, pH 8.2, 9.1, or 9.5, containing 1 mM magnesium chloride
3. Ethylene glycol monomethyl ether
4. Nitroblue tetrazolium salt
5. 5-Bromo-4-chloro-3-indoxyl phosphate
6. Counterstain
   a. Mayer's hematoxylin (Section 3.4)
   b. Buffered 0.5% neutral red solution (Section 3.2)
7. Mounting medium
   a. Glycerin jelly (Section 4.5)
   b. Permount or Diatex
8. Incubation medium
   a. Dissolve 5.0 mg nitroblue tetrazolium salt in 0.5 mL ethylene glycol monomethyl ether.
   b. Add 9.5 mL Tris-magnesium chloride buffer.
   c. Add 2.5 mg 5-bromo-4-chloro-3-indoxyl phosphate and dissolve completely.
   d. Use immediately.

Method

1. Fix smears in a cold fixative for 30 sec, rinse with water, and air-dry.
2. Incubate smears for 15 to 30 min in the incubation medium at room temperature.
3. Wash with several changes of water.
4. Counterstain with Mayer's hematoxylin or neutral red, wash with water, and air-dry.
5. Mount in a mounting medium.

Results

Enzyme activity is indicated by a dark blue to blue-black precipitate.

Comments

This method is as sensitive as, if not more sensitive than, other methods for alkaline phosphatase. It is particularly useful in immunocytochemistry and in situ hybridization.

The reaction product of this method is slightly to moderately soluble in synthetic mounting media. Therefore, mounting with glycerin jelly is recommended. Hematoxylin is used as the counterstain, although the color contrast between hematoxylin and the reaction product is low. However, the reaction product is unaffected by mounting in Crystal Mount (Biomeda Corp., Foster City, CA). When this material is used for mounting, water-soluble counterstains such as neutral red or buffered Giemsa stain may be used.

SUGGESTED READINGS

Chu NM, Janckila AJ, Wallace JH, et al: Assessment of a method for immunochemical detection of antigen on nitrocellulose membrane. *J Histochem Cytochem* 37:257–263, 1989.

Leary JJ, Brigati DJ, Ward DC: Rapid and sensitive colorimetric method for visualizing biotin-labeled DNA probes hybridized to DNA or RNA immobilized on nitrocellulose:bioblots. *Proc Natl Acad Sci USA* 80:4045–4049, 1983.

5.25 TOLUIDINE BLUE O STAIN FOR BASOPHILS

Reagents

1. Mota's fixative (Section 2.6)
2. Toluidine blue O (CI 52040)
3. Synthetic mounting medium (Section 4.5)
4. Toluidine blue solution
    a. Dissolve 0.1 g toluidine blue O in 100.0 mL 30% ethanol.
    b. Stored at room temperature, this solution is stable for 6 months.

Method

1. Fix smears for 1 min at room temperature and rinse with water.
2. Stain with toluidine blue solution at room temperature for 2 min.
3. Wash with water, dry, and mount with synthetic mounting medium.

Results

Metachromatic granules are present in the cytoplasm of the basophils, mast cells, and their precursors. Rarely, toxic granules in the neutrophils may also appear as small, metachromatic granules, but they can be differentiated from those in the basophils by the tiny size of the toxic granules.

SUGGESTED READING

Yam LT, Li CY, Crosby WH: Cytochemical identification of monocytes and granulocytes. *Am J Clin Pathol* 55:283–290, 1971.

5.26 β-GLUCURONIDASE (MODIFIED AFTER LORBACHER, ET AL)

Reagents

1. Fixative: cold buffered formol acetone (Section 2.1)
2. 0.1 M acetate buffer, pH 5.2 (Section 1.3)
3. Naphthol AS-BI β-D-glucuronic acid
4. 0.05 M sodium bicarbonate (420 mg $NaHCO_3$ in 100.0 mL water)
5. Fresh hexazotized 4% pararosaniline solution (Section 5.15)
6. a. Mayer's hematoxylin (Section 3.4)
    or
    b. Buffered 1% methyl green solution (3.1)
7. Synthetic mounting medium (Section 4.5)
8. Substrate solution
    a. Dissolve 14.0 mg naphthol AS-BI β-D-glucuronic acid in 1.0 mL 0.05 M sodium bicarbonate.
    b. Add 0.1 M acetate buffer to a final volume of 100.0 mL.
    c. Stored at 4°C to 10°C, this solution is stable for 1 to 2 months.
9. Incubating solution
    a. Mix 10.0 mL substrate solution and 0.05 mL fresh hexazotized pararosaniline solution.
    b. Use immediately.

Method

1. Fix fresh smears in cold buffered formol acetone for 30 sec. Wash briefly in distilled water and air-dry.
2. Incubate smears in the incubating solution for 1 to 2 hr in a water bath at 37°C.
3. Wash smears with water.
4. Counterstain with Mayer's hematoxylin or methyl green for 1 to 5 min.
5. Wash with water, dry, and mount with a synthetic mounting medium.

Results

Enzyme activity is bright red, strong in the monocytes, and moderate to weak in the neutrophils. Activity is diffuse in the monocytes and granulocytes and granular in the lymphocytes. Absence of activity in the neutrophils indicates either that the smears are aging or that staining conditions are less than optimal.

Comment

This modified method is more sensitive than the original method.

SUGGESTED READINGS

Hayashi M: Distribution of β-glucuronidase activity in rat tissues employing the naphthol AS-BI glucuronide hexazonium pararosaniline method. *J Histochem Cytochem* 12:659–669, 1964.

Lorbacher P, Yam LT, Mitus WJ: Cytochemical demonstration of β-glucuronidase activity in blood and bone marrow cells. *J Histochem Cytochem* 15:680–687, 1967.

5.27 IRON STAIN (PERLS' REACTION)

Reagents

1. Fixative: absolute methanol
2. Potassium ferrocyanide ($K_4Fe(CN)_6 \cdot 3H_2O$)
3. Concentrated hydrochloric acid
4. Buffered 0.5% neutral red solution, pH 5.0 (Section 3.2)
5. Synthetic mounting medium (Section 4.5)
6. 2% potassium ferrocyanide solution
   a. Dissolve 1.0 g potassium ferrocyanide in 50.0 mL distilled water.
   b. Stored refrigerated, this solution is stable for 1 to 3 months. Stored at room temperature, it is stable for 1 week.
7. 2% hydrochloric acid
   a. Add 2.0 mL concentrated hydrochloric acid to 98.0 mL distilled water.
   b. Mix well and store at room temperature. It is stable for 1 month.
8. Working staining solution
   a. Mix equal parts of solutions of potassium ferrocyanide and hydrochloric acid.
   b. Use mixture immediately after preparation.

Method

1. Fix smears in methanol for 5 min and air-dry.
2. Place smears in working staining solution for 10 min, incubate at 37°C, wash with distilled water, and air-dry.
3. Counterstain with 0.5% buffered neutral red solution for 1 min, wash with tap water, and air-dry.
4. Mount in synthetic mounting medium.

Results

Hemosiderin stains blue-green; nuclei of cells stain red.

Comments

For optimal preservation of cell morphology, smears are used at least 1 to 2 hr after preparation.

For proper assessment of iron content in marrow, thick smears with plenty of marrow particles should be chosen for staining. Marrow smears known to have adequate iron should always be stained and used as a control.

SUGGESTED READING

Perls M: Nachweis von Eisenoxyd in gewissen pigmentosen. *Virchows Arch [Pathol Anat]* 39:42–48, 1867.

5.28 AMINOCAPROATE ESTERASE (TRYPSIN-LIKE ENZYME)

Reagents

1. Fixative: cold buffered formol acetone (Section 2.1)
2. 0.067 M phosphate buffer, pH 7.4 (Section 1.1)
3. Naphthol AS aminocaproate (Pierce Chemical)
4. Ethylene glycol monomethyl ether
5. Fresh hexazotized 4% new fuchsin solution (Section 5.14)
6. a. Mayer's hematoxylin (Section 3.4)
      or
   b. Buffered 1% methyl green solution (Section 3.1)
7. Synthetic mounting medium (Section 4.5)
8. Substrate solution
   a. Dissolve 20.0 mg naphthol AS aminocaproate in 10.0 mL ethylene glycol monomethyl ether.
   b. Stored at 4°C to 10°C, this solution is stable for 2 to 3 months.
9. Incubating medium
   a. Mix 9.0 mL phosphate buffer, 0.1 mL fresh hexazotized new fuchsin solution, and 1.0 mL substrate solution.
   b. Filter.
   c. Use immediately.

Method

1. Fix smears with cold buffered formol acetone solution for 30 sec, rinse with water, and air-dry.
2. Incubate smears at room temperature for 30 to 60 min in the filtered incubating medium.
3. Rinse with water.
4. Counterstain with 1% methyl green for 5 min.
5. Wash with water, air-dry, and mount in synthetic mounting medium.

Results

Enzyme activity appears as bright red granules in the cytoplasm of the mast cells.

Comment

If a blue reaction product is desired, fast blue BB or RR may be used in place of hexazotized new fuchsin.

SUGGESTED READINGS

Hopsu VK, Glenner GG: Further observations on histochemical esterase and amidase activities with similarities to trypsin. *J Histochem Cytochem* 11:520–528, 1963.

Yam LT, Yam CF, Li CY: Eosinophilia in systemic mastocytosis. *Am J Clin Pathol* 73:48–54, 1980.

5.29 MONOAMINE OXIDASE (METHOD OF GLENNER ET AL.)

Reagents

1. Fixative: cold buffered methanol acetone (Section 2.2)
2. Tryptamine hydrochloride
3. Sodium sulfate
4. Nitroblue tetrazolium
5. Phosphate buffer, 0.067 M, pH 7.6 (Section 1.1)
6. Mayer's hematoxylin (Section 3.4)
7. Glycerin jelly (Section 4.5)
8. Incubating medium
    a. Dissolve 50.0 mg tryptamine hydrochloride, 8.0 mg sodium sulfate, and 10.0 mg nitroblue tetrazolium in 20.0 mL phosphate buffer.
    b. Add 20.0 mL distilled water.
    c. Use immediately.

Method

1. Fix fresh smears or imprints in cold buffered methanol acetone for 30 sec at 4°C to 10°C, wash briefly with water, and air-dry.
2. Incubate smears in the incubating medium for 90 min at 37°C.
3. Rinse briefly with water.
4. Counterstain with hematoxylin for 1 to 5 min.
5. Wash with water, air-dry, and mount with glycerin jelly.

Results

Enzyme activity appears as purple granules in the cytoplasm of cells of the nervous system, including the tumor cells of neuroblastoma.

SUGGESTED READING

Glenner CC, Barner HJ, Brown CW Jr: The histochemical demonstration of monoamine oxidase activity by tetrazolium salts. *J Histochem Cytochem* 5:591–600, 1957.

Section 6
HISTOLOGY AND HISTOCHEMISTRY

6.1 PREPARATION OF PARAFFIN-EMBEDDED TISSUE SECTIONS

Reagents and Equipment

1. 10% neutral-buffered formaldehyde (Section 2.7) or another suitable fixative
2. Ethanols (80%, 95%, and 100%)
3. Xylene
4. Paraplast or other suitable tissue-embedding paraffin
5. Gelatin (granular type)
6. Tissue cassettes
7. Automated tissue processor (optional)
8. Embedding instrument
9. Rotary microtome with steel knife
10. Water bath (37°C to 45°C)

Method

1. Trim tissue specimens to 2 to 3 mm in thickness and approximately 20 × 25 mm in length and width. Specimen size depends on the size of the cassettes and embedding forms. Smaller specimens will require shorter fixation and processing times.
2. Place tissue in an amount of neutral-buffered formaldehyde at least 20 times that of the tissue volume and allow to fix overnight.
3. Place specimens in cassettes and dehydrate in graded alcohols with agitation as follows: 80% ethanol 2 to 4 hr, 95% ethanol 2 hr, 95% ethanol 1 to 2 hr, 100% ethanol 1 hr, 100% ethanol 1 hr, and 100% ethanol 1 hr.
4. Clear in three changes of xylene, 1 to 2 hr each.
5. Infiltrate with paraffin (60°C to 65°C), two changes, 2 hr each.
6. Remove tissue specimens one at a time, quickly place them in prewarmed embedding molds, and fill the molds with paraffin. Allow to cool and harden thoroughly, with or without the aid of a refrigerated surface (optional embedding center), before removing the embedded specimen.
7. Cut sections 4 to 6 μm thick with a rotary microtome equipped with a steel knife and float onto a warm-water bath (37°C to 45°C) to which 1.0 to 2.0 g gelatin has been added (be sure gelatin has been completely dissolved).
8. Pick up sections from underneath with clean microscope slides and allow them to air-dry thoroughly. Adherence can be enhanced by placing the dried slides in a 56°C oven for 30 min to 2 hr. Allow to cool.
9. Store until ready to stain.
10. Sectioned tissue blocks can be resealed by briefly dipping in molten paraffin and allowed to cool. Sections and blocks may be stored indefinitely.

6.2 PREPARATION OF PLASTIC-EMBEDDED TISSUE SECTIONS

Reagents and Equipment

1. 10% neutral buffered formaldehyde (Section 2.7) or another suitable fixative
2. 0.1 M cacodylate buffer, pH 7.0 (Section 1.6)
3. Ethanols or acetones (70%, 85%, and 100%)
4. Embedding monomer, catalyst, and cross-linking agent (these are commonly supplied as kits containing all necessary chemicals, such as Dupont/Sorvall's embedding medium kit or Polysciences' JB-4 embedding kit).
5. Commercially available plastic embedding molds and aluminum block holders
6. Rotary microtome (Polysciences' JB-4, Dupont/Sorvall) or other similar instrument equipped with a 0.5-in. glass knife.

Method

1. Trim tissue specimen to 1 mm in thickness and no larger than 10 × 15 mm in length and width.
2. Place specimens in fixative for 4 to 24 hr, depending on the size and type of tissue.
3. If enzyme histochemistry is desired, it is best to fix the specimens at 4°C and to remove the fixative by placing specimens in cacodylate buffer for 18 to 24 hr prior to processing.
4. Dehydrate tissue in graded alcohols or acetones as follows (for preservation of enzyme activity, use acetones for dehydration at 4°C): 70% alcohol 1 hr, 85% alcohol 1 hr, and 100% alcohol 1 hr. Dehydration can be performed more quickly if done in vacuo, 20 to 30 min each.
5. Prepare fresh, catalyzed monomer according to the manufacturer's instructions and infiltrate tissue in vacuo with two changes of monomer, 1 hr each. For enzyme histochemistry, perform this step at 4°C.
6. Prepare fresh embedding medium of catalyzed monomer plus cross-linking agent according to the manufacturer's instructions.
7. Remove tissue and dab excess monomer from the specimen with tissue paper. Place the tissue in the embedding mold and add embedding medium. Place the aluminum block holder over the tissue in the mold. Allow to polymerize for 75 to 90 min. Remove the hardened tissue block.
8. Cut sections 1 to 3 μm thick on a microtome equipped with a glass knife. Float sections onto a distilled water bath at room temperature with the aid of extra-fine needlepoint forceps.
9. Pick up each section from beneath with a clean microscope slide; allow it to dry thoroughly. Better adhesion of the section to the slide can be achieved by placing the dried slide on a hot plate set at a low setting for 2 min (this procedure is not recommended for enzyme histochemistry). Allow it to cool before staining.

6.3 PREPARATION OF CRYOSTAT SECTIONS FOR ENZYME HISTOCHEMISTRY

Reagents

1. Baker's formol-calcium solution (Section 2.8)
2. Albuminized coverslips or slides
   a. Smear small amount of Mayer's albumin fixative on a coverslip or slide.
   b. Dry in an oven at 140°C overnight before use.
3. Holt's gum sucrose solution (Section 4.1)

Method

1. Obtain fresh tissue and trim into small pieces approximately 1 × 1 × 0.5 cm. Fix in cold Baker's formol calcium solution.
2. After 2 to 4 hr of fixation, trim tissue blocks down to 0.5 × 0.5 × 0.2 cm; continue to fix tissue in the cold Baker's formol calcium solution for 15 to 24 hr.
3. Wash blocks briefly in cold water for 5 min; blot with water-absorbing paper. Immerse blocks in cold gum sucrose solution and store at 4°C to 10°C for at least 24 hr before sectioning.
4. Cut specimens 6 μm thick in a cryostat. Mount sections on albuminized coverslips or slides and store sections at 4°C to 10°C in tightly sealed envelopes before histochemical staining.

Comments

Enzyme activity in tissue blocks kept in cold gum sucrose solution can be preserved for several months (except the activity of naphthol AS acetate esterase).

Tissues fixed in Baker's formol calcium solution and kept in gum sucrose solution are also suitable for paraffin-embedded sections for conventional histologic examination.

6.4 HEMATOXYLIN AND EOSIN (H&E) STAIN

Reagents

1. Mayer's hematoxylin, obtained from a commercial source or prepared (Section 3.4)
2. Eosin Y (CI 45380)
3. Ethanols (70%, 80%, and 95%)
4. Glacial acetic acid
5. Xylene
6. Synthetic mounting medium (Section 4.5)
7. Alcoholic eosin, 1% stock solution
   a. Dissolve 1.0 g eosin Y in 20.0 mL distilled water.
   b. Add 80.0 mL 95% ethanol.
   c. Stored at room temperature, this solution is stable for 2 months.
8. Working eosin stain
   a. Mix one part stock eosin and three parts 80% ethanol.
   b. Add 0.5 mL glacial acetic acid to each 100.0 mL of working eosin before use.

Method

1. Deparaffinize sections in two changes of xylene for 10 min each.
2. Hydrate through graded alochols and finally through distilled water for 2 min each.
3. Stain with hematoxylin for 5 to 10 min, rinse well, and soak in tap water for 5 min.
4. Stain with working eosin for 1 to 2 min; rinse with water.
5. Soak in two changes of 70% ethanol for 2 min each.
6. Dehydrate in graded alcohols, 10 dips each.
7. Clear in two changes of xylene; mount with synthetic mounting medium.

SUGGESTED READING

Preece A: *A Manual for Histologic Technicians,* ed. 3. Boston, Little, Brown, 1972, pp 232–234.

6.5   GIEMSA STAIN (PARAFFIN)

Reagents

1. Absolute methanol
2. 0.067 M phosphate buffer, pH 6.6 (Section 1.1)
3. Wright's stain, obtained from a commercial source or prepared (Section 5.7)
4. Giemsa stain, obtained from a commercial source or prepared stock Giemsa solution and working Giemsa stain (Reagents 10, 11)
5. Giemsa powder
6. Glycerol
7. 1% acetic acid
8. Xylene
9. Synthetic mounting medium (Section 4.5)
10. Stock Giemsa solution
    a. Dissolve, with aid of mild heat, 1.0 g Giemsa powder in 66.0 mL glycerol.
    b. Let stand in 60°C water bath for 2 hr.
    c. Add 66.0 mL absolute methanol by stirring.
    d. Filter and store at room temperature; stable for several months.
11. Working Giemsa stain
    a. Just before use, add 50 drops stock Giemsa to 50.0 mL phosphate buffer.
    b. Mix.

Method

1. Deparaffinize and hydrate sections.
2. Rinse sections in two changes of absolute methanol for, 3 min each.
3. Stain with Wright's stain for 6 min; rinse with water.
4. Stain with Giemsa stain for 45 min. Treat each slide individually thereafter.
5. Differentiate nuclei by several dips in 1% acetic acid until nucleoli and chromatin are clearly visible.
6. Rinse in water and dehydrate quickly (two to five dips) through alcohols; clear in two changes of xylene.
7. Mount in synthetic mounting medium.

6.6   GIEMSA STAIN (PLASTIC)

Reagents

1. Wright's stain (Section 5.7)
2. Stock Giemsa solution (Section 6.5)
3. 0.067 M phosphate buffer, pH 6.6 (Section 1.1)
4. Working Giemsa stain
    a. Dilute one unit of stock Giemsa solution to nine units of phosphate buffer.
5. 0.5% acetic acid
6. Alcohols (70%, 95%, and 100%)
7. Xylene
8. Synthetic mounting medium (Section 4.5)

Method

1. Stain with Wright's stain for 1 hr; rinse.
2. Stain with working Giemsa stain for 2 hr to overnight. Treat each slide individually thereafter.
3. Rinse in water; dip 6 to 12 times in 0.5% acetic acid.
4. Rinse; dehydrate quickly, five dips each, in graded alcohols (70%, 95%, and 100%).
5. Clear in two changes of xylene. Check differentiation of nuclei before mounting.
    a. If color is too dark, take section back to 100% alcohol until desired color is obtained.
    b. If color is too pale, take section back through alcohols to water and stain longer in Giemsa stain.
6. Mount in synthetic mounting medium.

6.7 METHYL GREEN–PYRONINE STAIN (PARAFFIN)

Reagents

1. Disodium phosphate (Na_2HPO_4)
2. Citric acid
3. Methanol
4. Concentrated hydrochloric acid
5. Concentrated sodium hydroxide
6. Pyronine Y (CI 45005)
7. Methyl green (CI 42585)
8. 0.5% phenol solution (w/v)
9. 1% fresh resorcinol (w/v)
10. Acetone
11. Xylene
12. Synthetic mounting medium (Section 4.5)
13. Citrate/phosphate buffer, pH 5.3
    a. Mix 2.84 g disodium phosphate and 2.1 g citric acid in 25.0 mL methanol.
    b. Add 50.0 mL distilled water to dissolve.
    c. Titrate with concentrated hydrochloric acid or sodium hydroxide to pH 5.3.
    d. Add enough water to bring volume to 100.0 mL.
    e. Stored at 4°C, this solution is stable for 3 months.
14. Methyl green–pyronine solution
    a. Dissolve 0.25 g pyronine Y and 0.75 g methyl green in 0.5 mL of 0.5% phenol solution.
    b. Add 2.5 mL fresh resorcinol solution and 100.0 mL citrate phosphate buffer.
    c. Mix well.
    d. Allow mixture to age at room temperature for 2 to 3 days.
    e. Filter and keep at room temperature. It will remain stable for at least 3 to 4 months.

Method

1. Hydrate sections through graded alcohols to water.
2. Stain in methyl green-pyronine solution for 1 to 5 min.
3. Rinse briefly in three changes of water.
4. Dehydrate rapidly in two changes of acetone; clear in xylene, and mount in synthetic mounting medium.

Results

Cytoplasmic and nucleolar RNA stains red. Most intense cytoplasmic staining is seen in the plasma cells.

Comments

To prove that the red color is due to RNA, a control section is prepared by preincubating a slide in a 0.1% ribonuclease solution at pH 6.6 for 3 hr before staining in the methyl green–pyronine solution.

RNA in paraffin-embedded tissue is best preserved if the tissue is fixed in Carnoy's solution (methanol-glacial acetic acid, 3:1) before embedding.

If the red color in both the cytoplasm and nucleolus is weak, and if acetone removes too much of the red stain, slides may be washed in water after staining in methyl green–pyronine solution, blotted dry with bibulous paper, cleared in xylene, and mounted in synthetic mounting medium.

SUGGESTED READING

Luna LG (ed): *Manual of Histologic Staining Methods of the Armed Forces Institute of Pathology*, ed 3. New York, McGraw-Hill, 1968.

6.8 PERIODIC ACID–SCHIFF (PAS) REACTION (PARAFFIN)

Reagents

1. Periodic acid
2. Malt diastase
3. Saline solution
4. Basic fuchsin (CI 42500)
5. 1 N hydrochloric acid
6. Anhydrous sodium bisulfite
7. Mayer's hematoxylin (Section 3.4)
8. Activated charcoal
9. Xylene
10. Synthetic mounting medium (Section 4.5)
11. 1% periodic acid
    a. Dissolve 1.0 g periodic acid in 100.0 mL distilled water.
    b. Mix well.
    c. Stored at 4°C to 10°C, this solution is stable for 3 to 7 days.
12. 0.1% diastase solution
    a. Dissolve 50.0 mg malt diastase in 50.0 mL saline.
    b. Use immediately.
13. Schiff's reagent
    a. Dissolve 1.0 g basic fuchsin in 200.0 mL boiling distilled water.
    b. Mix and cool to 50°C.
    c. Filter and add 20.0 mL of 1 N hydrochloric acid to the filtrate.

d. Cool to between 20°C and 30°C and add 1.0 g anydrous sodium bisulfite with gentle mixing.
e. Keep this solution in the dark for 1 to 3 days.
f. Add 2.0 g activated charcoal and shake for 1 min.
g. Filter and store the filtrate in the dark at 4°C to 10°C. Solution is stable for several months.

Method

1. Deparaffinize and hydrate sections to water.
2. Incubate at room temperature in periodic acid for 5 min; rinse in distilled water.
3. For selective demonstration of connective tissues, digest sections in diastase solution for 60 min.
4. Incubate in Schiff's reagent for 15 min.
5. Wash in running water for 10 min.
6. Counterstain with hematoxylin for 5 to 10 min; wash in tap water for 5 min.
7. Dehydrate in alcohols, clear in xylene, and mount in synthetic mounting medium.

Results

A positive reaction should appear rose to purple-red.

Comments

PAS stain is useful for the identification of various substances, such as glycogen, mucin, fibrin, colloid, and amyloid. In this atlas, the major purpose of using PAS is to distinguish different kinds of lymphomas and leukemias (for details, see Part 1, Tables 3-1 and 3-2).

SUGGESTED READING

Luna LG (ed): *Manual of Histologic Staining Methods of the Armed Forces Institute of Pathology*, ed 3. New York, McGraw-Hill, 1968.

6.9   IRON STAIN (PERLS' REACTION)

Reagents

1. Potassium ferrocyanide
2. 10 N hydrochloric acid (36%)
3. Buffered 0.5% neutral red solution (Section 3.2)
4. Alcohols (95% and 100%)
5. Xylene
6. Synthetic mounting medium (Section 4.5)
7. 2% aqueous potassium ferrocyanide
   a. Dissolve 20.0 g potassium ferrocyanide in 1.0 L distilled water.
   b. Stored refrigerated, this solution is stable for 3 months.
8. 2% hydrochloric acid
   a. Dilute 40.0 mL 10 N hydrochloric acid to a final volume of 720.0 mL with distilled water.
9. Working solution
   a. Mix equal parts of 2% hydrochloric acid and 2% potassium ferrocyanide.
   b. Use immediately.

Method

1. Deparaffinize and hydrate sections to distilled water.
2. Incubatein working solution for 15 to 30 min.
3. Rinse in distilled water.
4. Counterstain with 0.5% neutral red for 3 to 10 min.
5. Rinse in water.
6. Dehydrate quickly in 95% and 100% alcohol, clear in xylene, and mount in synthetic mounting medium.

Results

Ferric iron stains bright blue; nuclei stain red.

SUGGESTED READINGS

Luna LG (ed): *Manual of Histologic Staining Methods of the Armed Forces Institute of Pathology*, ed 3. New York, McGraw-Hill, 1968.

Perls M: Nachweis von Eisenoxyd in gewissen pigmentosen. *Virchows Arch* [*Pathol Anat*] 39:42, 1867.

6.10   TOLUIDINE BLUE O STAIN

Reagents

1. Toluidine blue O (CI 52040)
2. Absolute ethanol
3. Xylene
4. Synthetic mounting medium (Section 4.5)
5. 0.1% Toluidine blue O solution
   a. Dissolve 0.1 g toluidine blue O in 30.0 mL absolute ethanol.
   b. Add 70.0 mL distilled water and mix well.
   c. Filter
   d. Stored at room temperature, this solution is stable for several months.

Method

1. Stain sections with 0.1% toluidine blue O solution at room temperature for 5 min.
2. Wash with water, dehydrate, and clear in alcohols and xylene.
3. Mount in synthetic mounting medium.

Results

Metachromatic granules are visible in the cytoplasm of basophilic granulocytes and mast cells. Plasma cell cytoplasm and stimulated lymphocytes are diffusely metachromatic.

SUGGESTED READING

Luna LG (ed): *Manual of Histologic Staining Methods of the Armed Forces Institute of Pathology,* ed 3. New York, McGraw-Hill, 1968.

6.11 GOMORI'S METHOD FOR RETICULUM

Reagents

1. Potassium permanganate
2. Potassium metabisulfite
3. Ferric ammonium sulfate
4. 10% silver nitrate solution
5. 10% potassium hydroxide, aqueous solution
6. 28% ammonium hydroxide
7. Sodium thiosulfate
8. 20% formaldehyde solution
9. 0.2% gold chloride solution
10. Alcohols (95% and 100%)
11. Xylene
12. Synthetic mounting medium (Section 4.5)
13. 0.5% potassium permanganate solution
    a. Dissolve 0.5 g potassium permanganate in 100.0 mL distilled water.
14. 2% potassium metabisulfite solution
    a. Dissolve 2.0 g potassium metabisulfite in 100.0 mL distilled water.
15. 2% ferric ammonium sulfate solution
    a. Dissolve 2.0 g ferric ammonium sulfate in 100.0 mL distilled water.
16. Ammoniacal silver solution
    a. Use acid cleaned glassware.
    b. To 10.0 mL of a 10% silver nitrate solution, add 2.5 mL of a 10% aqueous solution of potassium hydroxide.
    c. Add 28% ammonium hydroxide drop by drop, with continuous mixing, until the precipitate is completely dissolved.
    d. Add four more drops of silver nitrate solution.
    e. Bring solution to twice its volume with distilled water.
    f. Stored refrigerated until needed.
17. 2% sodium thiosulfate solution
    a. Dissolve 2.0 g sodium thiosulfate in 100.0 mL distilled water.

Method

1. Deparaffinize the sections and hydrate to distilled water.
2. Oxidize in potassium permanganate solution for 1 min and wash in tape water for 2 min.
3. Differentiate with potassium metabisulfite solution for 1 min and wash in tap water for 2 min.
4. Sensitize in ferric ammonium sulfate solution for 1 min.
5. Wash in tap water for 2 min; follow with two changes of distilled water.
6. Impregnate in the ammoniacal silver solution for 1 min and rinse in distilled water for 20 sec.
7. Reduce in 20% formaldehyde solution for 3 min and wash in tap water for 3 min.
8. Tone in gold chloride solution for 10 min and rinse in distilled water.
9. Reduce in potassium metabisulfite solution in 1 min.
10. Fix in sodium thiosulfate solution for 1 min and wash in tap water for 2 min.
11. Dehydrate in 95% and 100% alcohol, clear in xylene, and mount in synthetic mounting medium.

Results

Reticulum fibers stain black.

Comment

Gomori's method is useful for demonstrating marrow reticulum in myelofibrosis or other diseases, such as hairy cell leukemia and mast cell disease.

SUGGESTED READING

Luna LG (ed): *Manual of Histologic Staining Methods of the Armed Forces Institute of Pathology,* ed 3. New York, McGraw-Hill, 1968.

6.12 METHENAMINE SILVER STAIN

Reagents

1. Periodic acid
2. Methenamine (hexamethylene-tetramine)
3. Silver nitrate
4. Borax
5. 0.2% gold chloride solution (w/v), stored at room temperature; can be reused.
6. 3% sodium thiosulfate (w/v)
7. Buffered 1% methyl green solution, pH 4.2 (Section 3.1)
8. Alcohol (95% and 100%)
9. Xylene
10. Synthetic mounting medium (Section 4.5)
11. Periodic acid solution
    a. Dissolve 0.5 g periodic acid in 100.0 mL distilled water.
    b. Mix well.
    c. Stored at 4°C to 10°C, this solution is stable for 3 to 7 days.
12. Methenamine solution
    a. Dissolve 3.0 g methenamine in 100.0 mL distilled water.
    b. Stored at 4°C to 10°C, this solution is stable for at least 1 week.
13. Silver nitrate solution
    a. Dissolve 5.0 g silver nitrate in 100.0 mL distilled water.
    b. Mix well.
    c. Kept in a cold dark place, this solution is stable for 2 months.
14. Borax solution
    a. Dissolve 5.0 g borax in 100.0 mL distilled water.
    b. Mix well.
    c. Stored at room temperature, this solution is stable for 2 months.
15. Incubating solution
    a. Mix 10.0 mL of 3% methenamine solution, 0.5 mL of 5% silver nitrate solution, and 1.2 mL of 5% borax solution.
    b. Use immediately.

Method

1. Place sections in periodic acid solution at room temperature for 15 min.
2. Wash well in several changes of distilled water.
3. Place sections in the incubating solution at 50°C for 1 to 2 hr. After incubation for 1 hr, check sections frequently for optimal staining.
4. Wash in several changes of distilled water.
5. Tone in gold chloride solution for 2 min.
6. Wash in distilled water.
7. Place in sodium thiosulfate solution for 2 min.
8. Wash in tap water.
9. Counterstain with methyl green solution for 5 to 10 min, if needed.
10. Dehydrate in 95% and 100% alcohol, clear in xylene, and mount in synthetic mounting medium.

Results

Reticulin framework stains dark brown. Eosinophilic granules and hemosiderin also stain dark brown. Nuclei of most cells stain light brown. Nonspecific staining is usually minimal. This stain also outlines the sinuses of spleen well.

Comments

Methenamine silver stain is the best choice for outlining sinuses of the spleen. It is applicable to both cryostat and paraffin-embedded sections.

SUGGESTED READING

Jones DB, Nephrotic glomerulonephritis. *Am J Pathol* 33:313–330, 1957.

6.13 PEROXIDASE AND CYANIDE-RESISTANT PEROXIDASE

Reagents

1. 3,3-Diaminobenzide tetrahydrochloride
2. 0.1% hydrogen peroxide
3. 0.05 M Tris buffer, pH 7.6 (Section 1.2)
4. Sodium cyanide
5. 1 N hydrochloric acid
6. Buffered 1% methyl green solution (Section 3.1)
7. Alcohols (95% & 100%)
8. Xylene
9. Synthetic mounting medium (Section 4.5)
10. Incubating medium
    a. Dissolve 5.0 mg 3,3-diaminobenzidine tetrahydrochloride in 10.0 mL Tris buffer.
    b. Add 0.1 mL of 0.1% hydrogen peroxide.
    c. For selective demonstration of cyanide-resistant peroxidase, add 5.0 mg sodium cyanide to the incubating medium and titrate the pH back to 7.6 with 1 N hydrochloric acid.
    d. Use immediately.

Method

1. Incubate sections at room temperature for 30 min in the incubating medium.
2. Wash with water.
3. Counterstain with 1% methyl green for 5 to 10 min.
4. Wash with water, dehydrate and clear in alcohols and xylene, and mount in a synthetic mounting medium.

Results

Enzyme activity appears as brown granules. Peroxidase is strongly positive in all granulocytes, including neutrophils, eosinophils, and basophils. Cyanide-resistant peroxidase is positive only in eosinophils.

Comment

3,3-Diaminobenzidine tetrahydrochloride may be a carcinogen and should be used with caution.

SUGGESTED READING

Li CY, Yam LT, Crosby WH: Histochemical characterization of cellular and structural elements of the human spleen. *J Histochem Cytochem* 20:1049–1058, 1972.

6.14 PSEUDOPEROXIDASE FOR HEMOGLOBIN

Reagents

1. 0.05 M Tris buffer, pH 7.6 (Section 1.2)
2. 3,3-Diaminobenzidine tetrahydrochloride
3. Methanol
4. 0.1% hydrogen peroxide
5. Buffered 1% methyl green solution (Section 3.1)
6. Alcohols (95% & 100%)
7. Xylene
8. Synthetic mounting medium (Section 4.5)
9. Incubating medium
   a. Dissolve 5.0 mg 3,3-diaminobenzidine tetrahydrochloride in 7.0 mL Tris buffer.
   b. Add 3.0 mL methanol and 0.1 mL of 0.1% hydrogen peroxide.

Method

1. Pretreat sections in boiling water for 2 min.
2. Incubate sections at 37°C for 2 to 4 hr in the incubating medium.
3. Wash with water.
4. Counterstain with 1% methyl green for 5 to 10 min.
5. Wash with water, dehydrate and clear in alcohols and xylene, and mount in a synthetic mounting medium.

Results

The hemoglobin in erythrocytes and late erythroblasts stain dark brown.

Comment

3,3-Diaminobenzidine tetrahydrochloride may be a carcinogen and should be used with caution.

SUGGESTED READING

Li CY, Yam LT, Crosby WH: Histochemical characterization of cellular and structural elements of the human spleen. *J Histochem Cytochem* 20:1049–1058, 1972.

6.15 CHLOROACETATE ESTERASE

Reagents

1. Napththol AS-D chloroacetate
2. N,N-dimethylformamide
3. 0.067 M phosphate buffer, pH 7.4 (Section 1.1)
4. Fast blue BBN or freshly prepared, hexazotized 4% new fuchsin solution (Section 5.14)
5. Buffered 1% methyl green solution (Section 3.1)
6. Alcohols (95% & 100%)
7. Synthetic mounting medium (Section 4.5)
8. Substrate solution
   a. Dissolve 20.0 mg naphthol AS-D chloroacetate in 10.0 mL N,N-dimethylformamide; mix well.
   b. Store at 4°C to 10° before use. This solution is stable for 1 month.
9. Incubating medium
   a. Mix 9.5 mL phosphate buffer, 0.05 mL hexazotized new fuchsin, and 0.5 mL substrate solution.
   b. Use immediately.

Method

1. Incubate sections at room temperature for 30 min in the incubating medium.
2. Wash with water.
3. Counterstain with 1% methyl green for 5 to 10 min.
4. Wash with water, dehydrate with alcohols, air-dry, and mount in synthetic mounting medium.

Results

Enzyme activity appears as bright red granules in the cytoplasm of the neutrophilic granules and the mast cells.

Comment

For a blue reaction product, use 5.0 mg fast blue BBN instead of hexazotized new fuchsin.

SUGGESTED READING

Yam LT, Li CY, Crosby WH: Cytochemical identification of monocytes and granulocytes. *Am J Clin Pathol* 55:283–290, 1971.

6.16 NONSPECIFIC ESTERASE AND FLUORIDE-RESISTANT ESTERASE

Reagents

1. α-Naphthyl butyrate
2. Ethylene glycol monomethyl ether
3. 0.067 M phosphate buffer, pH 6.6 (Section 1.1)
4. Fresh hexazotized 4% pararosaniline solution (Section 5.15)
5. Sodium fluoride
6. Buffered 1% methyl green solution (Section 3.1)
7. Alcohols (95% & 100%)
8. Xylene
9. Synthetic mounting medium (Section 4.5)
10. Substrate solution
    a. Dissolve 100.0 mg α-naphthyl butyrate in 5.0 mL ethylene glycol monomethyl ether.
    b. Stored refrigerated, this solution is stable for 2 months.
11. Incubating medium
    a. Mix 9.4 mL phosphate buffer, 0.1 mL fresh hexazotized pararosaniline, and 0.5 mL substrate solution.
    b. Filter before use.
    c. For selective demonstration of fluoride-resistant esterase, add 15.0 mg sodium fluoride.
    d. Use immediately.

Method

1. Incubate sections for 30 min at room temperature in the filtered incbuating medium.
2. Wash with water.
3. Counterstain with 1% methyl green for 5 to 10 min.
4. Wash with water, dehydrate and clear in alcohols and xylene, and mount in a synthetic mounting medium.

Results

Fluoride-resistant enzyme activity appears as dark red granules, mainly in the cytoplasm of macrophages. The enzyme activity in spleen monocytes and sinus lining cells is fluoride-sensitive. The granulocytes and megakaryocytes are almost devoid of enzyme activity by this method.

SUGGESTED READING

Li CY, Yam LT, Crosby WH: Histochemical characterization of cellular and structural elements of the human spleen. *J Histochem Cytochem* 20:1049–1058, 1972.

6.17 COMBINED METHOD FOR NONSPECIFIC ESTERASE AND CHLOROACETATE ESTERASE

Reagents

1. Naphthol AS-D chloroacetate
2. N,N-dimethylformamide
3. Fast blue BBN
4. 0.067 M phosphate buffer, pH 7.4 (Section 1.1)
5. Buffered 1% methyl green solution (Section 3.1)
6. Alcohols (95% & 100%)
7. Xylene
8. Synthetic mounting medium (Section 4.5)
9. Incubating medium for nonspecific esterase (Section 6.16)
10. Substrate solution
    a. Dissolve 20.0 mg naphthol AS-D chloroacetate in 10.0 mL N,N-dimethylformamide.
    b. Mix well.
    c. Stored refrigerated, this solution is stable for 1 month.
11. Fast blue BBN incubating medium for chloroacetate esterase
    a. Dissolve 5.0 mg fast blue BBN in 9.5 mL phosphate buffer.
    b. Add 0.5 mL substrate solution.
    c. Filter.
    d. Use immediately.

Method

1. Incubate sections in incubating medium for nonspecific esterase for 30 min.
2. Wash with three changes of distilled water.

3. Incubate sections in fast blue BBN incubating medium at room temperature for 15 min.
4. Wash with water.
5. Counterstain with 1% methyl green for 5 to 10 min.
6. Wash with water, dehydrate and clear in alcohol and xylene, and mount in a synthetic mounting medium.

Results

In the spleen, nonspecific esterase is indicated by dark red granules in the monocytes, macrophages, and sinus lining cells. Chloroacetate esterase activity is indicated by discrete blue granules in the cytoplasm of the granulocytes.

SUGGESTED READINGS

Li CY, Yam LT, Crosby WH: Histochemical characterization of cellular and structural elements of the human spleen. *J Histochem Cytochem* 20:1049–1058, 1972.
Stutte HJ: Nature of human spleen red pulp cells with special reference to sinus lining cells. *Z Zellforsch* 91:300–314, 1968.
Yam LT, Li CY, Crosby WH: Cytochemical identification of monocytes and granulocytes. *Am J Clin Pathol* 55:283–290, 1971.

6.18 α-NAPHTHYL ACETATE ESTERASE FOR T LYMPHOCYTES

Reagents

1. α-Naphthyl acetate
2. Ethylene glycol monomethyl ether
3. 0.067 M phosphate buffer, pH 6.3 (Section 1.1)
4. Freshly prepared hexazotized 4% pararosaniline solution (Section 5.15)
5. Buffered 1% methyl green solution (Section 3.1)
6. Alcohols (95% & 100%)
7. Xylene
8. Synthetic mounting medium (Section 4.5)
9. Substrate solution
   a. Dissolve 100.0 mg α-naphthyl acetate in 5.0 mL ethylene glycol monomethyl ether.
   b. Cool solution to 4°C to 10°C before use.
   c. Stored refrigerated, this solution is stable for 2 months.
10. Incubating medium
    a. Mix 35.1 mL phosphate buffer, 2.4 mL fresh hexazotized pararosaniline, and 2.0 mL substrate solution.
    b. Adjust to pH 5.8 with hydrochloric acid.
    c. Filter before use.
    d. Use immediately.

Method

1. Incubate sections in the incubating medium for 2 to 3 hr at room temperature.
2. Wash with water.
3. Counterstain with 1% methyl green for 5 to 10 min.
4. Wash with water, dehydrate and clear in alcohols and xylene, and mount in a synthetic mounting medium.

Results

Enzyme activity appears as dark red granules. T lymphocytes exhibit a focal globular staining pattern, and monocytes exhibit diffuse, strong cytoplasmic staining.

SUGGESTED READINGS

Knowles DM II, Halper JP, Machin GA, et al: Acid α-naphthyl acetate esterase activity in human neoplastic lymphoid cells: Usefulness as a T-cell marker. *Am J Pathol* 96:257–278, 1979.
Pinkus GS, Hargreaves HK, McLeoad TA, et al: α-Napthyl acetate esterase activity: A cytochemical marker for T lymphocytes. *Am J Pathol* 97:17–42, 1979.

6.19 ACID PHOSPHATASE AND TARTRATE-RESISTANT ACID PHOSPHATASE (TRAP)

Reagents

1. l(+)-Tartaric acid
2. 0.1 M acetate buffer, pH 5.2 (Section 1.3)
3. Concentrated sodium hydroxide
4. Naphthol AS-BI phosphoric acid
5. N,N-dimethylformamide
6. Fresh hexazotized 4% pararosaniline solution (Section 5.15)
7. Buffered 1% methyl green solution (Section 3.1)
8. Alcohols (95% & 100%)
9. Xylene
10. Synthetic mounting medium (Section 4.5)
11. Acetate-tartrate buffer
    a. Dissolve 750.0 mg l(+)-tartaric acid in 100.0 mL 0.1 M acetate buffer.
    b. Titrate pH to 5.2 with concetrated sodium hydroxide.
    c. Stored refrigerated, this solution is stable for 2 months.
12. Substrate solution
    a. Dissolve 100.0 mg naphthol AS-BI phosphoric acid in 10.0 mL N,N-dimethylformamide.
    b. Mix well.

c. Stored at 4°C to 10°C, this solution is stable for at least 2 to 3 months.
13. Incubating medium
   a. Mix 9.5 mL acetate buffer, 0.05 mL fresh hexazotized 4% pararosiniline, and 0.5 mL substrate solution.
   b. For selective demonstration of TRAP, use 9.5 mL acetate-tartrate buffer instead of the acetate buffer.
   c. Filter and use immediately.

Method

1. Incubate sections for 30 min at room tempearture in the incubating medium.
2. Wash with water.
3. Counterstain with 1% methyl green solution for 5 to 10 min.
4. Wash with water, dehydrate and clear in alcohols and xylene, and mount in a synthetic mounting medium.

Results

Enzyme activity appears as bright red granules, mainly in the cytoplasm of macrophages. Various degrees of weak activity are also present in granulocytes and other cells. TRAP is present only in some specialized macrophages, such as Gaucher's cells, epithelioid cells, and hairy cells.

SUGGESTED READINGS

Janckila AJ, Li CY, Lam KW, et al: The cytochemistry of tartrate-resistant acid phosphatase: Technical considerations. *Am J Clin Pathol* 70:45–55, 1978.

Li CY, Yam LT, Crosby WH: Histochemical characterization of cellular and structural elements of the human spleen. *J Histochem Cytochem* 20:1049–1058, 1972.

6.20 ALKALINE PHOSPHATASE

Reagents

1. Naphthol AS phosphate
2. *N,N*-dimethylformamide
3. 0.04 M veronal buffer, pH 8.0 (Section 1.7)
4. Fresh hexazotized 4% new fuchsin solution (Section 5.14) or fast blue BBN
5. Buffered 1% methyl green solution (Section 3.1)
6. Alcohols (95% & 100%)
7. Xylene
8. Synthetic mounting medium (Section 4.5)
9. Substrate solution
   a. Dissolve 30.0 mg naphthol AS phosphate in 3.0 mL *N,N*-dimethylformamide.
   b. Cool this solution to 4°C to 10°C before use. Stored at this temperature, this solution is stable for 2 months.
10. Incubating medium
    a. Mix 9.7 mL veronal buffer, 0.05 mL fresh hexazotized 4% new fuchsin, and 0.3 mL substrate solution.
    b. Use immediately.

Method

1. Incubate sections for 30 to 60 min at 37°C in the incubating medium.
2. Wash with water.
3. Counterstain with 1% methyl green for 1 to 2 min.
4. Wash with water, dehydrate and clear in alcohols and xylene, and mount in synthetic mounting medium.

Results

Enzyme activity appears as bright red granules in the cytoplasm of vascular endothelium. The enzyme activity is insignificant in the granulocytes.

Comments

Naphthol AS-BI phosphoric acid also can give a bright red reaction product. Prepare the incubating medium as follows: Dissolve 5.0 mg naphthol AS-BI phosphoric acid in 0.5 mL *N,N*-dimethylformamide. Add 9.5 mL Tris buffer (0.2 M, pH 9.1—Section 1.2) and 0.05 mL hexazotized 1% new fuchsin solution (Section 5.14). Incubate the sections in this solution for 1 to 2 hr at 37°C.

For a blue color, use 5.0 mg fast blue BBN instead of hexazotized new fuchsin.

SUGGESTED READINGS

Li CY, Yam LT, Crosby YH: Histochemical characterization of cellular and structural elements of the human spleen. *J Histochem Cytochem* 20:1049–1058, 1972.

Stutte HJ: Hexazotiertes triamino-tritolyl-methanchlorid (neufuchsin) als kupplungssalz in der fermenthistochemie. *Histochemie* 8:327–331, 1967.

6.21 AMINOCAPROATE ESTERASE (TRYPSIN-LIKE ENZYME)

Reagents

1. Naphthol AS aminocaproate (Pierce)
2. Ethylene glycol monomethyl ether
3. 0.067 M phosphate buffer, pH 7.4 (Section 1.1)
4. Fresh hexazotized 4% new fuchsin solution (Section 5.14)
5. Buffered 1% methyl green solution (Section 3.1)
6. Alcohols (95% & 100%)
7. Xylene
8. Synthetic mounting medium (Section 4.5)
9. Substrate solution
   a. Dissolve 20.0 mg naphthol AS aminocaproate in 10.0 mL ethylene glycol monomethyl ether.
   b. Stored at 4°C to 10°C, this solution remains stable for 2 to 3 months.
10. Incubating medium
    a. Mix 9.0 mL phosphate buffer, 0.1 mL fresh hexazotized 4% new fuchsin, and 1.0 mL substrate solution.
    b. Filter before use.
    c. Use immediately.

Method

1. Incubate sections at room temperature for 30 min in the filtered incubating medium.
2. Wash with water.
3. Counterstain with 1% methyl green for 5 min.
4. Wash with water, dehydrate and clear in alcohols and xylene, and mount in a synthetic mounting medium.

Results

Enzyme activity appears as bright red granules in the cytoplasm of the mast cells.

SUGGESTED READINGS

Hopsu VK, Glenner GG: Further observations on histochemical esterase and amidase activities with similarities to trypsin. *J Histochem Cytochem* 11:520–528, 1963.

Li CY, Yam LT, Crosby WH: Histochemical characterization of cellular and structural elements of the human spleen. *J Histochem Cytochem* 20:1049–1058, 1972.

Yam LT, Yam CF, Li CY: Eosinophilia in systemic mastocytosis. *Am J Clin Pathol* 73:48–54, 1980.

6.22 CHLORAZOL FAST PINK

Reagents

1. Chlorazol fast pink (CI 25380)
2. 50% ethanol
3. Buffered 1% methyl green solution (Section 3.1)
4. Alcohols (95% & 100%)
5. Xylene
6. Synthetic mounting medium (Section 4.5)
7. 1% chlorazol fast pink in 50% ethanol
   a. Dissolve 1.0 g chlorazol fast pink in 100.0 mL 50% ethanol.

Method

1. Hydrate deparaffinized section to water if a paraffin section is used.
2. Incubate section for 30 min at room temperature in 1% chlorazol fast pink in 50% ethanol.
3. Wash with water.
4. Counterstain with 1% methyl green for 5 to 10 min.
5. Wash with water, dehydrate and clear in alcohols and xylene, and mount in a synthetic mounting medium.

Results

Eosinophils stain reddish, whereas other cell types remain unstained.

SUGGESTED READING

Maeda R, Kanazawa K, Nakano E, et al: Studies on the specificity of the chlorazol fast pink staining method. *Acta Histochem Cytochem* 3:65–73, 1970.

6.23 NAPHTHOL AS ACETATE ESTERASE

Reagents

1. Naphthol AS acetate
2. Ethylene glycol monomethyl ether
3. Fast blue BBN
4. 0.067 M phosphate buffer, pH 7.0 (Section 1.1)
5. a. Buffered 1% methyl green solution (Section 3.1)
   or
   b. Buffered 0.5% neutral red solution (Section 3.2)
6. Alcohols (95% & 100%)
7. Xylene
8. Synthetic mounting medium (Section 4.5)
9. Substrate solution

a. Dissolve 25.0 mg naphthol AS acetate in 10.0 mL ethylene glycol monomethyl ether.
   b. Mix well.
   c. Stored at 4°C to 10°C, this solution is stable for 2 to 3 months.
10. Incubating medium
    a. Dissolve 5.0 mg fast blue BBN in 9.0 mL phosphate buffer.
    b. Add 1.0 mL substrate solution.
    c. Filter
    d. Use immediately.

Method

1. Incubate sections at 37°C for 15 min in the incubating medium.
2. Wash with water.
3. Counterstain with 1% methyl green for 5 to 10 min or with 1% neutral red for 2 min.
4. Wash with water, dehydrate, clear in alcohols and xylene briefly, and mount in a synthetic mounting medium.

Results

Enzyme activity appears as discrete blue granules. In the spleen, activity is seen in sinus lining cells. Some of the macrophages in the cords of Billroth and in megakaryocytes may also show various degrees of activity.

Comments

If a bright red naphthol AS acetate esterase stain is desired, the fast blue BBN can be replaced by 0.05 mL hexazotized 4% new fuchsin method is less sensitive than the fast blue BBN method.

SUGGESTED READINGS

Li CY, Yam LT, Crosby WH: Histochemical characterization of cellular and structural elements of the human spleen. *J Histochem Cytochem* 20:1049–1058, 1972.

Stutte HJ: Nature of human spleen red pulp cells with special reference to sinus lining cells. *Z Zellforsch* 91:300–314, 1968.

Section 7
IMMUNOLOGY AND IMMUNOFLUORESCENCE

7.1 T-CELL AND B-CELL IDENTIFICATION AND QUANTITATION

Preparation of Mononuclear Cell Suspension from Peripheral Blood or Bone Marrow Aspirate

Principle

The separation of cells on a Ficoll-Hypaque gradient is a method that is frequently used to obtain a mononuclear cell population. This technique is based on density gradient separation and involves careful layering of a diluted blood sample over a Ficoll and sodium diatrizoate solution (Lymphoprep). After the gradient is centrifuged, the mononuclear cells are removed at the resulting interface. Granulocytes, red blood cells, and dead cells aggregate and pellet at the bottom of the separation tube.

Specimen Requirement

Specimens of blood or bone marrow aspirate are collected in heparinized tubes or syringes. These specimens should be stored at room temperature and processed as soon as possible. At least 2.0 mL of bone marrow aspirate is usually needed to perform a monoclonal antibody panel. For a normal white blood cell count, 30.0 to 40.0 mL of peripheral blood is required to perform a SIg and monoclonal antibody profile.

Equipment and Materials

1. Polypropylene conical centrifuge tubes
2. 20.0 mL syringe
3. 18-gauge × 3½-in. spinal needle
4. Refrigerated centrifuge

Reagents

1. Lymphoprep (Ficoll-Hypaque)
2. 0.9% sodium chloride (room temperature)
3. RPMI-1640 with L-glutamine (4°C)

Method

1. Place blood or bone marrow into an appropriately sized conical centrifuge tube. Dilute with an equal volume of 0.9% sodium chloride at room temperature. Mix gently.
2. Using a syringe with an 18-gauge × 3½-in. spinal needle attached, carefully underlay the diluted specimen with a volume of Ficoll equal to the original sample volume. This method creates a cleaner interface than those obtained when blood is layered over Ficoll because of decreased disruption of the separation media.
3. Centrifuge at room temperature for 30 min at 400 g.
4. Erythrocytes, granulocytes, and dead cells will sink to the bottom of the tube. Mononuclear cells should form a visible layer at the plasma–Ficoll junction. Aspirate some of the plasma without disturbing the interface. Use a transfer pipette to remove the mononuclear layer, and place in a 17 × 100 mm centrifuge tube.
5. Centrifuge the cell suspension at 4°C for 5 min at 400 g. If the cell button is contaminated by red blood cells, treat with ammonium chloride (see "0.83% Ammonium Chloride Treatment for Red Blood Cell Lysis"). If no red cells are visible, continue with step 6.
6. Aspirate the supernatant. Add 10.0 mL of cold RPMI-1640 to the cell pellet. Vortex. Centrifuge at 4°C for 5 min at 400 g.
7. Repeat step 6.
8. Aspirate the supernatant and resuspend the cell pellet in RPMI-1640. The volume of the diluent will vary according to the size of the cell pellet. Count the cells

on a hemacytometer or automated cell counter. Adjust the final cell concentration to 10×10^6 cells/mL.
9. Determine cell viability (see "Determination of Cell Viability").

Note: Ficoll should be used at room temperature. Store at 4°C protected from light.

Preparation of Single Cell Suspensions from Lymphoid Tissue

Specimen Requirement

The specimen should be delivered fresh in saline from the operating room (tissue fixed in formalin cannot be used). Place a portion of tissue (0.5 cm diameter minimum) in a 17 × 100 mm tube containing 10.0 mL cold RPMI media and store at 4°C until ready to process. Do not freeze tissue. For overnight storage, immerse tissue in RPMI-1640 media was supplemented with 20% heat-inactivated fetal calf serum and 100.0 U/mL penicillin-streptomycin.

Materials and Equipment

1. 100 × 17 mm capped centrifuge tube
2. 100 × 15 mm Petri dish
3. 22-gauge × 1½-in. needle
4. Surgical blade
5. Transfer pipet
6. 53 μm nylon mesh
7. Refrigerated centrifuge

Reagents

1. RPMI-1640 with L-glutamine (Gibco)
2. RPMI complete (100.0 mL total volume); 79.0 mL RPMI-1640 with L-glutamine; 20.0 mL heat-inactivated fetal calf serum; 1.0 mL penicillin-streptomycin at 10,000 U/mL
3. 0.83% ammonium chloride (prepare up to 1000.0 mL with distilled water); 8.3 g ammonium chloride (NH_4CL); 1.0 g potassium carbonate ($KHCO_3$); 0.04 g EDTA

Method

1. Place the tissue specimen in a disposable Petri dish (100 × 15 mm) with approximately 5.0 mL of cold RPMI-1640 with L-glutamine.
2. Using a needle and scalpel blade, gently disrupt the tissue so that cells are released into the surrounding RPMI medium.
3. When all tissue has been dissociated, aspirate the RPMI-cell suspension with a transfer pipette and place into a 17 × 100 mm test tube.
4. Rinse the Petri dish with 1.0 to 2.0 mL of fresh RPMI medium to retrieve as many cells as possible. Add this volume to the tube from step 3.
5. Use a 53 μm nylon mesh filter to remove any small remaining pieces of tissue.
6. Centrifuge the cell suspension at 4°C at 400 g for 5 min.
7. If the cell button is contaminated by red blood cells, treat with ammonium chloride (see "0.83% Ammonium Chloride Treatment for Red Blood Cell Lysis").
8. Determine cell viability (see "Determination of Cell Viability"). Minimum acceptable viability for immunophenotyping is 80%.
9. Adjust cell concentration to 10.0×10^6 cells/mL.

Preparation of Cell Suspension from Body Fluids

Principle

In order to perform surface marker studies on pleural, pericardial, or cerebrospinal fluids, the lymphocytes in these fluids must be isolated, washed, and adjusted to the concentration necessary for testing.

Specimen Requirements

Pleural and pericardial fluids that have increased or abnormal lymphocyte populations can be tested for surface markers. A volume of 10.0 to 100.0 mL is required, depending on the cellularity of the specimen. The fluid must be submitted in a heparinized container and delivered to the laboratory immediately.

Spinal fluids that show a substantial lymphocyte population may be suitable for immunophenotyping. Unfortunately, because of the small volumes routinely collected, the number of markers that can be done is usually limited. Spinal fluids that are clear and colorless may be sent in a tube without an anticoagulant. When the specimen is turbid or bloody, the fluid should be placed in a heparinized tube. All fluids should be sent to the laboratory immediately.

Material and Equipment

1. Polypropylene conical centrifuge tubes (size depending on volume of fluid)
2. Refrigerated centrifuge

Reagents

1. RPMI-1640 with L-glutamine
2. 0.83% ammonium chloride

Method

1. Place fluid into polypropylene conical tubes.
2. Centrifuge at 400 g for 5 min at 4°C.
3. If the cell pellet is contaminated by red blood cells, treat with 0.83% ammonium chloride (see "0.83% Ammonium Chloride Treatment for Red Blood Cell Lysis"). If no red blood cell contamination is present, proceed to step 4.
4. Decant supernatant. Wash two times with RPMI-1640 and centrifuge as in step 2.
5. Adjust the cell concentration to 10.0×10^6 cells/mL.
6. Determine cell viability (see "Determination of Cell Viability").

Note: If the fluid specimen is extremely bloody or appears to have a large number of granulocytes, it may be advantageous to use a Ficoll-Hypaque gradient to process the specimen instead of the above procedure. (See "Preparation of Mononuclear Cell Suspension from Peripheral Blood and Bone Marrow Aspirate.")

0.83% Ammonium Chloride Treatment for Red Blood Cell Lysis

Method

1. Decant supernatant, resuspend cell button, and fill tube with 0.83% ammonium chloride.
2. Invert the tube several times to disperse the cells. Allow cells to lyse at room temperature for approximately 5 min.

Caution: Excess time in ammonium chloride results in cell death and unacceptable alteration of scatter patterns. The altered scatter pattern will complicate the identification and gating of cell populations during analysis. Cell percentages may be altered due to death and differential loss of some cells.

3. Centrifuge at 4°C at 200 g for 10 min.
4. Decant supernatant and wash cells in cold RPMI-1640 medium.
5. Repeat steps 3 and 4.
6. Occasionally cell or tissue debris may clump. This debris can be removed by filtering through a 53 μm nylon mesh filter.
7. Count and adjust cell concentration to 10×10^6 cells/mL.

Determination of Cell Viability

Principle

The viability of cells is an important factor in an immunofluorescence assay because dead cells tend to take up fluorescent dye nonspecifically, leading to false-positive results. The trypan blue exclusion assay is a common method used for cell viability determinations. In this method, an aliquot of cells is incubated with an equal volume of trypan blue dye. The cells are then examined under a phase microscope and scored according to dye uptake.

Materials and Equipment

1. 20.0 μL pipette
2. Pipette tips
3. Hemacytometer
4. Microscope

Reagents

1. 0.3% trypan blue

Method

1. Combine 20.0 μL cell suspension and 20.0 μL 0.3% trypan blue. Mix gently.
2. Charge hemacytometer.
3. Review 100 cells and quantitate the percentage of viable cells in the entire cell population.

Results

Dead cells have permeable membranes that permit uptake of the dye and appear blue. Viable cells exclude the dye and appear clear or unstained. A viability of ≥80% is recommended for immunofluorescence assays.

Comments

For samples that contain <80% viable cells, it is possible to increase the number of living cells by removing dead cells through more washing or reprocessing the cells over a Ficoll-Hypaque gradient.

Staining for T- and B-Cell Surface Markers

Principle

In patients with lymphoid malignancies, identification of the immunologic phenotype of the malignant cells can aid in the classification of the disease. Surface markers can define both biological and prognostic characteristics of leukemias and lymphomas.

Cells are combined with fluorescent antibodies against human leukocytes. The procedure yields fluorescent-labeled cell surface antigens for analysis by FCM.

Quality Control Materials

Cryopreserved cells obtained by leukapheresis of a normal individual are run with each day's work. Cryopreserved lymphocytes from a known abnormal patient are used as abnormal controls whenever they are available.

B-Cell SIg

Principle

Serum immunoglobulin may adhere to leukocytes nonspecifically by cytophilic and Fc receptor binding. The polyclonal antibody may recognize this nonspecifically bound immunoglobulin. The use of a second color monoclonal antibody specific for B cells will help overcome this interference. During analysis, only dual-labeled cells will be counted as true positives.

Materials and Equipment

1. 50.0 µL, 100.0 µL, and 1.0 mL pipettes
2. Pipette tips
3. 12 × 75 mm capped centrifuge tubes
4. Magnetic stir plate and stir bar
5. Whatman No. 1 filter paper
6. pH meter
7. Fume hood
8. Vortex
9. Refrigerated centrifuge

Reagents

1. RPMI-1640 with L-glutamine
2. Phosphate buffered saline (PBS)
    a. 0.01 M PBS with 0.1% NaN_3 (pH 7.2 ± 0.2)
        i. 0.856 g $NaH_2PO_2 \cdot H_2O$ (6 mM)
        ii. 0.540 g Na_2HPO_4 (4 mM)
        iii. 8.0 g NaCl
        iv. 1.0 g NaN_3
    b. QS to 1.0 L with distilled water
    c. Adjust pH to 7.2 ± 0.2.
    d. Stored at room temperature, this solution is stable for 3 months.
3. PBS with 2% bovine serum albumin (PBS-BSA)
    a. Dissolve 20.0 g of BSA in 400.0 mL of 0.01 M PBS with 0.1% NaN_3.
    b. QS to 1.0 L with 0.01 M PBS.
    c. Filter with Whatman No. 1 filter paper.
    d. Stored at 4°C, this solution is stable for 2 months.
4. Fluorescein-conjugated $F(ab')_2$ fragments of polyclonal antisera monospecific for IgG, IgA, IgM, κ, and λ light chains and polyvalent anti-IgGAM. The antisera are diluted with PBS to a concentration that gives maximum fluorescence with minimal nonspecific background staining.
5. Phycoerythrin-conjugated anti-CD19
6. 2% paraformaldehyde
    a. Add 2.0 g paraformaldehyde to 100.0 mL PBS.
    b. Heat to 70°C under a fume hood.
    c. Remove from heat source and cool to room temperature (solution may still be slightly turbid).
    d. Add one to two drops of 1 N NaOH to dissolve paraformaldehyde completely (should be clear).
    e. Adjust to pH 7.4 using 1 N NaOH.
    f. Stored at 4°C, this solution is stable for 1 month.

Caution: Overheating will result in the formation of formaldehyde.

Method

1. Aliquot 1×10^6 cells for each antibody to be tested into individual 12 × 75 mm tubes (100.0 µL of a 10×10^6 cell/mL suspension). Include a negative patient control, to be used to measure autofluorescence. Use a fluorochrome-conjugated immunoglobulin of the same species and isotype as that of the antibody in use.
2. Add 2.0 mL PBS to each tube. Vortex.
3. Centrifuge at 400 g for 5 min at 4°C.
4. Aspirate the supernatant from the cell pellet.
5. Add the FITC-conjugated, titered polyclonal antibody and the phycoerythrin-conjugated CD19 antibody at a concentration recommended by the antibody manufacturer. Mix gently.
6. Incubate at 4°C for 30 min.
7. Add 2.0 mL PBS-BSA to each tube. Vortex.
8. Repeat steps 3 and 4.
9. Add 50.0 µL 2% paraformaldehyde. Vortex.
10. Store at 4°C in the dark until analyzed.

Reference Values

1. Surface immunoglobulin in reactive lymph nodes:
    a. polyvalent   26 ± 14%
    b. IgM   15 ± 9%
    c. IgD   10 ± 9%
    d. IgG   8 ± 7%
    e. IgA   3 ± 5%
    f. κ   17 ± 11%
    g. λ   13 ± 9%

2. Critera for monoclonality
   a. κ/λ >3:1
   b. λ/κ >2:1
   c. Predominant heavy chain: sum of other heavy chain >3:1

Monoclonal Antibody Panel

Materials and Equipment

1. 50.0 μL, 100.0 μL, and 1.0 mL pipettes
2. Pipette tips
3. 12 × 75 mm capped tubes
4. Vortex
5. Refrigerated centrifuge

Reagents

1. Phosphate buffered saline (PBS)
   a. 0.01 M PBS with 0.1% NaN_3 (pH 7.2 ± 0.2)
      i. 0.856 g $NaH_2PO_2 \cdot H_2O$ (6 mM)
      ii. 0.540 g Na_2HPO_4 (4 mM)
      iii. 8.0 g NaCl
      iv. 1.0 g NaN_3
   b. QS to 1.0 L with distilled water
   c. Adjust pH to 7.2 ± 0.2
   d. Stored at room temperature, this solution is stable for 3 months.
2. PBS with 2% bovine serum albumin (PBS-BSA)
   a. Dissolve 20.0 g of BSA in 400.0 mL of 0.01 M PBS with 0.1% NaN_3.
   b. QS to 1.0 L with 0.01 M PBS.
   c. Filter with Whatman No. 1 filter paper.
   d. Stored at 4°C, this solution is stable for 2 months.
3. a. Fluorescein isothiocyanate (FITC) or phycoerythrin (PE) conjugated monoclonal antibodies to human antigens (direct staining)
        or
   b. Purified unconjugated mouse anti-human primary antibodies
   c. Fluorescein or phycoerythrin conjugated goat anti-mouse (GAM-FITC or GAM-PE) secondary antibody (indirect staining)
4. Negative patient control. Use species-specific allotype.
5. 2% paraformaldehyde
   a. Add 2.0 g paraformaldehyde to 100.0 mL PBS.
   b. Heat to 70°C under a fume hood.
   c. Remove from heat source and cool to room temperature (solution may still be slightly turbid).
   d. Add one to two drops of 1 N NaOH to dissolve paraformaldehyde completely (should be clear).
   e. Adjust to pH 7.4 using 1 N NaOH.
   f. Stored at 4°C, this solution is stable for 1 month.
   Caution: Overheating will result in the formation of formaldehyde.

Method

1. For each antibody to be used, pipette 100.0 μL of a 10×10^6 cell/mL suspension into a 12 × 75 mm test tube.
2. Add 2.0 mL PBS-BSA to each test tube. Vortex.
3. Centrifuge at 400 g for 5 min at 4°C.
4. Aspirate the supernatant from the cell pellet.
5. Add the appropriate antibody and diluent to each tube of cells. Follow the antibody manufacturer's suggested concentrations. Mix gently.
6. Incubate at 4°C for 30 min.
7. Add 2.0 mL PBS-BSA to each tube. Vortex.
8. Repeat steps 3 and 4.
9. To the cells stained directly with antibodies conjugated with a fluorochrome, add 50.0 μL 2% paraformaldehyde; vortex; and store at 4°C in the dark until analyzed.
10. To the tubes containing cells stained with an unconjugated primary antibody, add 2.0 mL PBS-BSA and vortex.
11. Repeat steps 3 and 4.
12. Add GAM-FITC (secondary antibody) and diluent in a volume suggested by the antibody manufacturer.
13. Incubate at 4°C for 30 min.
14. Add 2.0 mL PBS-BSA to each test tube and vortex.
15. Repeat steps 3 and 4.
16. Add 50.0 μL 2% paraformaldehyde; vortex; and store at 4°C in the dark until analyzed.

Whole Blood Lysis Technique

Principle

An alternative method of staining is the whole blood lysis technique. This method involves the addition of a lytic agent to blood that has been stained with antibody, resulting in the lysis of red blood cells and leaving a leukocyte population. It is sometimes preferable to the density gradient separation method in that it deters selective cell loss.

Materials and Equipment

1. 100.0 μL and 1.0 mL pipettes
2. Pipette tips
3. 12 × 75 mm capped tubes

4. Vortex
5. Refrigerated centrifuge

Reagents

1. 0.9% sodium chloride
2. 0.83% ammonium chloride or commercial lysing solution
3. Phosphate buffered saline (PBS)
   a. 0.01 M PBS with 0.1% NaN_3 (pH 7.2 ± 0.2)
      i. 0.856 g $NaH_2PO_2 \cdot H_2O$ (6 mM)
      ii. 0.540 g Na_2HPO_4 (4 mM)
      iii. 8.0 g NaCl
      iv. 1.0 g NaN_3
   b. QS to 1.0 L with distilled water
   c. Adjust pH to 7.2 ± 0.2.
   d. Stored at room temperature, this solution is stable for 3 months.
4. PBS with 2% bovine serum albumin (PBS-BSA)
   a. Dissolve 20.0 g of BSA in 400.0 mL of 0.01 M PBS with 0.1% NaN_3.
   b. QS to 1.0 L with 0.01 M PBS.
   c. Filter with Whatman No. 1 filter paper.
   d. Stored at 4°C, this solution is stable for 2 months.
5. 2% paraformaldehyde
   a. Add 2.0 g paraformaldehyde to 100.0 mL PBS.
   b. Heat to 7°C under a fume hood.
   c. Remove from heat source and cool to room temperature (solution may still be slightly turbid).
   d. Add one to two drops of 1 N NaOH to dissolve paraformaldehyde completely (should be clear).
   e. Adjust to pH 7.4 using 1 N NaOH.
   f. Stored at 4°C, this solution is stable for 1 month.

Caution: Overheating will result in the formation of formaldehyde.

Specimen Requirements

1. 2.0 mL of either EDTA or ACD anticoagulated peripheral blood

Method

1. Determine white blood cell count and, if necessary, dilute blood with 0.9% sodium chloride to a concentration of approximately 5.0×10^6 leukocytes/mL.
2. Pipette 100.0 μL blood for each antibody to be tested into 12 × 75 mm tubes. Include a negative patient control, to be used to measure autofluorescence. Use a fluorochrome-conjugated antibody of the same species and isotype as that of the antibody being used.
3. Add antibody according to the manufacturer's suggested concentration. Mix gently.
4. Incubate for 30 min at room temperature in the dark.
5. Add lysing solution according to the manufacturer's instructions. Vortex immediately. (If using 0.83% ammonium chloride, the lysing volume is 2.0 mL.)
6. Hold tubes at room temperature and keep away from light until the solution's turbidity clears and lysing is complete (approximately 10 min).
7. Centrifuge at 4°C for 10 min at 200 g.
8. Aspirate supernatant and add 2.0 mL PBS-BSA. Vortex.
9. Repeat step 7.
10. Aspirate supernatant and add 50.0 μL 2% paraformaldehyde; vortex; and store at 4°C until analyzed.

Cell Cryopreservation

Materials and Equipment

1. 2.0 mL high-density polyethylene storage vial
2. 1.0 mL and 10.0 mL pipettes
3. Refrigerated centrifuge
4. Vortex
5. −80°C freezer
6. Liquid nitrogen (N_2) storage tank

Reagents

1. RPMI-1640 with L-glutamine
2. Heat-inactivated fetal calf serum (FCS)
3. Dimethyl sulfoxide (DMSO)
4. Liquid nitrogen (N_2)

Freezing Procedure

1. Adjust cells to be frozen to a concentration of 10.0×10^6 cells/mL in RPMI-1640.
2. Centrifuge cells at 400 g for 5 min at 4°C.
3. Remove 20% of RPMI supernatant and discard. Be careful not to disturb cell pellet.
4. Replace the volume removed with a comparable amount of heat-inactivated FCS.
5. Resuspend cell pellet.
6. Prepare a solution containing 20% DMSO in RPMI. Chill on ice for 10 min.
7. Combine 1.0 mL of 10.0×10^6 cell suspension in 20% heat-inactivated FCS in RPMI with 1.0 mL 20% DMSO in RPMI in a storage vial. Cap tightly and vortex. Label vial with specimen number.
8. Freeze at −80°C overnight and then transfer into liquid N_2.

Thawing Procedure

1. Immediately after removing a vial of cells from N_2, place in a 37°C water bath and gently invert until specimen begins to thaw.
   Caution: Do not keep tube in water bath long enough to warm the cell suspension. Proper thawing of the cell suspension is critical for optimal cell viability.
2. Transfer contents to a 12 × 75 mm test tube and wash three times with RPMI (400 g for 5 min at 4°C).
3. Perform cell viability (see procedure for "Determination of Cell Viability").

SUGGESTED READINGS

Ault K: Applications in immunology and lymphocyte analysis. In Melamed M (ed): *Flow Cytometry and Sorting*. New York, Wiley-Liss, 1990, pp 685–696.

Boyum A: Separation of leukocytes from blood and bone marrow. *Scand J Clin Lab Invest* 21(Suppl 97):77, 1968.

Carey J, Zarbo J: Clinical flow cytometry: State of the art analysis of carcinomas, leukemias, and lymphomas. *American Society for Clinical Pathologists' Workshop Manual*. 1993.

Dugue R, Everette E, Iturraspl J: Flow cytometric analysis of acute leukemias. *Clin Immunol Newsletter*, vol 10, No 4, April 1990.

Gjerset G, Nelson KA, Strong MD: Methods for cryopreserving cells. *Manual of Clinical Immunology*. Washington, DC, American Society for Microbiology, 1986.

Jackson A: Basic phenotyping of lymphocytes: Selection and testing of reagents and interpretation of data. *Clin Immunol Newsletter*, vol 10, No 4, April 1990.

Jackson AL, Warner NL: Preparation, staining and analysis by flow cytometry of peripheral blood leukocytes. *Manual of Clinical Laboratory Immunology*. Washington DC, American Society for Microbiology, 1986.

Lewis D: Cytochemistry I: Cell surface immunofluorescence. In Bauer K, Duque R, Shakey TV (eds): *Clinical Flow Cytometry, Principles and Application*. Baltimore, Williams & Wilkins, 1993, pp 143–158.

Technical Bulletin, Proper performance of Glen Cove Kappa/19 and Glen Cove Lambda/19. Gen Trak, Inc. Plymouth Meeting, PA, 1992.

7.2 INDIRECT IMMUNOFLUORESCENCE TECHNIQUE FOR TERMINAL DEOXYNUCLEOTIDYL TRANSFERASE (TdT)

Specimen Requirements

Smears of bone marrow, peripheral blood, or sediment of body fluids and touch preparations of bone marrow, lymph node, or solid tumors can be used for staining. A more satisfactory result can be obtained by cytocentrifugation of the leukocyte fraction separated by the Ficoll-Hypaque gradient technique. Specimens should be air-dried and processed as soon as possible. Otherwise, they should be stored at room temperature or in a vacuum desiccator at −70°C.

Materials and Equipment

1. Epifluorescence microscope
2. Coplin jar
3. Humid chamber
4. Mixer and magnetic stir bar
5. 15.0 μL micropipette
6. Diamond-tipped marking pen
7. Microscope slides (1 × 3 in.) and coverslips (18 × 18 mm)

Reagents

1. Rabbit anti-calf TdT antiserum
2. Fluorescein isothiocyanate conjugated F(ab')$_2$ goat anti-rabbit IgG antiserum
3. Normal rabbit IgG
4. Phosphate buffered saline (PBS), pH 7.4 (Section 1.8), stored at room temperature
5. Absolute methanol, stored at 0°C to 4°C
6. FA mounting F101P, pH 9.0 (Difco)

Method

1. Prepare two slides: a test slide and a negative control slide. On each slide, circle with a diamond-tipped marking pen the area where the cells are found. If material is available, also prepare a positive control either from a TdT-positive specimen from a leukemia or lymphoma patient or from a section of thymus.
2. Fix slides in absolute methanol for 30 min at 4°C.
3. Air-dry.
4. Carefully wipe off excess sample outside the circle with filter paper.
5. Apply 15.0 μL rabbit anti-calf TdT antiserum over the entire circled area of both the test slide and the positive control.
6. Apply 15.0 μL rabbit IgG over the entire circled area of the negative control slide.
7. Incubate all slides for 30 min at room temperature in a humid chamber.
8. Wash slides for 15 min in a Coplin jar with several changes of PBS.
9. Wipe off all excess PBS outside the circle, being careful not to let the sample dry out.
10. Apply 15.0 μL of fluorescein isothiocyanate-conju-

gated F(ab')₂ goat anti-rabbit IgG antiserum over the entire circled area of each slide.
11. Incubate for 30 min at room temperature in a humid chamber.
12. Repeat washing procedure as in step 8.
13. Place a small drop of FA mounting medium on a coverslip. Invert the circled area onto the drop to pick up the coverslip.
14. Use an epifluorescence microscope to examine the slides. Count the total number of nucleated cells in a bright field first, and then count the number of cells with fluorescent nuclei under fluorescence. Count a total of 200 to 500 cells and report the percentage of TdT-positive cells.

Interpretation

TdT-positive lymphocytes or thymocytes are present in the thymus, as well as 1% to 2% of bone marrow cells, which represent prothymocytes and pre-B cells. TdT is not normally seen in peripheral lymphocytes or in lymph nodes. Therefore, the presence of TdT-positive cells is helpful in the diagnosis of lymphomas and leukemias of T-cell origin, but TdT is also present in null-ALL and pre-B-ALL, as well as in chronic myelocytic leukemia with lymphoblast crisis.

SUGGESTED READINGS

Bollum FJ: Terminal deoxynucleotidyl transferase as a hematopoietic cell marker. *Blood* 54:1203–1215, 1979.

Donlon JA, Jaffe ES, Braylan RC: Terminal deoxynucleotidyl transferase activity in malignant lymphomas. *N Engl J Med* 297:461–464, 1977.

Habeshaw JA, Catley PF, Stansfield AG, et al: Terminal deoxynucleotidyl transferase activity in lymphoma. *Br J Cancer* 39:566–569, 1979.

Kung PD, Long JC, McCaffrey RP, et al: Terminal deoxynucleotidyl transferase in the diagnosis of leukemia and malignant lymphoma. *Am J Med* 64:788–794, 1978.

7.3 IMMUNOFLUORESCENCE TECHNIQUE FOR CIg

Specimen Requirement

Although this technique is applicable to smears and touch preparations, cytocentrifuge preparations are preferred.

Materials and Equipment

1. Fluorescence microscope
2. Mixer and magnetic stir bar
3. Humid chamber
4. Coplin jar
5. 20.0 μL micropipette
6. Microscope slides and coverslips
7. Diamond-tipped marking pen.

Reagents

1. Fixative: 95% ethanol-5% glacial acetic acid, stored at −20°C
2. Phosphate buffered saline (PBS), pH 7.4 (Section 1.8), stored at room temperature
3. Fluorescein-conjugated or rhodamine-conjugated immunoglobulin antisera
4. FA mounting fluid, pH 9.0 (Difco)

Method

1. On slides, circle with a diamond-tipped marking pen an area containing cells.
2. Fix slides for 15 min in ethanol-acetic acid fixative at −20°C.
3. Hydrate slides with PBS for 15 min.
4. Wipe off excess PBS outside the circle with filter paper.
5. Apply 20.0 μL immunoglobulin antiserum to the circled area. (Antibodies should be titered to the highest concentration that gives maximum fluorescence with minimal background staining.)
6. Incubate slides for 30 min at 4°C in a humid chamber.
7. Wash slides for 15 min in a Coplin jar with several changes of PBS.
8. Place a drop of mounting medium on a coverslip. Place the circled area over the drop and pick up the coverslip.
9. Examine the slides under a fluorescence microscope. Count 200 cells under regular light and cells with cytoplasmic fluorescence under ultraviolet light.
10. Calculate the percentage of positive cells.

Interpretation

Pre-B lymphocytes carry only a cytoplasmic μ heavy chain; occasionally, a corresponding light chain may be present. Pre-B cells are usually seen in pre-B acute lymphocytic leukemia and chronic myelocytic leukemia in lymphoblast crisis. Plasma cells also contain CIg, which can be of any class. The cytoplasmic immunoglobulins in plasma cells are only usually intact molecules or light chains. The identification of CIg in plasma cells is needed only in nonsecretory myeloma or biclonal gammopathy. Two paraproteins can be produced by the same clone or by two different clones of plasma cells.

Comments

Proper fixation to make the cell membrane permeable to fluorochrome-conjugated antisera is essential for the demonstration of CIg in cytologic preparations.

SUGGESTED READINGS

LeBien TW, Hozier J, Minowada J, et al: Origin of chronic myelocytic leukemia in a precursor of pre-B lymphocytes. *N Engl J Med* 301:144–147, 1979.

Seligmann M, Vogler LB, Preud'Homme JL, et al: Immunological phenotypes of human leukemias in the B-cell lineage. *Blood Cells* 7:237–246, 1981.

Vogler LB, Crist WM, Bookman DE, et al: Pre-B cell leukemia: A new phenotype of childhood lymphoblastic leukemia. *N Engl J Med* 298:872–878, 1978.

Section 8
IMMUNOCYTOCHEMISTRY AND IMMUNOHISTOCHEMISTRY

8.1 IMMUNOPEROXIDASE METHOD

Principle

The basic principle of the immunoperoxidase method is to use peroxidase to label a specific antiserum that reacts to the particular antigen of interest. The peroxidase reacts with a chromogenic substrate, giving a colored reaction product that indicates the location of the antigen of interest. Based on this principle, many methods are devised by adding a series of antibodies to bridge the reactions. Our method uses rabbit antiserum as the primary antiserum specific for the antigen of interest (e.g., esterase). A secondary antiserum (goat anti-rabbit immunoglobulin) is used to bridge the first reaction and the rabbit antiperoxidase–peroxidase complex. When a chromogenic substrate for peroxidase is added, a colored reaction product appears to indicate the location of the antigen of interest (e.g., esterase). An example of this principle is as follows:

Antigen (esterase)
↓
Rabbit anti-esterase (primary antiserum)
↓
Goat anti-rabbit immunoglobulin (secondary antiserum)
↓
Rabbit antiperoxidase
↓
Peroxidase + Substrate → Colored reaction product

Specimen Requirements

Paraffin-embedded tissue sections can be used. Cut sections 6 μm thick, deparaffinize, and rehydrate before use.

Plastic-embedded tissue sections can also be used. Cut sections 2 μm thick and air-dry.

Reagents

1. Sodium phosphate (Na_2HPO_4)
2. Potassium phosphate (KH_2PO_4)
3. Sodium chloride
4. Pepsin
5. 0.01 N hydrochloric acid
6. Egg albumin
7. Absolute methanol
8. Hydrogen peroxide (0.6% and 3%)
9. 3-Amino-9-ethylcarbazole
10. N,N-dimethylformamide
11. 0.1 M acetate buffer, pH 5.2 (Section 1.3)
12. Normal goat serum, 1:20 dilution
13. Specific primary rabbit antisera
14. Secondary goat or swine antisera with specificity for immunoglobulin of rabbit
15. Horseradish peroxidase–anti-horseradish peroxidase (rabbit PAP complexes)
16. Mayer's hematoxylin (Section 3.4)
17. Glycerin jelly (Section 4.5)
18. Phosphate-buffered saline (PBS, Section 1.8)
19. Pepsin solution
    a. Dissolve 200.0 mg pepsin in 50.0 mL 0.01 N hydrochloric acid.
20. 1% egg albumin solution
    a. Dissolve 1.0 g egg albumin in 100.0 mL PBS.
    b. Stored at 4°C to 10°C, this solution is stable for 2 months.
21. Incubating medium
    a. Dissolve 10.0 mg 3-amino-9-ethylcarbazole in 2.5 mL N,N-dimethylformamide.
    b. Add 47.0 mL acetate buffer.
    c. Add 0.5 mL 3% hydrogen peroxide.
    d. Filter.
    e. Use immediately.

Method

1. Deparaffinize and hydrate sections to water. If pepsin treatment is desired, incubate slides in pepsin solution for 20 min in 37°C and rinse in distilled water.
2. Block endogenous peroxidase by incubating the sections in methanol containing 0.6% hydrogen peroxide for 30 min. Rinse in PBS.
3. Incubate with 1% egg albumin or dilute normal goat serum (1:20) at room temperature for 10 min. Discard excess serum.
4. Incubate with properly diluted specific primary antibody in a moist chamber for 60 min at room temperature. Prepare controls using normal rabbit serum instead of specific primary antibody from a rabbit.
5. Wash with three changes of PBS, 5 min each.
6. Incubate with diluted secondary goat or swine anti-rabbit immunoglobulin (1:20) for 30 min.
7. Wash with three changes of PBS, 5 min each.
8. Incubate with diluted rabbit PAP complexes (1:20) for 30 min in the dark.
9. Wash with three changes of PBS, 5 min each.
10. Incubate in the filtered incubating solution for 30 min at room temperature.
11. Wash with water.
12. Counterstain with Mayer's hematoxylin for 1 to 5 min.
13. Wash with water and mount in glycerine jelly.

Results

Positive staining appears as bright red granules in the cytoplasm of the cells.

Comments

This staining method for peroxidase yields a highly chromogenic reaction product and appears more sensitive than the method using 3,3-diaminobenzidine hydrochloride as the indicator.

The peroxidase method of Hanker et al (2) yields a dark brown to black reaction product that is insoluble in organic solvent. Tissue stained by this method at pH 5.2 can be mounted in synthetic medium and kept permanently.

We use the immunoperoxidase method to examine antigens in paraffin-embedded or plastic-embedded tissues. Antigens in these tissues that have been successfully demonstrated include lysozyme, hemoglobin, cytoplasmic immunoglobulins, prostatic and neutrophilic acid phosphatase, and factor VIII antigen.

Fresh blood films and frozen tissue sections also may be used for study. The smears may be fixed with the general cytochemical fixative for 30 secs, and the tissue sections may be fixed in citrate-buffered 60% acetone for 30 secs followed by a brief rinse in water before they are used for staining.

Most surface markers are sensitive to fixation, tissue embedding, and the process for inactivation of endogenous peroxidase. Therefore, tissues that either have been embedded in paraffin and plastics or contain cells with strong endogenous peroxidase activity are not suitable for surface marker studies.

SUGGESTED READINGS

Graham RC Jr, Lundholm V, Karnovsky MJ: Cytochemical demonstration of peroxidase activity with 3-amino-9-ethylcarbazole. *J Histochem Cytochem* 13:150–152, 1965.

Hanker JS, Yates PE, Metz CB, et al: A new specific, sensitive and noncarcinogenic reagent for the demonstration of horseradish peroxidase. *Histochem J* 9:789–792, 1977.

Sternberger LA, Hardy PH, Cuculis JJ, et al: The unlabelled antibody enzyme method of immunochemistry. *J Histochem Cytochem* 18:315–338, 1970.

Yam LT, Janckila AJ, Lam KW, et al: Immunochemistry of prostatic acid phosphatase. *Prostate* 2:97–107, 1981.

8.2 IMMUNOALKALINE PHOSPHATASE METHOD

Reagents

1. Fixative: buffered 60% acetone in citrate (Section 2.3)
2. RPMI-1640 (Gibco)
3. Ficoll-Hypaque solution
4. Normal goat, swine, or rabbit sera
5. Specific antibodies
6. a. F(ab')$_2$ fraction of goat anti-mouse IgG conjugated with calf intestinal alkaline phosphatase
   or
   b. F(ab')$_2$ fraction of goat anti-rabbit IgG conjugated with calf intestinal alkaline phosphatase
7. 10% fetal calf serum
8. Naphthol AS phosphate
9. N,N-dimethylformamide
10. 0.04 M veronal buffer, pH 7.6 (Section 1.7)
11. Fast violet LB salt (CI 37150)
12. Levamisole hydrochloride
13. Mayer's hematoxylin (Section 3.4)
14. Glycerin jelly (Section 4.5)
15. Incubating medium
    a. Dissolve 15.0 mg naphthol AS phosphate in 0.5 mL N,N-dimethylformamide.
    b. Add 50.0 mL veronal buffer, 20.0 mg fast violet LB salt, and 12.0 mg levamisole; mix until dissolved.

c. Filter before use.
d. Use immediately.

Method

1. Prepare mononuclear cell suspensions by centrifuging 5.0 to 10.0 mL of heparinized venous blood diluted with RPMI-1640 medium (1:1) over a cushion of Ficoll-Hypaque solution at 400 g for 40 min. Harvest the cells, wash three times with RPMI-1640 medium, and adjust to a concentration of 2×10^6 cells/mL. Prepare blood smears or buffy coat smears of blood and marrow by conventional methods.
2. Add 1.0 mL of cells to each of a series of 1.5 mL conical centrifuge tubes (one tube per antibody or antiserum). Centrifuge and discard supernatant.
3. Suspend sediment in 0.2 mL of a 1:20 dilution of normal goat serum for 10 min at 4°C. Centrifuge and discard supernatant.
4. Suspend in 0.2 mL of antibody of appropriate dilution for 30 min at 4°C. Centrifuge and discard supernatant. Controls are prepared by substituting mouse ascites for monoclonal antibody or normal rabbit serum for serum with specific antibody activity.
5. Wash three times in RPMI-1640 by centrifugation.
6. Suspend in 0.2 mL of properly diluted goat anti-mouse IgG conjugated with alkaline phosphatase (1:20 or 1:40) for 30 min at 4°C. Centrifuge and discard supernatant.
7. Wash three times in RPMI-1640 by centrifugation.
8. Suspend in 1.0 mL RPMI-1640 with 10% fetal calf serum. Prepare smears with a cytocentrifuge. Air-dry.
9. Fix smears with fixative for 30 secs, wash in water, and air-dry.
10. Incubate smears in the filtered incubating medium for 30 to 45 min.
11. Wash smears with water.
12. Counterstain with Mayer's hematoxylin for 1 to 5 min.
13. Wash in water, dry, and mount in glycerin jelly.

Results

Activity of alkaline phosphatase appears as discrete bright red granules on the surface of the cells.

Comments

Fresh blood smears and frozen tissue sections may be labeled and stained in a manner similar to that for the cell suspensions, but with the following modifications. Fix the blood smears or sections for 30 secs, wash in water, and air-dry. Use the same dilutions of serum or antibodies as indicated for the cell suspensions. Incubate for 30 min at 10°C in a humidified chamber. Wash the slides by soaking them in three changes of isotonic solution for 5 min each.

If a blue reaction product is desired, naphthol AS phosphate and fast blue BBN can be used as the substrate/coupler combination. Other staining methods using naphthol AS-TR phosphate/fast violet B salt and naphthol AS phosphate/fast violet B salt are also useful.

This technique may not be as sensitive as the immunoperoxidase technique in demonstrating minute amounts of tissue antigens, but it is most suitable for use in the study of the surface markers. We use this technique almost exclusively for this purpose. Antigens on the cell surface that have been successfully demonstrated include HLA-DR antigens, pan-T antigens, helper T antigens, suppressor T antigens, B-cell antigens, common ALL antigens, and myeloid antigens.

SUGGESTED READINGS

Janckila AJ, Stelzer GT, Wallace JH, et al: Phenotype of the hairy cells of leukemic reticuloendotheliosis defined by monoclonal antibodies. *Am J Clin Pathol* 79:431–437, 1983.

Mason DY, Sammons R: Alkaline phosphatase and peroxidase for double immunoenzymatic labelling of cellular constituents. *J Clin Pathol* 31:454–460, 1978.

Ponder BA, Wilkinson MM: Inhibition of endogenous tissue alkaline phosphatase with the use of alkaline phosphatase conjugates in immunohistochemistry. *J Histochem Cytochem* 29:981–984, 1981.

8.3 IMMUNOALKALINE PHOSPHATASE METHOD FOR SMEARS AND IMPRINTS

Specimen Preparation

1. Collect blood samples in heparin to prepare standard "wedge" smears (Section 5.1, slide method).
2. For specimens with white blood cell counts less than $20 \times 10^3/\mu L$, use the buffy coat portions to ensure that a sufficient number of cells are present on the smear.
3. Prepare smears of marrow aspirates (Section 5.2) and tissue imprints (Section 5.3) in the usual manner. Air-dry them at room temperature for at least 2 hr before fixation.

Reagents

1. Fixative: cold buffered formol acetone (Section 2.1)
2. Phosphate buffered saline (PBS), pH 7.2 (Section 1.8)
3. Specific antibodies

4. a. F(ab')₂ fraction of goat anti-mouse IgG
   or
   b. F(ab')₂ fraction of goat anti-rabbit IgG, conjugated with calf intestinal alkaline phosphatase.
5. Naphthol AS phosphoric acid
6. *N,N*-dimethylformamide
7. 0.05 M Tris buffer, pH 8.2 (Section 1.2)
8. Fast red violet LB salt
9. Levamisole hydrochloride
10. Mayer's hematoxylin (Section 3.4)
11. Glycerin jelly (Section 4.5)
12. Incubating medium
    a. Dissolve 15.0 mg naphthol AS phosphoric acid in 0.5 mL *N,N*-dimethylformamide.
    b. Add 50.0 mL Tris buffer, 40.0 mg fast red violet LB salt, and 12.0 mg levamisole (1 mM); mix until dissolved.
    c. Filter.
    d. Use immediately.

Method

1. Fix air-dried smears or imprints in cold fixative for 30 sec and rinse for 15 min with three changes of PBS.
2. Add 0.2 mL of a 1:20 dilution of specific antibody to cover the smears. Incubate in a humid chamber for 30 min at room temperature. Controls are prepared by substituting nonimmune mouse ascites for monoclonal antibody or normal rabbit serum for serum with specific antibody activity.
3. Wash with three changes of PBS, 5 min each.
4. Add 0.2 mL of a 1:30 dilution of alkaline phosphatase–conjugated goat anti-mouse (or rabbit) IgG. Incubate in a humid chamber for 20 min at room temperature.
5. Wash with three changes of PBS, 5 min each.
6. Incubate smears or imprints in the filtered incubating medium for 30 to 45 min at 37°C.
7. Wash smears with water.
8. Counterstain with Mayer's hematoxylin for 5 to 10 mins.
9. Wash in running tap water for 10 mins, air-dry, and mount in glycerin jelly.

Results

Activity of alkaline phosphatase appears as discrete bright red granules arranged in a ring-like fashion on the surface of the cells.

Comments

This method is less sensitive but more practical than the method for cell suspensions.

The intensity of the staining may be determined by several factors, including the stability of the antigen, the density of the antigen distribution on the cell surface, and the binding affinity of the antibodies.

Monoclonal antibodies of comparable dilution can be divided into three groups according to staining intensity. These include the following: strong (HLA-DR, CD2, CD3, CD5, CD8, CD41a), moderate (CD4, CD10, CD11b, CD11c, CD13, CD20, CD22), and weak (CD14, CD33, CD19, CD21). The antibodies in the strong and moderate groups are more suitable in practical applications for cell identification on air-dried smears.

Staining intensity also varies according to the location of the cells in the "wedge" smears. Staining is stronger in cells at the thick end and weaker in cells at the thin end of the smear. Therefore, the middle portion of a smear should be used for evaluation.

Combined cytochemical enzymatic marker staining is possible. Smears should be stained for cytochemical markers before the addition of the monoclonal antibodies (step 2) because commercially available products containing sodium azide as a preservative may inhibit enzymatic (particularly peroxidase) activity.

With the development of an effective method of inhibiting endogenous peroxidase activity, the immunoperoxidase method can also be used for immunocytochemical evaluation of cells in peripheral blood, bone marrow, and other specimens (smears, imprints, or cytospins) that contain hematopoietic cells with endogenous peroxidase activity.

SUGGESTED READINGS

Li CY, Ziesmer SC, Lazcano-Villareal O: Use of azide and hydrogen peroxide as an inhibitor for endogenous peroxidase in the immunoperoxidase method. *J Histochem Cytochem* 35:1457–1460, 1987.

Li CY, Ziesmer SC, Yam LT, et al: Practical immunocytochemical identification of human blood cells. *Am J Clin Pathol* 81:204–212, 1984.

8.4 ALKALINE PHOSPHATASE–ANTI-ALKALINE PHOSPHATASE (APAAP) METHOD FOR CYTOLOGIC MATERIALS

Specimen Preparation

1. Prepare smears of blood, buffy coat, and marrow aspirate and cytospins (Sections 5.1, 5.2, 5.3, 5.4, and 5.6). Air-dry. Store overnight at room temperature in a dust-free container if necessary.
2. When paraffin-embedded tissues are used, cut sections at 6 μm, deparaffinize, and rehydrate before use.

Cryostat sections are cut at 6 μm, fixed in cold acetone for 5 to 10 min, and air-dried before use (Section 8.5).

Reagents

1. Fixatives
   a. Buffered formol acetone solution (Section 2.1)
   or
   b. Fresh cold acetone (4°C to 10°C, HPLC grade)
2. 0.05 M Tris buffer, pH 7.6, 8.0, or 8.2 (Section 1.2)
3. 0.05% Tween 20 in phosphate-buffered saline (PBS), pH 7.2
   a. Add 5.0 mL of 10% Tween 20 to 95.0 mL PBS, pH 7.2.
   b. Mix well.
   c. Stored at room temperature, this solution is stable for at least 3 months.
4. 5% normal goat serum (NGS)/PBS/Tween 20
   a. Add 0.05 mL NGS to 9.5 mL of 0.05% Tween 20 in PBS and 8.5 mL PBS.
   b. Stored at 4°C to 10°C, this solution is stable for 2 months.
5. Primary antibodies (mouse IgG)
6. F(ab')$_2$ fraction of goat anti-mouse IgG
7. Alkaline phosphatase–anti-alkaline phosphatase (APAAP) complexes
8. PBS 1/15 M, pH 7.2 (Section 1.1)
9. Reagents for alkaline phosphate staining reactions (Sections 5.22, 5.23 or 5.24)
10. N,N-dimethylformamide
11. Mayer's hematoxylin (Section 3.4)
12. Levamisole (12.0 mg/50.0 mL incubation solution)
13. Synthetic mounting medium (Section 4.5)
14. Pepsin solution (Section 8.1)

Method

1. Fix smears with buffered formol acetone for 30 sec at 4°C to 10°C and rinse briefly in three changes of PBS. Air-dry. If cold acetone is used for fixation, fix smears for 5 min and air-dry at room temperature for 1 hr.
2. Incubate slides in 5% NGS/PBS/Tween 20 for 10 min at room temperature.
3. Shake off excess serum. Do not rinse.
4. Add 0.05 to 0.2 mL primary antibody in appropriate dilution to cover the smear. Incubate in a humidified chamber at room temperature for 30 to 60 min.
5. Drain off antibody and rinse slides two to three times in PBS; then wash in two changes of tap water, 3 min each.
6. Add 0.05 to 0.2 mL of diluted goat anti-mouse IgG solution and incubate for 15 to 30 min in a humidified chamber at room temperature.
7. Drain off antibody and rinse slides two to three times in PBS; then wash in two changes of tap water, 3 min each.
8. Add 0.05 to 0.2 mL of diluted solution of APAAP complex. Incubate for 15 to 30 min in a humidified chamber at room temperature.
9. Drain off solution and rinse slides two to three times in PBS; then wash in two changes of tap water, 3 min each.
10. Incubate slides in one of the incubation media in the presence of levamisole (Sections 5.22 and 5.23) for alkaline phosphatase for 15 to 45 min at room temperature.
11. Rinse in tap water for 2 min and counterstain with Mayer's hematoxylin for 5 to 10 minutes.
12. Wash in tap water, dry, mount in synthetic mounting medium, and examine.
13. Controls are prepared by substituting nonimmune mouse ascites for primary antibody in step 4.
14. Tissue sections may be processed in an identical fashion. If pepsin treatment is desired, incubate slides after step 1 in pepsin solution for 10 to 20 min at 37°C and wash in three changes of distilled water, 3 min each. Dry thoroughly.

Results

Enzyme activity is seen as red (or blue) granules on the surface or in the cytoplasm of the cells.

Comments

This method is more sensitive than the indirect immunoalkaline phosphatase method and is most suitable for staining smears and tissue sections. However, the sensitivity of this method and of the indirect alkaline phosphatase method for staining cells in suspensions is the same.

Endogenous levamisole-resistant alkaline phosphatase activity may be seen in intestinal epithelial cells, placental tissues, and, on rare occasions, epithelial tumor cells. We frequently use this and other methods for alkaline phosphatase to study hematopoietic cells and tissues, and we use the immunoperoxidase methods for nonhematopoietic cells and tissues.

SUGGESTED READINGS

Cordell JL, Falini B, Erber WN, et al: Immunoenzymatic labeling of monoclonal antibodies using immune complexes of alkaline phosphatase and monoclonal antialkaline phosphatase (APAAP) complex. *J Histochem Cytochem* 32:219–229, 1984.

Yam LT, Janckila AJ, Epremian BE, et al: Diagnostic significance of levamisole-resistant alkaline phosphatase cytochemistry and immunocytochemistry. *Am J Clin Pathol* 91:31–36, 1989.

Yam LT, Janckila AJ, Li CY: The immuno-alkaline phosphatase methods. In DeLellis RA (ed): *Advances in Immunohistochemistry*. New York, Raven Press, 1988, pp 1–29.

8.5 LABELED STREPTAVIDIN-BIOTIN (LSAB) METHOD FOR TISSUE SECTIONS

Specimen Preparation

Prepare either paraffin-embedded sections or cryostat sections (Sections 6.1 and 6.3)

Reagents

1. Fresh cold acetone (4°C to 10°C, HPLC grade)
2. Phosphate buffered saline (PBS), pH 7.2 (Section 1.8)
3. 0.1% sodium azide in distilled water or PBS (store at room temperature; make fresh every 2 weeks)
4. Ethylene-diamine tetraacetate/PBS (no Tween) solution
   a. Add 0.36 g ethylene diamine tetraacetate to 1000.0 mL PBS, pH 7.2.
   b. Mix well.
   c. Stored at room temperature, this solution is stable for 1 month.
5. 3% hydrogen peroxide
6. 0.05% Tween 20 in PBS, pH 7.2
   a. Add 5.0 mL 10% Tween 20 in 95.0 mL PBS, pH 7.2.
   b. Mix well.
   c. Stored at room temperature, this solution is stable for 1 month.
7. 5% normal goat serum (NGS)/PBS/Tween 20
   a. Add 0.5 mL NGS to 1.0 mL of 0.05% Tween 20 in PBS and 8.5 mL PBS.
   b. Stored at 4°C to 10°C, this solution is stable for 1 month.
8. 1% normal human AB serum/Tween 20/PBS buffer
9. Primary antibodies
10. Biotinylated goat–anti-mouse IgG of proper dilution in 1% normal human AB serum/Tween 20/PBS buffer
11. Peroxidase-labeled streptavidin of proper dilution in 1% normal human AB serum/Tween 20/PBS buffer
12. Reagents for peroxidase staining reactions (Sections 5.0 or 5.10)
13. 0.1 M acetate buffer, pH 5.2 (Section 1.3)
14. Alcohols (95% and 100%)
15. Xylene
16. Mayer's hematoxylin (Section 3.4)
17. Synthetic mounting medium (Section 4.5)
18. Pepsin solution (Section 8.1)

Method

1. For paraffin-embedded sections, dewax in three changes of xylene, 10 min each. Hydrate sections in three changes of alcohol and finally in water. For cryostat sections, fix tissue in cold acetone in Coplin jars for 5 to 10 min. Air-dry for 1 hr at room temperature.
2. If pepsin treatment is desired, incubate slides in pepsin solution for 10 to 20 min in 37°C and rinse in distilled water.
3. Block endogenous peroxidase by incubating the sections in fresh, 0.1% azide, and 3% hydrogen peroxide (azide:peroxide = 9:1) for 10 to 30 min. Rinse in tap water for 1 min.
4. Incubate slides in 5% NGS/PBS/0.5% Tween 20 buffer for 10 min.
5. Blot off the NGS solution. Do not rinse.
6. Add 0.05 to 0.2 mL of primary antibody appropriately diluted in 1% NGS/PBS/Tween 20 buffer. Incubate for 30 to 60 min at room temperature.
7. Drain off antibody and rinse slides two to three times in PBS; then wash in two changes of tap water, 3 min each.
8. Add diluted biotinylated goat–anti-mouse IgG solution. Incubate for 15 to 30 min at room temperature.
9. Drain off antibody and rinse slides two to three times in PBS; then wash in two changes of tap water, 3 min each.
10. Add diluted peroxidase-labeled streptavidin solution and incubate for 15 min at room temperature.
11. Drain off streptavidin solution and rinse two to three times in PBS; then wash in two changes of tap water, 3 min each.
12. Incubate slides for 2 min in 0.1 M sodium acetate buffer. Place slides in chromogen solution (Section 5.10 or 5.12) and incubate for 15 min at room temperature.
13. Rinse in tap water for 2 min.
14. Counterstain in Mayer's hematoxylin for 5 to 10 min.
15. For sections stained with amino-ethylcarbazole as the chromogen, mount sections in glycerin jelly. For sections stained with diaminobenzidine, dehydrate in three changes of alcohol, clear in xylene, and mount in a synthetic medium.

16. Controls are prepared by substituting nonimmune mouse ascites for primary antibody in step 6.

Results

Enzyme activity varies according to the chromogen used. The reaction product is bright red when aminocarbazole is used. It is dark brown when diaminobenzidine is used.

Comments

The choice of tissue sections is determined by the stability of antigens during tissue processing. The cryostat sections are used for demonstration of antigens that may become attenuated during the process of paraffin embedding.

Intestinal alkaline phosphatase can be used as an alternative to horseradish peroxidase. Simply replace the peroxidase-labeled streptavidin with alkaline phosphatase-labeled streptavidin. Also, delete the step of peroxidase inactivation with azide and hydrogen peroxide. After enzyme labeling, stain for alkaline phosphatase activity (Section 5.22 or 5.23).

SUGGESTED READINGS

Hsu SM, Raine L, Fanger H: Use of avidin–biotin–peroxidase complex (ABC) in immunoperoxidase technique: A comparison between ABC and unlabeled antibody (PAP) procedures. *J Histochem Cytochem* 29:577–580, 1981.

Li CY, Ziesmer SC, Lazcano-Villareal O: Use of azide and hydrogen peroxide as an inhibitor for endogenous peroxidase in the immunoperoxidase method. *J Histochem Cytochem* 35:1457–1460, 1987.

Shi ZR, Itzkowitz SH, Kim YS: A comparison of three immunoperoxidase techniques for antigen detection in colorectal carcinoma tissues. *J Histochem Cytochem* 36:317–322, 1988.

Wood GS, Warnke R: Suppression of endogenous avidin–biotin activity in tissues and its relevance to biotin–avidin detection system. *J Histochem Cytochem* 10:1196–1204, 1981.

8.6 LABELED STREPTAVIDIN-BIOTIN (LSAB) METHOD FOR CYTOLOGIC MATERIALS

Specimen Preparation

1. Prepare smears of blood, buffy coat, or marrow aspirate (Sections 5.1, 5.2, 5.3, and 5.4).
2. Prepare cytospins on silanized glass slides (Section 5.6). Air-dry. Store overnight at room temperature in a dust-free container if necessary.

Reagents

1. Fixative
   a. Cold buffered formol acetone (Section 2.1)
      or
   b. Fresh cold acetone (4°C to 10°C, HPLC grade)
2. Phosphate buffered saline (PBS), pH 7.2 (Section 1.8)
3. 0.1% sodium azide in distilled water or PBS
4. 3% hydrogen peroxide
5. 0.05% Tween 20 in PBS, pH 7.2 (Sections 1.8 and 8.5)
6. 5% normal goat serum (NGS) in PBS, pH 7.2/Tween 20 (Section 8.5)
7. 1% normal human AB serum/Tween 20 PBS buffer
8. Primary antibodies
9. Biotinylated goat anti-mouse IgG of proper dilution in 1% normal human AB serum/Tween 20 PBS buffer
10. Peroxidase-labeled streptavidin of proper dilution in 1% normal human AB serum/Tween 20 PBS buffer
11. Reagents for peroxidase staining reactions (Section 5.9 or 5.10)
12. Ethylene diamine tetraacetate/PBS (No Tween) solution (Section 8.5)
13. 0.1 M acetate buffer, pH 5.2 (Section 1.3)
14. Mayer's hematoxylin (Section 3.4)
15. Synthetic mounting medium (Section 4.5)

Method

1. Fix air-dried smears or cytospins in cold buffered formol acetone for 30 sec and rinse briefly in three changes of deionized water. Air-dry. If cold acetone is used, fix for 5 min and air-dry at room temperature for 1 hr.
2. Block endogenous peroxidase with 0.1% sodium azide and 3% hydrogen peroxide (azide:peroxide = 9:1) for 10 to 30 min.
3. Rinse in tap water for 1 min.
4. Incubate slides in 5% NGS/PBS/0.5% Tween 20 buffer for 10 min.
5. Blot off the 5% NGS solution. Do not rinse.
6. Add 0.05 to 0.2 mL primary antibody appropriately diluted in 1% NGS/PBS/Tween 20 buffer and incubate for 30 to 60 min at room temperature.
7. Drain off antibody and rinse slides two to three times in PBS; then wash in two changes of tap water, 3 min each.
8. Add diluted biotinylated goat-anti-mouse IgG solution and incubate for 15 min at room temperature.
9. Drain off antibody and rinse slides two to three times in PBS; then wash in two changes of tap water, 3 min each.

10. Add diluted peroxidase-labeled streptavidin solution and incubate for 15 min at room temperature.
11. Drain off streptavidin solution and rinse slides two to three times in PBS; then wash in two changes of tap water, 3 min each.
12. Incubate slides for 2 min in 0.1 M sodium acetate buffer, pH 5.2. Place slides in chromogen solution (Section 5.10 or 5.12) and incubate for 15 min at room temperature.
13. Rinse in tap water for 2 min.
14. Counterstain with Mayer's hematoxylin for 5 to 10 min.
15. Wash in tap water 5 to 10 min, air-dry, and mount in synthetic mounting medium.
16. Controls are prepared by substituting nonimmune mouse ascites for primary antibody in step 6.

Results

Enzymic activity varies according to the chromogen used. The reaction product is bright red with the 3-amino-9-ethylcarbazole method (Section 5.10) and dark brown with the 3,3'-diaminobenzidine method (Section 5.9).

Comments

When the peroxidase reactions (Sections 5.9 and 5.10) are used in the immunoperoxidase procedures at pH 5.2, replace the Tris buffer, pH 7.6, with sodium acetate buffer, pH 5.2.

Calf intestinal alkaline phosphatase may be used as the labeling enzyme in this LSAB method. The LSAB-alkaline phosphatase method is identical to the LSAB-peroxidase method except that streptavidin-labeled alkaline phosphatase (method section, step 10) is used instead of streptavidin-labeled peroxidase. Activity of alkaline phosphatase can be demonstrated cytochemically (Sections 5.22, 5.23, 5.24, or 8.3) at pH 8.2 in the presence of levamisole.

SUGGESTED READINGS

Shi ZR, Itzkowitz SH, Kim YS: A comparison of three immunoperoxidase techniques for antigen detection in colorectal carcinoma tissues. *J Histochem Cytochem* 36:317–322, 1988.

Li CY, Ziesman SC, Lazcano-Villareal O: Use of azide and hydrogen peroxide as an inhibitor for endogenous peroxidase in the immunoperoxidase method. *J Histochem Cytochem* 35:1457–1460, 1987.

Section 9
CYTOGENETICS

9.1 PREPARATION OF REAGENTS FOR CYTOGENETIC STUDIES

Reagents

1. Democolcine (Colcemid) (10.0 µg/mL) solution
   a. Dilute 1.0 mg of Democolcine (Sigma, St. Louis) with 100.0 mL balanced salt solution (Eagle's essential medium, RPMI-1640, or others).
   b. Mix well.
   c. Stored at 4°C to 10°C, this solution is stable for 1 month.
2. 0.075 M hypotonic potassium chloride solution
   a. Dissolve 2.8 g potassium chloride in 500.0 mL distilled water.
   b. Mix well.
   c. Stored at room temperature, this solution is stable for several months.
3. Carnoy solution
   a. Mix three parts methanol (or ethanol) with one part glacial acetic acid.
   b. Prepare immediate before use.
4. Decomplemented fetal calf serum
   a. Incubate 100.0 mL fetal calf serum in a water bath at 56°C for 30 min.
   b. Shake container periodically.
   c. Stored frozen, this solution is stable for several months. Stored refrigerated, this solution is stable for 1 month. Keep refrigerated or frozen before use.
5. Culture medium
   a. To 100.0 mL balanced salt solution add 1.0 mL penicillin (100.0 µg/mL)-streptomycin (100.0 µg/mL) and 2.0 mL 0.2 M glutamine.
   b. Stored frozen, this solution is stable for several months. Stored refrigerated, this solution is stable for 1 month. Keep refrigerated or frozen before use.
6. Phytohemagglutinin (PHA) solution
   a. Rehydrate one ampule of phytohemagglutinin (Burroughs-Wellcome, Triangle Park, N.C.) with 5.0 mL distilled water.
   b. Stored at 4°C to 10°C, this solution is stable for about 1 month.

9.2 CYTOGENETIC STUDIES OF BONE MARROW (DIRECT METHOD)

Reagents and Equipment

1. Colcemid solution, 10.0 µg/mL (Section 9.1)
2. Heparin (preservative-free, 1000 units/mg)
3. 0.075 M hypotonic potassium chloride solution (Section 9.1)
4. Fresh Carnoy solution (Section 9.1)
5. Stains (Giemsa, quinacrine, or others)
6. Balanced salt solution (Eagle's essential medium, RPMI-1640, or others)
7. Pasteur pipettes
8. Alcohol-cleaned slides in cold 20% ethanol (4°C to 10°C)
9. 15.0 mL plastic conical centrifuge tube and/or tissue culture flasks
10. Alcohol lamp
11. Tabletop centrifuge

Method

1. Place 0.5 to 1.0 mL fresh marrow aspirate into a plastic tube containing two to three drops of heparin. Shake well. Transport specimen to cytogenetic laboratory immediately.
2. Add an equal volume of colcemid solution to the marrow aspirate. Mix gently with a Pasteur pipette to break up the marrow particles. Centrifuge at room temperature for 7 min at 700 rpm.

3. Use a Pasteur pipette to remove as much of the supernatant plasma as possible. Transfer the thin cell layer (buffy coat layer) at the interface between the plasma and the erythrocytes to another plastic conical tube containing 4.0 to 5.0 mL colcemid solution. Mix cells gently with a Pasteur pipette. Keep cells at room temperature for 60 to 90 min.
4. Centrifuge at 700 rpm for 7 min at room temperature. Remove supernate and mix cells gently with a Pasteur pipette.
5. Add 10.0 mL hypotonic potassium chloride solution to cells. Mix gently with a Pasteur pipette. Incubate at 37°C for 10 min.
6. Centrifuge at 700 rpm for 7 min. Remove supernate with a Pasteur pipette. Shake tube gently to resuspend cells.
7. Add 5.0 mL fresh Carnoy solution to cells. Mix gently with a Pasteur pipette. Let cell suspension stand at room temperature for 10 min.
8. Centrifuge at 700 rpm for 7 min. Remove supernate. Resuspend and fix cells with fresh Carnoy solution for 5 min.
9. Repeat step 8 until the supernate becomes clear and the cell pellet appears white.
10. Remove supernate. Suspend cells with fresh Carnoy solution so that the cell suspension appears slightly turbid.
11. With a Pasteur pipette, place two to three drops of the cell suspension on a wet slide immersed in cold 20% ethanol. Flame slide gently over alcohol burner to ensure spreading and drying of cells.
12. Dry slides at room temperature or in a drying oven at 60°C to 65°C for 1 to 24 hr before staining.

Comments

Slides prepared through flaming with an alcohol burner or heat may not stain well with the trypsin banding method.

The fixative, Carnoy solution, should be prepared fresh immediately before use.

9.3 CYTOGENETIC STUDIES OF PERIPHERAL BLOOD

Reagents and Equipment

1. Sterile plastic tube (15.0 mL, 16 × 125 mm)
2. Sterile tissue culture flasks
3. Phytohemagglutinin A (PHA) (Section 9.1)
4. Decomplemented fetal calf serum (Section 9.1)
5. Plastic syringes (10.0 to 20.0 mL)
6. 22-Gauge needles
7. Heparin (preservative-free, 1000 units/mL)
8. Colcemid solution (10.0 µg/mL) (Section 9.1)
9. 0.075 M hypotonic potassium chloride solution (Section 9.1)
10. Fresh Carnoy solution (Section 9.1)
11. Balanced salt solution (Eagle's essential medium, RPMI-1640, or others)
12. Pasteur pipettes
13. Alcohol-cleaned slides in cold 20% ethanol (4°C to 10°C)
14. Alcohol lamp
15. Tabletop centrifuge
16. Incubator

Method

1. Draw desired amount of peripheral blood (10.0 to 20.0 mL) into a plastic syringe containing 0.2 mL heparin. Invert syringe several times to ensure mixing of blood and heparin.
2. Place syringe into incubator at 37°C in an upright position for 30 to 60 min.
3. Use the needle cap to bend the needle into a U shape and push the plunger to transfer the leukocyte-rich plasma from the syringe into a plastic tube.
4. Determine the number of cells per cubic millimeter in the leukocyte-rich plasma.
5. Add a sufficient number of cells (e.g., 10^6 cells/mL) to the tissue culture flask containing approximately 8.0 to 10.0 mL culture medium (balanced salt solution with 20% fetal calf serum). Add more culture medium to bring the final volume to 12.0 mL if necessary. The desirable final cell concentration is 1000 to 2000 cells per milliliter of culture medium. Add 0.2 mL PHA to each flask. Culture cells for 2 to 7 days as needed.
6. One hour before harvesting, add 0.2 mL colcemid solution to each culture. Mix well by gentle shaking. Return cultures to incubator.
7. Remove cultures from incubator; mix by shaking flasks. Transfer cell suspension to a plastic tube.
8. Centrifuge at 700 rpm for 7 min at room temperature. Remove supernate and mix cells gently with a Pasteur pipette.
9. Add 10.0 mL hypotonic potassium chloride solution to cells. Mix gently with a Pasteur pipette. Incubate at 37°C for 10 min.
10. Centrifuge at 700 rpm for 7 min. Remove supernate with a Pasteur pipette. Shake tube gently to resuspend cells.
11. Add 5.0 mL fresh Carnoy solution to cells. Mix gently with a Pasteur pipette. Let cell suspension stand at room temperature for 10 min.

12. Centrifuge at 700 rpm for 7 min. Remove supernate. Resuspend and fix cells with fresh Carnoy solution for 5 min.
13. Repeat step 12 until cell pellet appears white.
14. Remove supernate. Suspend cells with fresh Carnoy solution so that the cell suspension appears slightly turbid.
15. With a Pasteur pipette, place two to three drops of the cell suspension on a wet slide immersed in cold 20% ethanol. Flame slide gently over alcohol burner to ensure spreading and drying of cells.
16. Dry slides at room temperature or in a drying oven at 60°C to 65°C for 1 to 24 hr before staining.

Comments

Do not add PHA to short-term (24 hr or less) cultures. Slides prepared through flaming with an alcohol burner or heat may not stain well with the trypsin banding method.

9.4 GIEMSA STAIN

Reagents and Equipment

1. Giemsa stock solution (Section 3.3)
2. Phosphate buffer, M/15, pH 6.4–6.6 (Section 1.1)
3. Staining jars
4. Decolorizing solution
   a. Add two to three drops of glacial acetic acid in 100.0 mL of 10% ethanol.
5. Permount or Diatex (Section 4.5)

Method

1. Stain slides for 10 min at room temperature with buffered Giemsa solution (Giemsa:buffer = 1:10 or 1:15).
2. Rinse slides with running tap water.
3. Examine wet slides under a microscope for staining intensity and background staining. Decolorize slides for 5 to 10 sec with the decolorizing solution.
4. Wash slides with running tap water. Air-dry before mounting in Permount or Diatex.

9.5 GIEMSA-TRYPSIN BANDING

Reagents and Equipment

1. Giemsa stain (Section 3.3)
2. Phosphate buffer, M/15, pH 6.8 (Section 1.1)
3. Trypsin EDTA solution (Gibco, Grand Island, N.Y.)
4. Normal saline (0.85% sodium chloride)
5. Working trypsin solution
   a. Thaw stock trypsin solution before use.
   b. Dilute trypsin solution 1:10 with normal saline at room temperature immediately before use.
6. Decomplemented fetal calf serum (Section 9.1)
7. Permount or Diatex (Section 4.5)

Method

1. Place air-dried smears (1 to 2 weeks old) in an oven at 37°C for 4 to 5 hr.
2. Immerse slides, while still warm, in 0.025% trypsin (dilute stock trypsin with normal saline at 1:10) at room temperature for desired time.
3. Rinse slides in two changes of cold saline containing a small amount of fetal calf serum.
4. Stain with diluted Giemsa solution (Giemsa:phosphate buffer = 1:50) for 15 to 20 min.
5. Rinse with water and air-dry overnight before mounting with synthetic mounting medium.

Comments

Stock trypsin solution should be stored at −5°C to −20°C and thawed immediately before use. The diluted trypsin solution may be stored for 2 to 3 days at 4°C without apparent loss of activity; it should not be refrozen or reused.

Chromosome slides that are prepared through flaming with an alcohol burner or heat do not band well.

9.6 GIEMSA C-BANDING

Reagents and Equipment

1. Diluted hydrochloric acid solution (0.2 N)
2. Diluted barium hydroxide solution [0.07 N Ba(OH)$_2$]
3. Saline sodium citrate (17.53 g sodium chloride; 8.82 g trisodium citrate dihydrate and distilled water to 1000.0 mL)
4. Giemsa stain (Section 3.3)
5. Phosphate buffer, M/15, pH 6.8 (Section 1.1)
6. Permount or Diatex (Section 4.5)

Method

1. Incubate aged (1 to 2 weeks old), air-dried slides in 0.2 N hydrochloric acid at room temperature for 30 min.
2. Rinse thoroughly with distilled water.
3. Place slides in warmed barium hydroxide solution in a water bath at 37°C for 5 to 10 min.

4. Rinse slides in distilled water.
5. Incubate slides in saline-sodium citrate solution at 65°C for 2 hr.
6. Rinse with distilled water.
7. Stain with diluted Giemsa (Giemsa:phosphate buffer = 1:50) for 1 to 2 hr.
8. Rinse slides with distilled water. Air-dry before mounting with synthetic medium.

Comments

If chromosomes are swollen and/or C bands are faint, decrease the time of exposure to barium hydroxide.

9.7 QUINACRINE FLUORESCENT STAIN

Reagents

1. Quinacrine mustard dihydrochloride working solution (50.0 μg/mL of modified McIlvaine's buffer)
2. Stock solutions for modified McIlvaine's working buffer, pH 7.0
   a. Stock solution A: 0.1 M citric acid ($H_3C_6H_5O_7 \cdot H_2O$) (21.0 g citric acid/1.0 L water)
   b. Stock solution B: 0.2 M disodium phosphate (Na_2HPO_4 28.4 g/1.0 L H_2O)
3. Working buffer solution
   a. Add 86.3 mL stock solution A to 453.7 mL stock solution B.
   b. Add distilled water to make 1.0 L.
4. Synthetic mounting medium (Section 4.5)

Method

1. Immerse slides into a staining jar containing the working solution of quinacrine mustard dihydrochloride stain in the dark at room temperature for 20 min.
2. Rinse slides with three changes of distilled water. Leave slides in distilled water for 3 min.
3. Air-dry. Mount in buffer or distilled water before examination. Seal edges of coverslips with synthetic mounting medium.

Comments

Both the quinacrine mustard dihydrochloride and its working solution should be stored in the dark. The stability of the working solution is variable.

The fluorescence in the chromosomes will fade with exposure to fluorescent excitation. It may or may not be revived by placing the slides in the dark again.

SUGGESTED READINGS FOR SECTIONS 9.1 THROUGH 9.7

Caspersson T, Zech L, Johansson C: Differential binding of alkylating fluorochromes in human chromosomes. *Exp Cell Res* 60:315–319, 1970.

Dewald G, Allen JE, Strutzenberg DK, et al: A cytogenetic method for mailed-in bone marrow specimens for the study of hematologic disorders. *Lab Med* 13:225–229, 1982.

Lam-Po-Tang PRLC: An improved method of processing bone marrow for chromosomes. *Scand J Haematol* 5:158–160, 1968.

Seabright M: A rapid banding technique for human chromosomes (letter to the editor). *Lancet* 2:971–972, 1971.

9.8 DNA PLOIDY ANALYSIS: RAPID NUCLEAR ISOLATION AND STAINING

Principle

Utilizing flow cytometry, DNA content can be measured to determine the ploidy status, DNA index, and cell cycle statistics of cells from tissue samples. The correlation of these data with disease type and staging can yield valuable information on the prognosis of various malignancies. The following method is designed for the fluorescent staining of DNA in isolated nuclei from tissue specimens. The tissue is minced directly in the media, which (1) provides a preparation of isolated nuclei (due to detergent); (2) hydrolyzes the RNA to eliminate unwanted RNA staining (RNAse); and (3) contains the dye to stain the nuclei (propidium iodide). The propidium iodide (PI) intercalates between the base pairs of double-stranded DNA. The amount of bound PI is directly proportional to the amount of DNA present.

Specimen Requirements

Approximately 0.1 to 0.2 g of fresh or frozen tissue is required for DNA analysis. Fresh tissue must be placed in RPMI medium and stored at 4°C for up to 24 hr prior to processing. Frozen specimens must be snap-frozen in liquid nitrogen and stored at −75°C until processing.

Quality Control Materials

1. Normal human mononuclear cells are used to establish the location of the diploid population. Mononuclear cells are separated from peripheral blood using the density gradient technique. The cell suspension must be adjusted to a concentration of 2.0×10^6 cells/mL for DNA analysis. Cells may be frozen in DMSO according to the procedure for cell cryopreservation.

Frozen cells must be thawed and washed twice with RPMI; add 1.0 mL of PI staining buffer; then proceed to step 3 of the method.
2. Chicken erythrocyte nuclei (CEN), calf thymocyte nuclei (CTN), and 2.0 micro beads of QC material are used for instrument calibration.

Materials and Equipment

1. Petri dish
2. Fluorescent microscope
3. Scalpel
4. Transfer pipette
5. Nylon mesh (53 μm)
6. Pipettes (1.0 and 10.0 mL)
7. Falcon tubes (12 × 75 mm)
8. Vortex mixer
9. Tuberculin syringe with a 27-gauge needle
10. 15.0 mL conical tube
11. Hemocytometer
12. Tissue forceps
13. Freezer (−70°C)

Reagents

1. 4 mM sodium citrate buffer, pH 7.8 ± 0.2
   a. 1.17 g sodium citrate
   b. 1.0 L distilled water
   c. Adjust pH to 7.8 ± 0.2
   d. Stored at 4°C, this solution is stable for up to 1 year.
2. PI staining buffer, pH 7.2 ± 0.2
   a. 480.0 mL 4 mM sodium citrate buffer, pH 7.8
   b. 25.0 mg PI
   c. 5.0 mL 10% triton X-100
   d. Adjust pH to 7.2 ± 0.2.
   e. QS to 500.0 mL with 4 mM sodium citrate buffer
   f. Stored in a foil-wrapped bottle at 4°C, this solution is stable for up to 3 months.
3. RNase reagent
   a. RNase, DNAse free (Boehringer Mannheim, Indianapolis, IN)
   Note: Level of activity may vary from one lot to another.
   b. Use amount recommended for 2×10^6 cells/mL
   c. Stored at 4°C, this reagent is stable until the expiration date on the label.
4. 0.9% sodium chloride
   a. Stored at room temperature, this reagent is stable until the expiration date on the label.

Method

1. Place the tissue in a Petri dish, add 2.0 mL 0.9% saline to rinse and, if frozen, to thaw the tissue. Transfer the tissue to a clean Petri dish with tissue forceps.
2. Add 1.0 mL PI staining buffer to the Petri dish. Mince the tissue with the scalpel, using the forceps to immobilize the tissue. This process should be completed within 1–2 min; a cloudy solution of free cells will result.
   Note: Exhaustive mincing is not necessary; tumor cells will generally be released more readily than normal cellular components or fibrous tissue. To maintain a high ratio of tumor cells to normal cells, avoid exceeding the 2-min time limit.
3. Filter the solution through 53 μm nylon mesh into a 12 × 75 mm test tube.
4. Add 5.0 μL RNase to the tube.
5. Incubate for 20 min at 37°C in the dark.
6. Incubate for 30 min at 4°C in the dark.
7. Prior to running specimens on the flow cytometer, draw the cell suspension up and down four or five times into the tuberculin syringe with the needle attached. This will disaggregate clumped nuclei.
8. Count the nuclei on a hemocytometer using a fluorescent microscope. Adjust the cell concentration to 2.0×10^6 cells/mL.
9. Keep tubes on ice in the dark until analyzed. Specimens must be analyzed within 24 hr of staining.

SUGGESTED READINGS

Becton Dickinson Procedures in Becton Dickinson Sourcebook. San Jose, CA, Becton Dickinson Immunocytometry Systems, 1990.

Darzynkiewicz Z, Crissman HA (eds): *Flow Cytometry*. San Diego, Academic Press, 1990, pp 121–125.

Thornthwaite JT, Sugarbaker EV, Temple WJ: Preparation of tissue for DNA flow cytometric analysis. *Cytometry* 1:229–237, 1980.

Section 10
IN SITU HYBRIDIZATION

Materials and Equipment

1. Thermal plate

Reagents

1. Ethanols (70%, 95%, and 100%)
2. Aminopropyl triethoxysilane (AES) (Section 4.6)
3. Xylene
4. 0.1% sodium azide
5. Phosphate buffered saline (PBS)
6. 0.01% Triton X-100 (Sigma)
7. DNase/RNase-free proteinase K (0.1 mg/mL; Boehringer-Mannheim, Indianapolis, IN)
8. 50% formamide
9. Saline-sodium citrate (SSC)
10. 0.25% nonfat dry milk
11. Brij 35 (Sigma, St. Louis, MO)
12. 5% goat serum
13. Peroxidase-conjugated mouse monoclonal anti-digoxigenin antibody (1:300 in 0.5% goat serum; Boehringer-Mannheim)
14. 0.1 M sodium acetate pH 6.0
15. Diaminobenzidine (DAB, Sigma)
16. 3% hydrogen peroxide

Preparation of Slide and Section

1. Wash clean slides on the slide rack once with 95% ethanol and once with 100% ethanol.
2. Treat slides with 2% AES in absolute alcohol for 2 min and air-dry. (Section 4.6)
3. Cut 3- to 5-μm sections of tissue in paraffin and mount them onto the AES-treated slides. Melt the paraffin in an oven at 80°C for 45 min or at 65°C overnight.

Preparation of the Probe

Plasmid DNA probe (modified from Genius™ 4 manual from Boehriner-Mannheim)

1. Prepare and purify plasmid DNA by cesium chloride gradient and G-50 sepharose column or commercial plasmid prep kits.
2. Digest plasmid DNA with the appropriate restriction enzyme(s) and isolate the needed DNA fragment by gel electrophoresis. Commercially prepared DNA fragments may also be used for probe synthesis.
3. The probe is prepared by the random primed method, with digoxigenin-11-dUTP (Boehringer-Mannheim) as the label.
4. Denature 5.0 μg DNA fragment along with approx 500 ng of hexanucleotide primers at 95°C for 10 min in a 1.5 mL Eppendorf tube and then place on ice for 1 min.
5. Centrifuge this solution briefly; add the appropriate amount of digoxigenin-11-dUTP, deoxynucleotide triphosphates (dNTPs), buffer, and Klenow fragment to a final volume of 50 ul; incubate the reaction mixture in a 37°C water bath for 18 to 24 hr.
6. Precipitate DNA probe with 0.1 vol of 4 M lithium chloride and 2.5–3 vols of ethanol at −20°C for at least 2 hr, and centrifuge the DNA pellet.
7. Remove the residual nucleotides by washing the DNA pellet three times with 70% ethanol.
8. Resuspend the DNA probe in double-distilled water and boil the probe at 100°C for 15 min. Melt it into single strands and determine the length of the probe by agarose gel electrophoresis. Approximately 100 to 300 bases is the optimal length.

Plasmid/RNA probe (modified with Genius 4 manual from Boehringer-Mannheim)

1. Linearize the template DNA with the appropriate restriction enzyme. Orientation of the template insert

with respect to the promoter of the vector must be determined to ascertain whether sense or anti-sense probes will be produced using a given promoter in the labeling reaction. When the template insert is downstream of the selected promoter, it will yield a sense probe if oriented in the forward direction; an antisense probe if oriented in the reverse direction. Sense probe serves as a negative control in the detection of mRNA.

2. Purify linearized DNA with phenol/chloroform extraction, and precipitate template DNA with ethanol.
3. Add the following to a microcentrifuge tube on ice: 1.0 μg DNA template, 2.0 μL NTP labeling mixture (10 mM ATP, 10 mM CTP, 10 mM GTP, 6.5 mM UTP, and 3.5 mM dig-11-UTP), and 2.0 μL 10× transcription buffer (0.4 M Tris, pH 8.0; 60 mM magnesium chloride; 0.1 M dithiothreitol; 20 mM spermidine; 0.1 M sodium chloride; and 1.0 U/μL RNase inhibitor).
4. Adjust volume to 18.0 μL with sterile diethylpyrocarbonate (DEPC)-treated distilled water and add 2.0 μL of either SP6 or T7 RNA polymerase, depending on the orientation of the template insert.
5. Centrifuge briefly and incubate at 37°C for 2 hr.
6. Precipitate the labeled RNA probe with .1 vol 4M lithium chloride and 2.5-3 vol ethanol.
7. Rinse RNA pellet twice with 70% ethanol and then dissolve RNA in 100.0 μL sterile, DEPC-treated distilled water at 37°C for 30 min.
8. Determine the amount of newly synthesized RNA probe by spectrophotometry.
9. Adjust RNA concentration to 0.5 μg/μL and add an equal volume of 60 mM sodium carbonate/40 mM sodium bicarbonate, pH 10.2.
10. Hydrolyze digoxygenin-labeled RNA at 60°C for 10 min.
11. Stop RNA hydrolysis by adding an equal volume of 0.2 M sodium acetate/1% acetic acid, pH 6.0.
12. Precipitate partially hydrolyzed RNA probe with 1/20 volume of glycogen (20 mg/mL) and 3 volumes of ethanol.
13. Resuspend the RNA probe in DEPC-treated, double-distilled water. Determine the probe length by 1% denaturing agarose gel electrophoresis and transfer to nylon with direct immunodetection. The appropriate probe length should be approximately 150 to 300 bases for obtaining the optimal in situ signal.

Oligonucleotide Probe

1. Purify the synthesized oligonucleotide probe by the denaturing gel (20% polyacrylamide with 8 M urea) and passing it through a G-25 column.
2. Mix 100 pmol of oligonucleotide with 4.0 μL of tailing buffer (1 M potassium cacodylate, 125 mM Tris, pH 6.6, and 1.25 mg/mL bovine serum albumin); 4.0 μL of 25 mM cobalt chloride; 1.0 μL of 1 mM dig-11-dUTP; 50 units of terminal transferase; and redistilled water to make a volume of 20.0 μL.
3. Incubate the reaction mixture at 37°C for 15 min and then stop the reaction with 2.0 μL of 0.2 M EDTA. Determine the length of the probe by polyacrylamide gel electrophoresis.

In Situ Hybridization

1. Deparaffinize the tissue in xylene and hydrate through graded alcohols.
2. Air-dry slide(s)
3. Inactivate the endogenous peroxidase with 0.1% sodium azide and 0.3% hydrogen peroxide.
4. Following a brief wash in PBS, treat slide(s) with 0.01% Triton X-100 for 5 min and digest specimen with DNase-free proteinase K at room temperature for 30 min.
5. Wash slide(s) with PBS three times, rinse with 70% alcohol once, and air-dry.
6. Mix 250.0 ng/mL DNA probe with the hybridization buffer that contains 50% formamide, 3× SCC, and 0.25% nonfat dry milk; add the hybridization mixture to the tissue section.
7. Place a coverslip carefully on the hybridization mixture to avoid trapping air bubbles between tissue specimen and coverslip.
8. Denature the prepared slide on a thermal plate at 100 ± 3°C for 10 min and then move the slide(s) to a moist chamber at 37°C for 45 min.
9. Following hybridization, dip the slide(s) briefly into 2× SSC/0.25% Brij 35 to remove excess hybridization mixture and coverslip.
10. Wash slide(s) consecutively with 2× SSC/0.25% Brij 35 at room temperature, 2× SSC/0.25% Brij 35 at 52°C, and 0.1× SSC/0.25% Brij 35 at 52°C, each for 30 min.
11. Rinse slide(s) with PBS and block with PBS/5% goat serum for 5 to 10 min, before adding peroxidase-conjugated mouse monoclonal anti-digoxigenin antibody (1:300 in 0.5% goat serum); incubate the reaction mixture are room temperature for 30 min. If the biotinylated probe is used, use peroxidase-conjugated streptavidin instead.
12. Wash off the residual antibodies with three changes of PBS and rinse slide(s) with 0.1 M sodium acetate.
13. Process chromogenic development in DAB solution (20.0 mg diaminobenzidine and 20.0 μL of 3% hydro-

gen peroxide in 40.0 mL of 0.1 M sodium acetate, pH 6.0) for 10 min or in nickel chloride–enhanced DAB solution (20 mg DAB, 0.1% nickel chloride, 0.07% imidazole, 0.8% sodium chloride, and 120.0 µL of 3% hydrogen peroxide in 40.0 mL of 0.1 M sodium acetate, pH 6.0) for 5 min; and then 5 min in 0.5% cobalt chloride/50 mM Tris, pH 7.2.

14. Rinse slide(s) three times with distilled water and counterstain in Schmidt's hematoxylin (when DAB is used) or in nuclear fast red (when nickel chloride–enhanced DAB is used) for 30 sec. The Schmidt's light blue nuclear stain is developed in running tap water for 15 min. The excess nuclear fast red is washed away with water.

SUGGESTED READINGS

1. Chow K-C, Li C-Y: Nonisotopic detection methods for *in situ* hybridization cytochemistry. In Avrameas S, Papamichail M, Nakane PK, Pesce A (Committee) *Twenty-Five Years of Immunoenzymatic Techniques.* Athens, International Congress Abstract Book, Triaena Congress, 1991, pp 85
2. Chow K-C, Nacilla JQ, Witzig T, et al: Is persistent polyclonal B lymphocytosis caused by Epstein-Barr virus? A study with polymerase chain reaction and *in situ* hybridization. *Am J Hematol* 41:270–275, 1992.
3. Kessler C, Holtke H-J, Seibl R, et al: Nonradioactive labeling and detection of nucleic acids, I: A novel DNA labeling and detection system based on digoxigenin:anti-digoxigenin

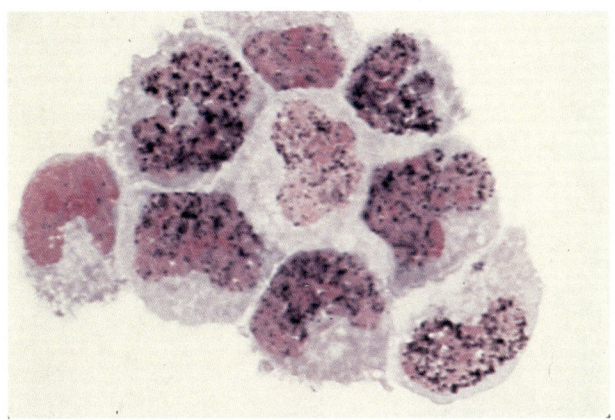

FIGURE A. Epstein-Barr virus gene detected in Daudi cell line. Peroxidase-conjugated oligoprobe and diaminobenzedine/H_2O_2 (DAB/H_2O_2) were used to identify the viral signal. The signal is black dots in the nucleus. (Giemsa counterstain).

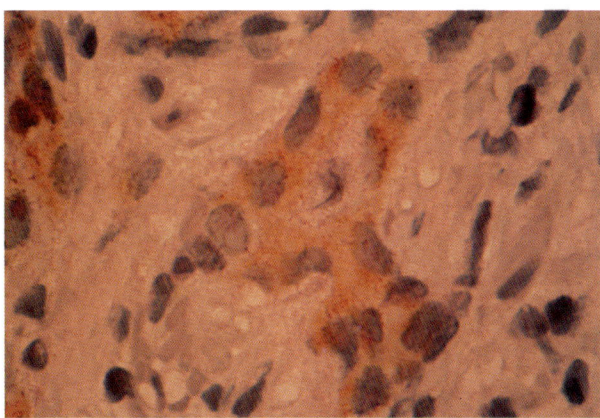

FIGURE C. Detection of prostatic specific antigen (PSA) mRNA in prostate carcinoma. The digoxigenin-labeled antisense oligoprobe was recognized by peroxidase-conjugated antibody and DAB/H_2O_2. The signal is brown granules in the perinuclear cytoplasm of tumor cells. (Schmidt's hematoxylin counterstain).

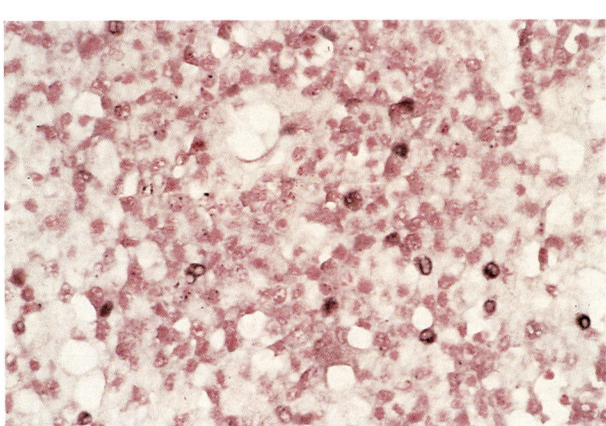

FIGURE B. Epstein-Barr virus in brain lymphoma from a transplant patient with an immunosuppressive regimen. Digoxigenin-labeled Bam HI W fragment probe and DAB/H_2O_2 with nickel enhancement were used to detect the viral signal. (Nuclear fast red counterstain).

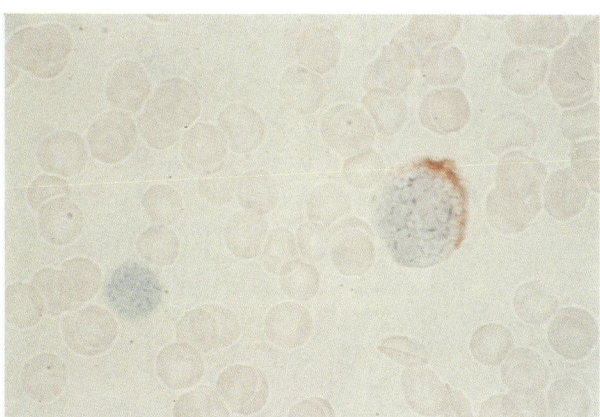

FIGURE D. Detection of topoisomerase II mRNA in a blood smear from a patient with acute myelocytic leukemia. The digoxigenin-labeled probe was detected by alkaline phosphatase–conjugated antibody and iodonitro tetrazolium. The signal is a red precipitate in the cytoplasm of the blast cell. (Schmidt's hematoxylin counterstain).

ELISA principle (digoxigenin system). *Biol Chem Hoppe-Seyler* 371:917, 1990.

Holtke H-J, Seibl R, Burg J, et al: Nonradioactive labeling and detection of nucleic acids, II: Optimization of the digoxigenin system. *Biol Chem Hoppe-Seyler* 371:929, 1990.

Seibl R, Holtke H-J, Ruger R, et al: Nonradioactive labeling and detection of nucleic acids, III: Application of the digoxigenin system. *Biol Chem Hoppe-Seyler* 371:939, 1990.

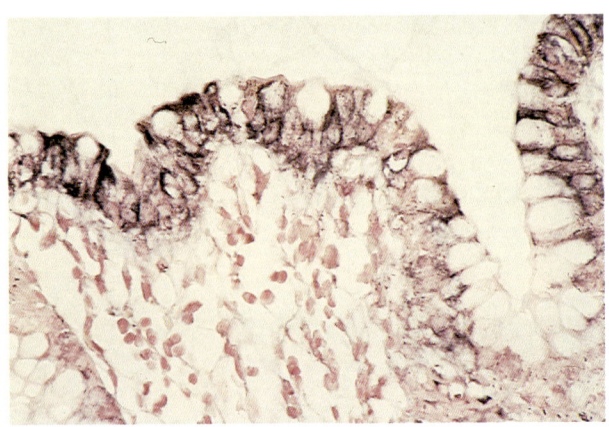

FIGURE E. Detection of TGFβ-1 message in Bouin's-fixed, paraffin-embedded colon tissue. The digoxigenein-labeled anti-sense riboprobe was recognized by peroxidase-conjugated antibody and DAB/H_2O_2 with nickel enhancement. The signal is a black/blue precipitate in the cytoplasm of colonic epithelial cells. (Nuclear fast red counterstain).

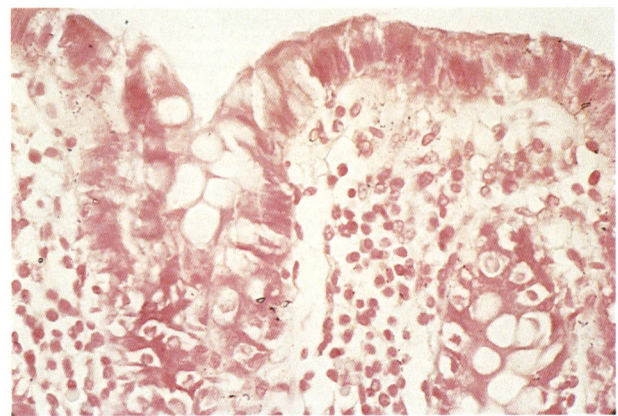

FIGURE F. Colon tissue was hybridized with a sense riboprobe (as the negative control of Figure E). Other conditions were identical to those of Figure E.

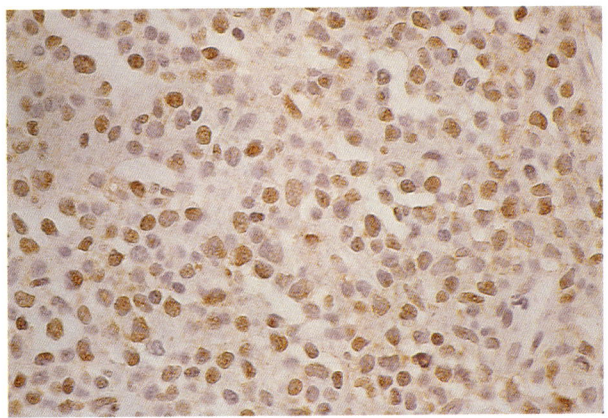
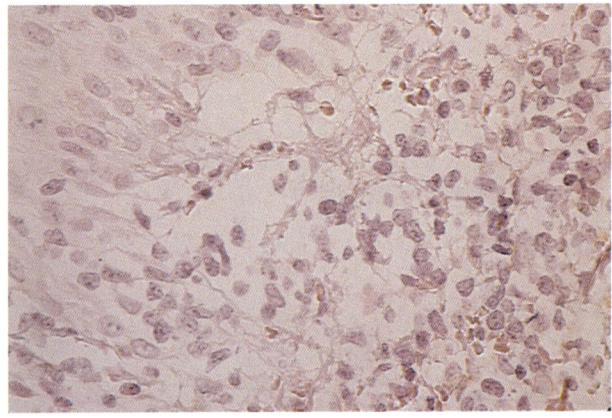

FIGURE G AND H. Detection of a human T-cell lymphotropic virus type I (HTLV-I) signal in a skin biopsy specimen from a patient with adult T-cell leukemia/lymphoma (Figure G) but not in a patient with mycosis fungoides (Figure H). A digoxigenin-labeled DNA fragment (Eco RI and Hind III fragments from pHT-1 [M]3.9 that contains LTR, pX, and env of HTLV-I) was recognized by peroxidase-conjugated antibody and DAB. The signal is a brown precipitate within the nuclei. (Schmidt's hematoxylin counterstain).

Part Three
CASE HISTORIES WITH COLOR ILLUSTRATIONS

CASE 1 Acute Myeloid Leukemia

A 12-year-old boy was experiencing easy fatigability and had had two episodes of epistaxis in the past 2 months. Blood examination yielded the following data: RBC $2.34 \times 10^{12}/L$ ($2.34 \times 10^6/\mu L$); hemoglobin 84.0 g/L (8.4 g/dL); hematocrit 0.253 (25.3%); platelets $180.0 \times 10^9/L$ ($180.0 \times 10^3/\mu L$); and WBC $24.3 \times 10^9/L$ ($24.3 \times 10^3/\mu L$) with 60% blasts.

Comments. This case illustrates the difficulty in differentiating among the subtypes of acute leukemias, granulocytic sarcoma, and large-cell lymphoma when morphologic studies alone are used. In addition, the morphology of leukemic blasts may change significantly in relapse after chemotherapy. Consequently, confirmation of leukemia cell type by cytochemical and immunocytochemical studies is essential for accurate diagnosis and proper mangement of the hematologic malignancies.

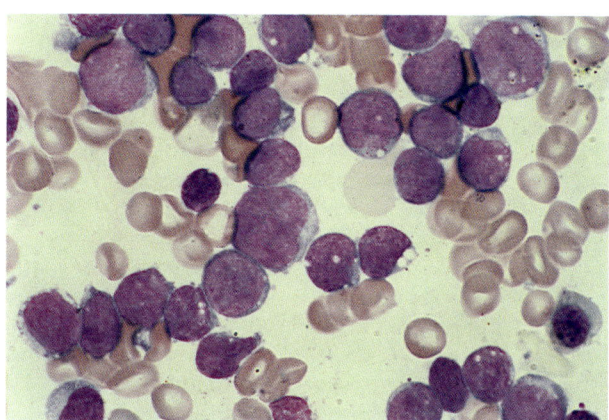

CASE 1-1. A marrow smear showed features consistent with acute lymphoblastic leukemia (ALL) (Wright's stain, ×1000). The patient was then treated with vincristine, prednisone, and intrathecal methotrexate, followed by L-asparaginase, central nervous system (CNS) radiation, and methotrexate maintenance.
Eighteen months later, although the bone marrow still showed no evidence of leukemia, he developed pain in the right testis and some nodularity at its distal pole. Right orchiectomy was performed.

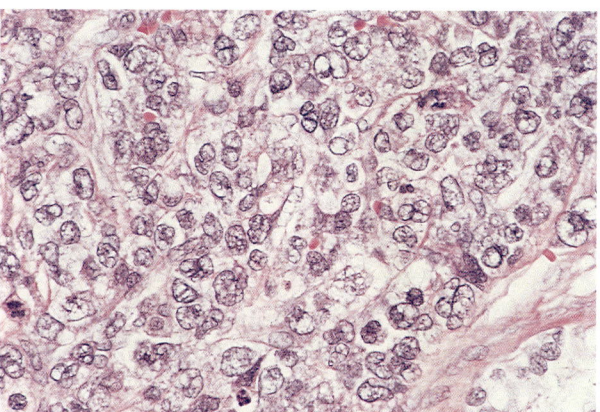

CASE 1-3. A section of the right testis showed extensive interstitial pleomorphic large-cell infiltration sparing the testicular tubules (H&E stain, ×400). This morphologic feature is similar to that of non-Hodgkin's lymphoma. However, because of the previous history of ALL, the infiltration was considered to be testicular relapse of acute leukemia.

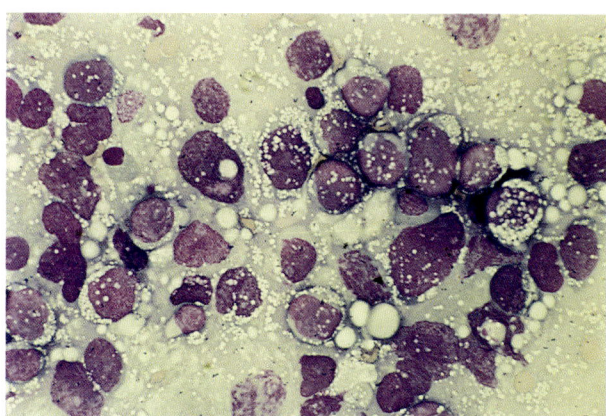

CASE 1-2. A touch imprint preparation of the right testis showed large "blasts" with prominent cytoplasmic vacuolization (Giemsa stain, ×400).

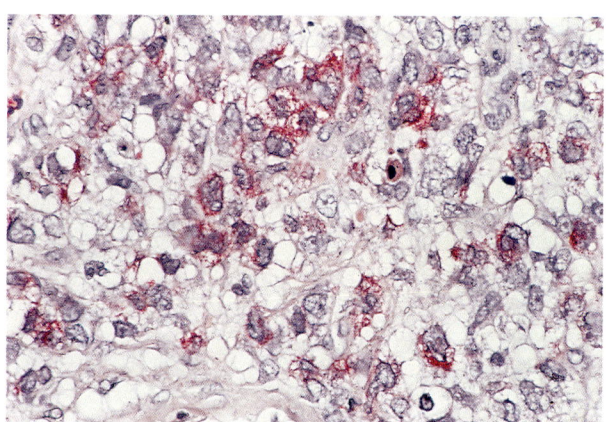

CASE 1-4. The cells from the testicular tumor were then studied histochemically (chloroacetate esterase, ×400). Many of the tumor cells were positive (reddish cytoplasmic staining) for chloroacetate esterase.

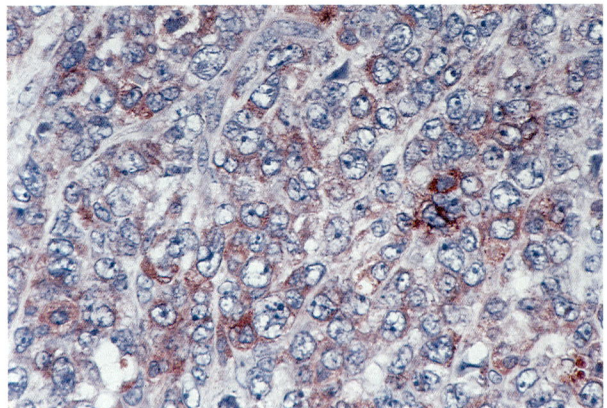

CASE 1-5. Many of the tumor cells were also positive (reddish brown cytoplasmic staining) for lysozyme (immunoperoxidase stain for lysozyme, ×400). The presence of lysozyme and chloroacetate esterase indicated that the tumor cells were myeloid rather than lymphoid. This finding raised the question: Was this testicular lesion a second neoplasm or a relapse of the same acute myeloid leukemia (AML) that was originally misdiagnosed as ALL because of the morphologic similarity of these two leukemias?

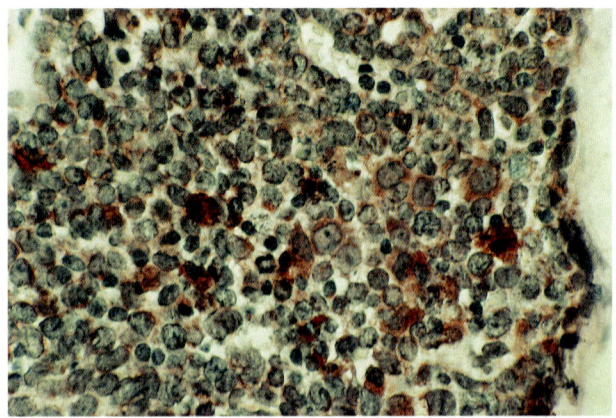

CASE 1-6. To answer this question, the original bone marrow biopsy section was restained with immunohistochemical stain (immunoperoxidase stain for lysozyme, ×400). This stain showed that the leukemic blasts were positive (reddish brown cytoplasmic staining) for lysozyme, a finding that confirmed the suspicion that the original disease was AML.

Four months later, the patient developed bone marrow and CNS relapse. The morphology of the leukemic blasts examined at that time was similar to that of the testicular imprints, and the blasts were positive for the peroxidase stain. The patient eventually died of refractory progressive leukemia complicated with infection 4 months after bone marrow and CNS relapse.

CASE 2 Acute Myeloblastic Leukemia (M1)

A 54-year-old woman was initially seen because of increasing fatigue and easy bruising of 3 weeks' duration. Positive physical findings included pale, scattered ecchymoses and petechiae and mild hepatosplenomegaly. Blood examination yielded the following data: RBC 2.55×10^{12}/L ($2.55 \times 10^{6}/\mu$L); hemoglobin 73.0 g/L (7.3 g/dL); hematocrit 0.20 (20%); platelets 23.0×10^{9}/L ($23.0 \times 10^{3}/\mu$L); and WBC 162.0×10^{9}/L ($162.0 \times 10^{3}/\mu$L) with 82% blasts.

Comments. This patient's blasts contained Auer rods, the classic morphologic and cytochemical features of acute myeloblastic leukemia (AML, M1, type according to the French-American-British [FAB] classification). The peroxidase-positive rods (phi bodies) are usually much more numerous and prominent than the Auer rods that are visualized with Wright's stain. Peroxidase stain is useful in confirming the myeloid cell type. Chloroacetate esterase stain is a good marker for neutrophilic precursors but is generally less sensitive than peroxidase stain for identification of early myeloblasts. Staining with α-naphthyl butyrate esterase was negative in this case.

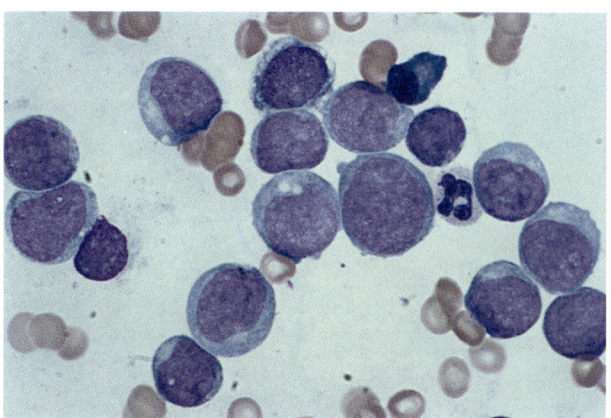

CASE 2-1. A marrow smear showed extensive replacement of the marrow by myeloblasts (Wright's stain, ×1000).

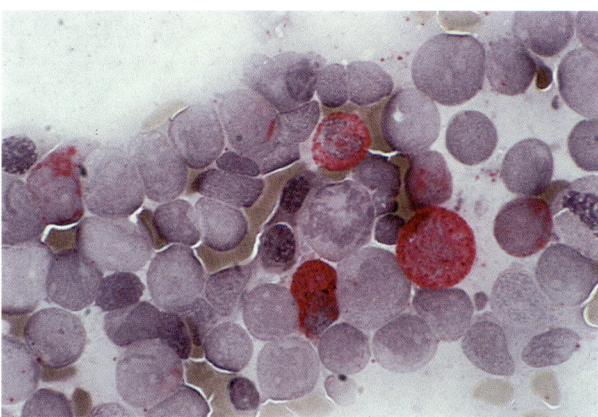

CASE 2-3. A marrow smear showed positive chloroacetate esterase staining (bright red granular staining) in the cytoplasm of a few leukemic blasts (chloroacetate esterase stain, ×1000). A chloroacetate esterase–positive Auer rod was present in one blast in this field.

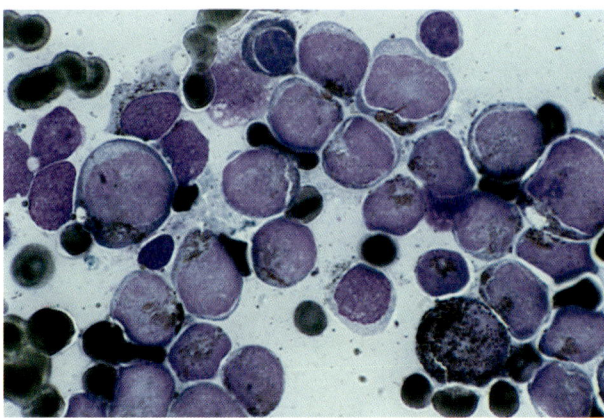

CASE 2-2. A marrow smear showed positive peroxidase staining (dark brownish granular staining) in the cytoplasm of most of the leukemic blasts (peroxidase stain, ×1000). Peroxidase-positive Auer rods (phi bodies); were present in three blasts. Peroxidase-positive, atypical large granules were also present in the cytoplasm of some leukemic blasts.

CASE 3 Acute Promyelocytic Leukemia (M3)

A 45-year-old man was initially seen because of a 3-week history of easy bruising and bleeding gums. Physical examination revealed multiple ecchymoses and petechiae. Blood examination yielded the following data: RBC 3.45×10^{12}/L ($3.45 \times 10^6/\mu L$); hemoglobin 106.0 g/L (10.6 g/dL); hematocrit 0.301 (30.1%); platelets 26.0×10^9/L ($26.0 \times 10^3/\mu L$); WBC 1.3×10^9/L ($1.3 \times 10^3/\mu L$) with 21.5% neutrophils, 42% lymphocytes, 1.5% monocytes, 2.5% eosinophils, 32.5% promyelocytes, and 2.5% normoblasts; fibrinogen 1.11 g/L (111 mg/dL); and fibrin split product 80 µg/mL.

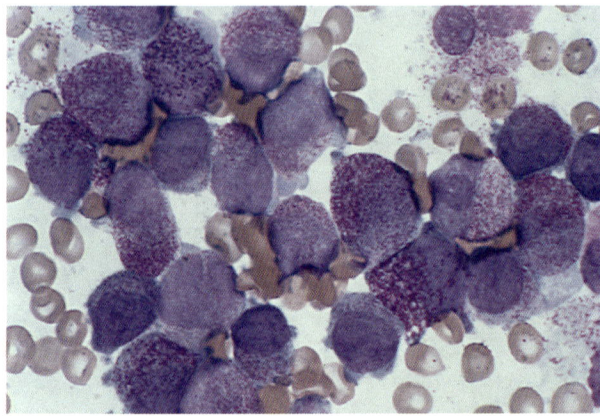

CASE 3-1. A marrow smear showed markedly hypercellular marrow with numerous abnormal, hypergranular promyelocytes (Wright's stain, ×1000). This finding is characteristic of hypergranular promyelocytic leukemia (M3 type of the FAB classification). However, a few "hypogranular," monocytoid cells with bilobed nuclei were also noted.

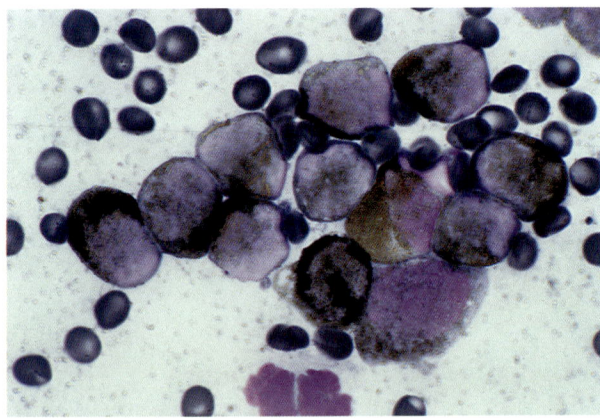

CASE 3-2. A marrow smear showed positive peroxidase staining (dark brownish granular staining) in the cytoplasm of most of the leukemic cells (peroxidase stain, ×1000). Multiple peroxidase-positive Auer rods were present in one of the leukemic cells at the 11 o'clock position of the field. Further staining with α-naphthyl butyrate esterase was negative.

Comments. This case illustrates the characteristic morphologic and cytochemical features of hypergranular promyelocytic leukemia (M3). The abnormal promyelocytes usually show intense positive staining for both peroxidase and chloroacetate esterase stains. The intensity of peroxidase staining is often too strong, and it may become difficult to see the individual granules or Auer rods in the cytoplasm of leukemic cells. The presence of multiple Auer rods in the leukemic cells is best demonstrated by chloroacetate esterase stain. This type of leukemia is commonly associated with episodes of hemorrhage and disseminated intravascular coagulation (DIC), which require induction chemotherapy and administration of heparin to control the coagulopathy.

In the atypical form of acute promyelocytic leukemia (hypogranular variant of M3), the hypogranular monocytoid cells are predominant and are morphologically similar to those of acute monocytic leukemia (AMoL, M5). The majority of cells in the peripheral blood are either devoid of granules or contain only a few fine azurophilic granules. The nuclei of these cells are unusually bilobed, multilobed, or reniform. The findings of a few cells with characteristic hypergranular cytoplasm or multiple Auer rods ("faggot" cells) is important in establishing the diagnosis.

The chromosomal translocation t(15;17) has been associated with cases of typical M3 and with the cases of the M3 variant that have been studied.

This variant of acute promyelocytic leukemia must be recognized as being in the M3 category because its treatment is the same as the treatment for typical M3.

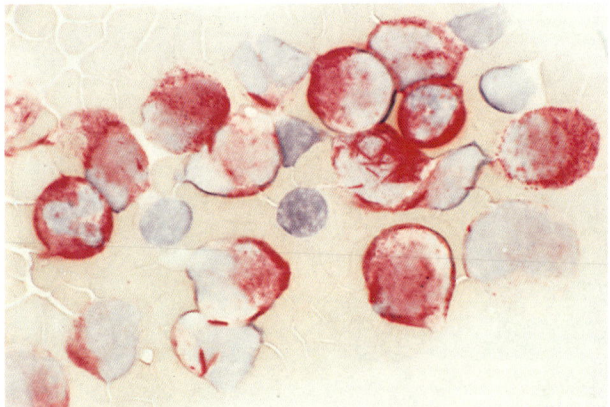

CASE 3-3. A marrow smear from a similar patient showed positive chloroacetate esterase staining (bright red granular staining) in the cytoplasm of most of the leukemic cells (chloroacetate esterase stain, ×1000). Multiple chloroacetate esterase–positive Auer rods were easily seen in two of the leukemic cells in this field.

CASE 4 Acute Myelomonocytic Leukemia (M4)

A 58-year-old man was initially seen because of a 5-month history of fatigue associated with mild leukocytosis and thrombocytopenia. Physical examination revealed moderate hepatomegaly (3 cm below the right costal margin) and splenomegaly (2 cm below the left costal margin). Blood examination yielded the following data: RBC 4.65×10^{12}/L ($4.65 \times 10^6/\mu L$); hemoglobin 127.0 g/L (12.7 g/dL); hematocrit 0.399 (39.9%); platelets 99.0×10^9/L ($99.0 \times 10^3/\mu L$); and WBC 82.0×10^9/L ($82.0 \times 10^3/\mu L$) with 27% neutrophils, 14% lymphocytes, 30% monocytes, 6.5% metamyelocytes, 11.5% myelocytes, 3.5% promyelocytes, and 7% blasts.

Comments. This case illustrates the characteristic morphologic and cytochemical features of acute myelomonocytic leukemia (M4 type according to the FAB classification).

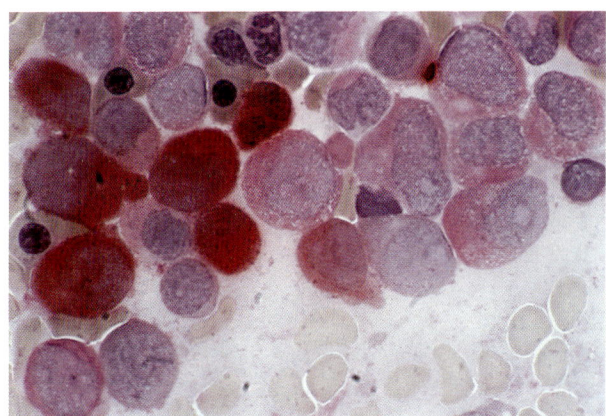

CASE 4-2. A marrow smear showed aggregates of immature cells positive for chloroacetate esterase (pink cytoplasmic staining) on the right side of the field and immature cells positive for α-naphthyl butyrate esterase (brownish red cytoplasmic staining) on the left side of the field (combined chloroacetate esterase and α-naphthyl butyrate esterase stains, ×1000). Most of the immature cells in this case were also positive for peroxidase stain.

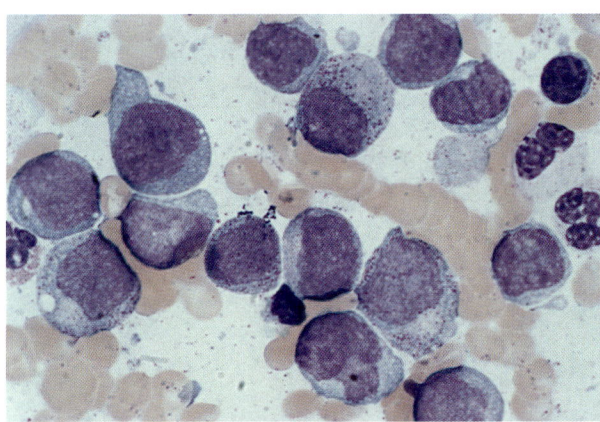

CASE 4-1. A marrow smear showed marked hypercellularity with abnormal myeloid maturation and the presence of many monocytoid cells (Wright's stain, ×1000). Approximately 30% blasts were present.

CASE 5 — Acute Myelomonocytic Leukemia (M4 Variant)

A 79-year-old woman was admitted to the hospital with a history of vague abdominal pain for more than 10 years and a new onset of nausea, vomiting, and easy bruising. Physical examination revealed mild splenomegaly 1 cm below the left costal margin. Blood examination yielded the following data: RBC 3.24×10^{12}/L (3.24×10^{6}/μL); hemoglobin 101.0 g/L (10.1 g/dL); hematocrit 0.291 (29.1%); mean corpuscular volume 89.8 fL (89.8 μm^3); platelets 79.0×10^{9}/L (79.0×10^{3}/μL); and WBC 56.6×10^{9}/L (56.6×10^{3}/μL) with 48.5% neutrophils, 4.5% lymphocytes, 23% monocytes, 2% metamyelocytes, 6% myelocytes, 16% promyelocytes, and 0.5% nucleated RBCs.

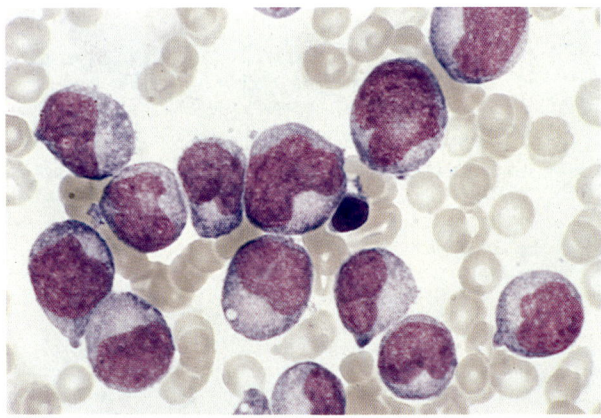

CASE 5-1. A marrow smear showed marked hypercellularity with abnormal myeloid maturation and the presence of immature monocytoid cells (Wright's stain, ×1000). Peroxidase stain was positive in most leukemic cells.

Comments. This case illustrates the characteristic cytochemical features of an unusual variant of acute myelomonocytic leukemia with both granulocytic and monocytic esterases in the leukemic cells.

Cytogenetic study of the bone marrow showed the following karyotype:
8 = 45,XX,−10,del(9)(q?22q?34)/11 = 46,XX[AN].

The patient was initially treated with hydration and hydroxyurea for control of the WBC count followed by a 5-day course of etoposide, with a good response. Results of blood studies 2 weeks after chemotherapy revealed the following data: hemoglobin 121.0 g/L (12.1 g/dL); platelets 45.0×10^{9}/L (45.0×10^{3}/μL); and WBC 8.4×10^{9}/L (8.4×10^{3}/μL) with 63% neutrophils, 16% lymphocytes, 18% monocytes, 1% basophils, 1% metamyelocytes, and 1% blasts.

The patient returned to her local hospital for continuing supportive care.

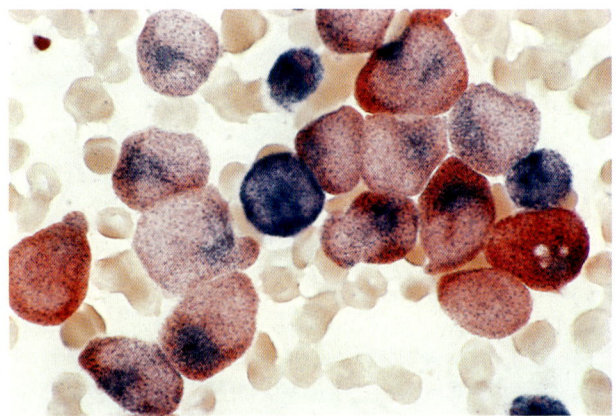

CASE 5-2. A marrow smear showed positive staining for both chloroacetate esterase (blue granular staining) and α-naphthyl butyrate esterase (brownish red cytoplasmic staining) in the cytoplasm of most leukemic cells (combined α-naphthyl butyrate esterase and chloroacetate esterase stains, ×1000).

CASE 6 Acute Monoblastic Leukemia (M5a)

A 62-year-old man was found to be thrombocytopenic during an examination for left buttock pain of 3 weeks' duration. Physical examination revealed marked hepatomegaly to the level of the umbilicus and splenomegaly to 3 cm below the left costal margin. Right axillary lymphadenopathy and a few ecchymoses over the extremities were also noted. Blood examination yielded the following data: RBC 3.27×10^{12}/L ($3.27 \times 10^6/\mu$L); hemoglobin 104.0 g/L (10.4 g/dL); hematocrit 0.306 (30.6%); platelets 31.0×10^9/L ($31.0 \times 10^3/\mu$L); WBC 45.7×10^9/L ($45.7 \times 10^3/\mu$L) with 11% neutrophils, 6% lymphocytes, 0.5% metamyelocytes, 71% blasts, 11.5% promonocytes, and 0.5% normoblasts; and fibrinogen 1.13 g/L (113 mg/dL). The fibrin split product level was markedly elevated (>300 μ/mL), and the protamine gel test result was positive. Both prothrombin time and partial thromboplastin time were prolonged.

Comments. This case illustrates the characteristic morphologic and cytochemical features of acute monoblastic leukemia (M5a). A coagulation disorder is also commonly associated with this type of leukemia, as was found in this case. Previous studies have shown that acute monoblastic leukemia may respond to therapeutic agents differently from the way other nonlymphoblastic leukemias respond. Recognition of the entity is important for determination of optimal therapy.

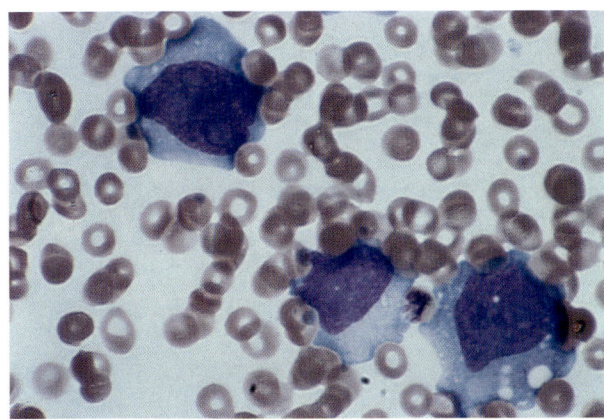

CASE 6-1. A blood smear showed the presence of blasts containing abundant cytoplasm and prominent nucleoli (Wright's stain, ×1000). This finding was consistent with acute monoblastic leukemia (M5a type of the FAB classification).

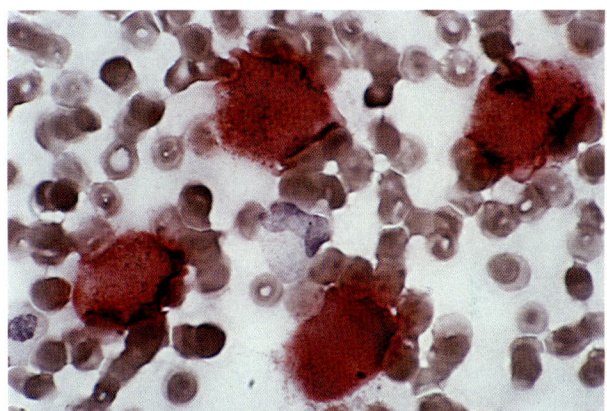

CASE 6-2. Another blood smear showed strong α-naphthyl butyrate esterase staining (brownish red staining) in the cytoplasm of all leukemic blasts (α-naphthyl butyrate esterase stain, ×1000). This finding confirmed the diagnosis of acute monoblastic leukemia.

CASE 7 Acute Erythroleukemia (M6)

A 45-year-old man was initially seen because of recent onset of blurred vision with hemorrhage of the right fundi. He had a 2-month history of increasing fatigue, dyspnea on exertion, and pallor. Physical examination revealed a right fundic hemorrhage at the 1 to 2 o'clock position. Blood examination yielded the following data: RBC $1.8 \times 10^{12}/L$ ($1.8 \times 10^{6}/\mu L$); hemoglobin 69.0 g/L (6.9 g/dL); hematocrit 0.20 (20.0%); mean corpuscular volume 111 fL (111 μm^3); reticulocytes 0.018 (1.8%); platelets $35.0 \times 10^{9}/L$ ($35.0 \times 10^{3}/\mu L$); and WBC $6.4 \times 10^{9}/L$ ($6.4 \times 10^{3}/\mu L$) with 12% neutrophils, 38% lymphocytes, 9.5% monocytes, 0.5% metamyelocytes, 40% blasts, and 21.5% nucleated RBCs. Vitamin B_{12} was 203.0 ng/L and folate was 5.0 $\mu g/L$. A blood smear showed a leukoerythroblastic picture and the presence of microcytic hypochromic RBCs.

Comments. This case illustrates the characteristic morphologic, cytochemical, and immunocytochemical features in a case of acute erythroleukemia (M6) with an unusual monocytic component instead of the usual granulocytic component. The patient received induction chemotherapy with doxorubicin hydrochloride, cytarabine hydrochloride, and thioguanine. He achieved complete remission and remained in remission at the last follow-up 5 1/2 years later.

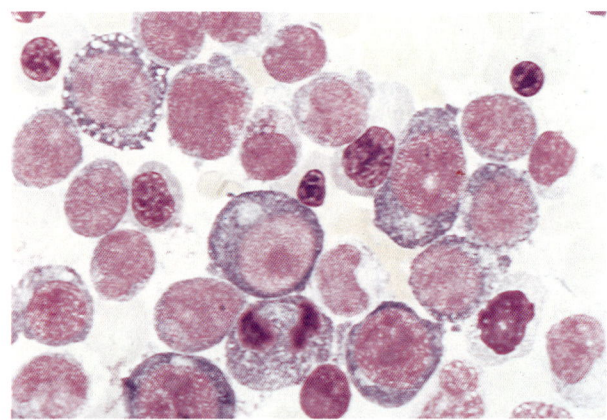

CASE 7-1. A marrow smear showed marked erythroid hyperplasia with an erythroid:granulocyte ratio of >2:1 (Wright's stain, ×1000). Erythroid maturation was abnormal, with megaloblastoid features. More than 30% blast cells were present among the nonerythroid cells, and this could be classified as M6 of the FAB classification.

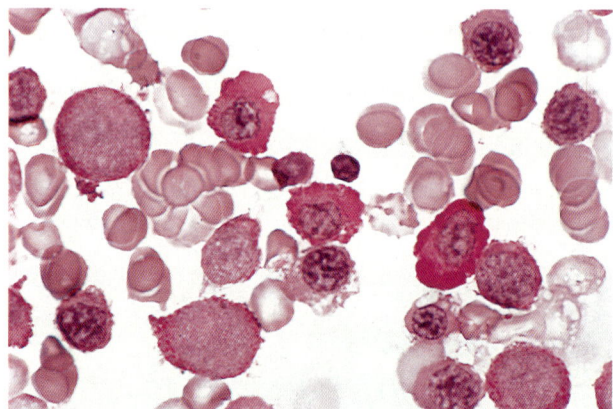

CASE 7-2. A marrow smear showed PAS positivity (reddish staining) in the cytoplasm of some red blood cell precursors (PAS stain, ×1000).

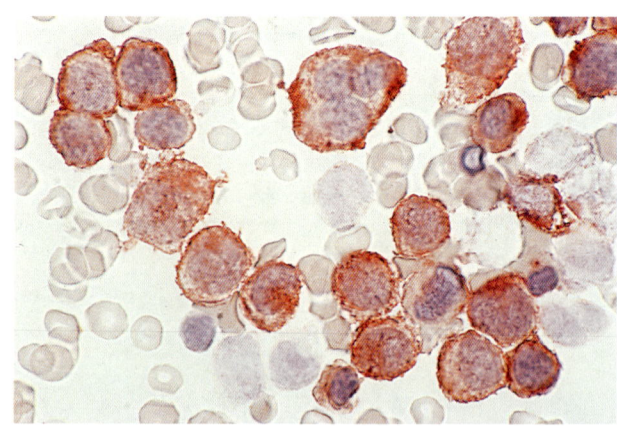

CASE 7-3. A marrow smear showed positive immunostaining of early erythroid antigen on the surface and cytoplasm of atypical erythroblasts, including multinucleated cells at the 12 o'clock position of the field (indirect immunoperoxidase stain for early erythroid antigen using monoclonal antibody RC 82.4, ×1000). Most of the other immature monocytoid cells were positive for α-naphthyl butyrate esterase staining but negative for peroxidase and chloroacetate esterase staining.

CASE 8 Acute Myeloid Leukemia—Basophilic Differentiation

A 57-year-old man was initially seen because of a 2-week history of fatigue and epistaxis. Physical examination revealed numerous mucosal petechiae. Blood examination yielded the following data: RBC 3.13×10^{12}/L (3.13×10^6/µL); hemoglobin 95.0 g/L (9.5 g/dL); hematocrit 0.274 (27.4%); platelets 11.0×10^9/L (11.0×10^3/µL); and WBC 10.1×10^9/L (10.1×10^3/µL) with 60% blasts, 6% neutrophils, 32.5% lymphocytes, and 1.5% eosinophils.

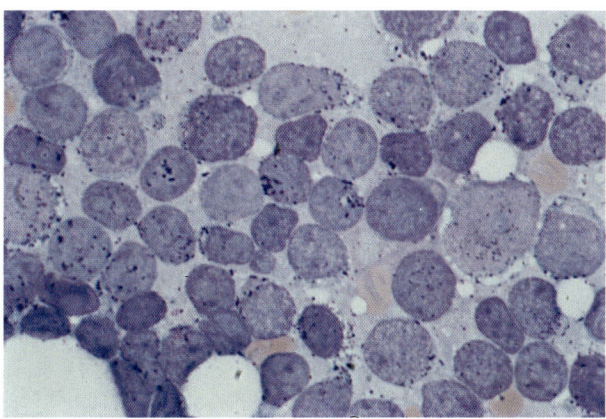

CASE 8-1. A marrow smear showed extensive replacement of marrow by blasts (Wright's stain, ×1000). Most of the leukemic blasts contained various-sized basophilic granules, which was suggestive of acute granulocytic leukemia. However, the peroxidase stain was negative in most of the leukemic blasts. Chromosomal analysis of these cells showed a normal 46,XY, Ph[1]-negative karyotype.

Comments. This case represents a rare type of acute myeloid leukemia with primitive basophilic differentiation. Leukemic blasts usually contain granules that either stain very weakly or are negative for peroxidase but stain positively with toluidine blue, as also occurs in normal basophils. It is important to consider this rare type of acute leukemia as a possible diagnosis when using the peroxidase stain to differentiate nonlymphoblastic from lymphoblastic leukemia.

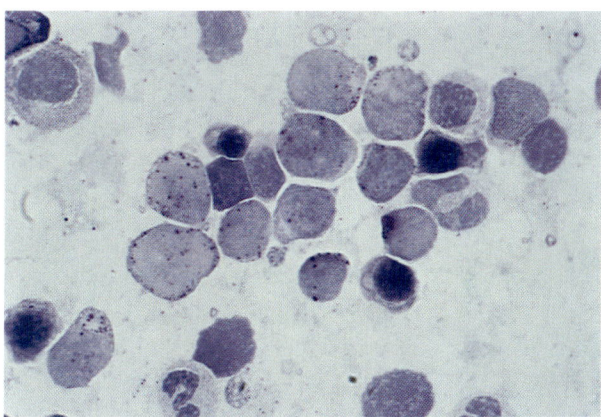

CASE 8-2. A marrow smear showed positive toluidine blue staining (purple granular staining) in the cytoplasm (toluidine blue stain, ×1000). Metachromatic granules were present in many of the leukemic blasts.

CASE 9 Acute Myeloid Leukemia—Eosinophilic Differentiation

A 62-year-old man was examined for a 6-week history of painful swelling over his right foot and ankle. He had a 1-year history of myelodysplastic syndrome with pancytopenia. Six months ago he had noticed a small, firm, erythematous, circular lesion on his right upper arm; the biopsy specimen of the lesion was interpreted as large-cell lymphoma. Physical examination revealed numerous circular, red, raised, firm skin nodules over his face, chest, abdomen, back, and right arm. There was mild pretibial edema and right ankle edema with tenderness over the dorsum of the right foot. Results of roentgenographic examination of the right foot were negative. Magnetic resonance imaging (MRI) examination of the right foot showed an abnormal bone marrow signal in the second metatarsal head and distal half of the second metatarsal shaft and edema surrounding the distal second metatarsal and dorsum of the foot. A bone scan showed a significant increase in vascularity to the forefoot on the right, with a focal intense vascular blush related to the region of the second metatarsal phalangeal joint on the right. Results of a skin biopsy from the right arm were consistent with leukemia cutis. Blood examination yielded the following data: RBC $3.17 \times 10^{12}/L$ ($3.17 \times 10^{6}/\mu L$); hemoglobin 82.0 g/L (8.2 g/dL); hematocrit 0.259 (25.9%); mean corpuscular volume 82.9 fL (82.9 μm^3); reticulocytes 0.0195 (1.95%); platelets $107.0 \times 10^{9}/L$ ($10.7 \times 10^{3}/\mu L$); and WBC $6.0 \times 10^{9}/L$ ($6.0 \times 10^{3}/\mu L$) with 2.5% neutrophils, 26% lymphocytes, 2.5% monocytes, 69% blasts, and 2.5% nucleated RBCs.

Comments. The patient received induction chemotherapy with idarubicin hydrochloride, cytarabine hydrochloride, vincristine, and prednisone. He achieved complete remission but relapsed 7 months later. The reinduction therapy achieved only temporary partial remission. He died of leukemia 10 months after the diagnosis.

Other morphologic variations of acute eosinophilic leukemia may include the presence of poorly stained vacuole-like granules in the cytoplasm of the leukemic cells.

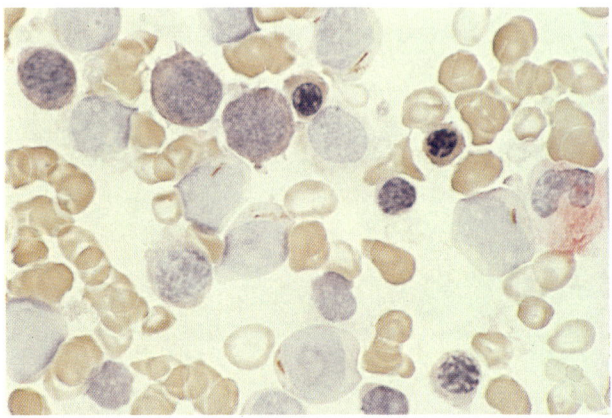

CASE 9-2. A marrow smear showed positive cyanide-resistant peroxidase staining (dark brownish staining) of Auer rods in the cytoplasm of some leukemic blasts. A normal band form neutrophil near the right margin of the field was positive for chloroacetate esterase (red granular cytoplasmic staining) and negative for cyanide-resistant peroxidase stain (combined chloroacetate esterase and cyanide-resistant peroxidase stains with hematoxylin counterstain, ×1000). This finding confirmed the diagnosis of acute myeloid leukemia with early eosinophilic differentiation.

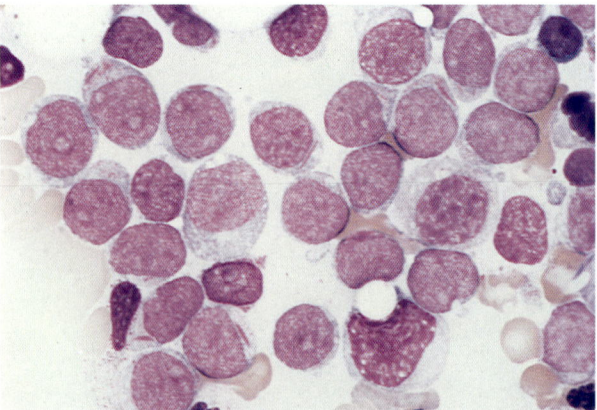

CASE 9-1. A marrow smear showed replacement of marrrow by leukemic blasts (Wright's stain, ×1000). Some of the leukemic cells contained various-sized orange-red granules and Auer rods, which is suggestive of early eosinophilic differentiation. Leukemic blasts were positive for peroxidase and negative for both α-naphthyl butyrate esterase and chloroacetate esterase.

CASE 10 Acute Megakaryocytic Leukemia (M7)

A 57-year-old woman had a 2-year history of a myelodysplastic syndrome requiring frequent transfusion and iron-chelating therapy because of iron overload. She underwent splenectomy 3 months ago because of pain over the left upper quadrant of the abdomen. Physical examination revealed no petechiae or peripheral adenopathy. Blood examination yielded the following data: RBC 3.23×10^{12}/L (3.23×10^{6}/µL); hemoglobin 98.0 g/L (9.8 g/dL); hematocrit 0.278 (27.8%); mean corpuscular volume 86 fL (86 µm^3); platelets 447.0×10^{9}/L (447.0×10^{3}/µL); and WBC 138.9×10^{9}/L (138.9×10^{3}/µL) with 6% neutrophils, 6.5% lymphocytes, 2.5% monocytes, 0.5% myelocytes, and 83% blasts.

Comments. Cytogenetic study of the bone marrow showed the following karyotype: 4 = 46,XX,del(5)(q22q33)/14 = 47,XX, +21,del(5)(q22q33)/2 = 47,XX, −13,+21, +21, del (5) (q22q33), der (12) t (12;?13) (p1?3; q1?4)[AA].

Repeat marrow examination after two cycles of chemotherapy with daunorubicin, cytarabine hydrochloride, and thioguanine revealed residual leukemia. The patient declined further chemotherapy and eventually died 6 months later.

This case illustrates the characteristic morphologic, cytochemical, and immunocytochemical features of acute megakaryocytic leukemia (M7). Other morphologic variations of M7 include the presence of cytoplasmic granules and vacuoles in leukemic blasts, marked variation in the size of leukemic cells, and clustering of leukemic blasts simulating other round cell tumors.

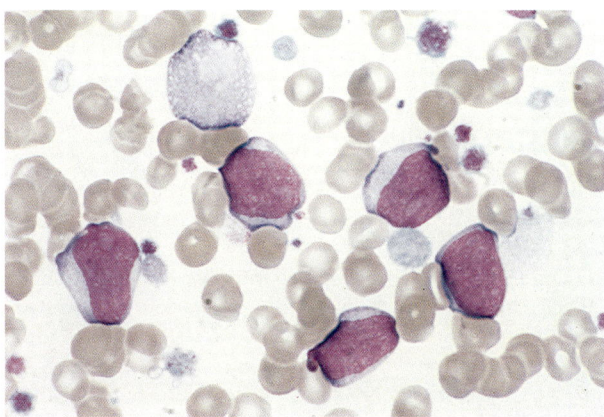

CASE 10-1. A blood smear showed many blasts and increased numbers of platelets, including some unusually large but hypogranular platelets (Wright's stain, ×1000). These leukemic blasts were negative for peroxidase stain.

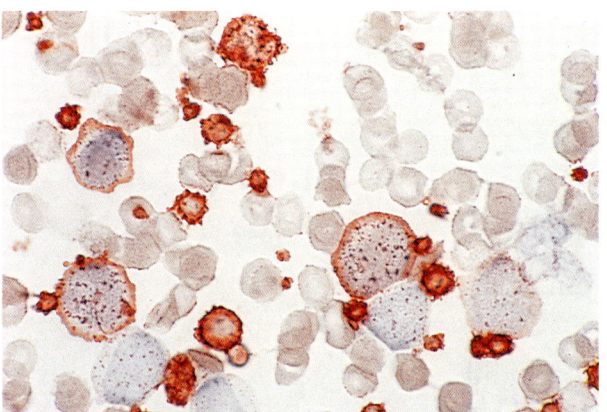

CASE 10-2. A blood smear showed strong, positive immunostaining of glycoprotein IIb/IIIa (CD41A) complex on the surface of most of the leukemic blasts and platelets (indirect immunoperoxidase stain for glycoprotein IIb/IIIa complex using monoclonal antibody HP1-1D, ×1000). This finding established the diagnosis of acute megakaryocytic leukemia (M7).

CASE 11 Intravascular Lymphomatosis

A 52-year-old woman was initially seen because of a 3-month history of anemia that required repeated blood transfusions and a 1-month history of a slowly progressive change in mental status, which was characterized by inappropriate behavior and a declining level of consciousness. She was unconscious at the time of admission. Physical examination revealed spontaneous head turning with roving eye movements. She responded to painful stimuli but not to verbal stimuli. Cheyne-Stokes respirations, meningismus, and positive Kernig's and Brudzinski's signs were noted. A computed tomographic (CT) scan revealed a zone of infarction in the posterior portion of the right temporal lobe. Blood examination yielded the following data: RBC 3.77×10^{12}/L (3.77×10^6/µL); hemoglobin 117.0 g/L (11.7 g/dL); hematocrit 0.344 (34.4%); platelets 69.0×10^9/L (69.0×10^3/µL); and WBC 6.8×10^9/L (6.8×10^3/µL) with 66% neutrophils, 27% lymphocytes, 5% monocytes, 1% eosinophils, and 1% basophils. She remained unconscious and died on the seventh day after admission to the hospital.

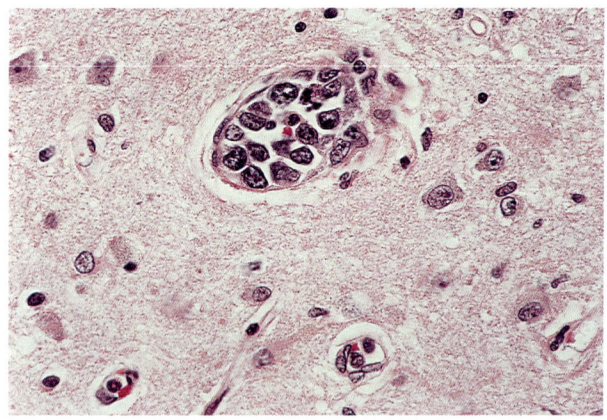

CASE 11-1. A section of the brain showed many blast-like neoplastic cells within the lumina of the cerebral vessels (H&E stain, ×400). Similar vascualr involvement was also seen in the kidney, adrenal glands, and lungs, but no involvement of the marrow, lymph nodes, or spleen was apparent. The neoplastic cells stained negatively for chloroacetate esterase, cytoplasmic immunoglobulin, and lysozyme.

Comments. Until recently, *systemic angioendotheliomatosis* was originally considered to be an endothelial cell–derived tumor. This theory had been supported by the characteristic intravascular confinement of the tumor in conjunction with electron microscopic features and positive immunostaining of factor VIII–related antigen, as illustrated in this case. However, the histogenesis has recently been reassessed as being of a lymphoid nature based on positive staining of newly available immunohistochemical markers, including leukocyte common antigen (CD45) and CD20 (as shown in this case). The term used to describe this disease has been changed to *intravascular lymphomatosis*. The inappropriate presence of factor VIII–related antigen in the intravascular tumor cells and CD20 in the endothelial cells lining the tumor-containing vessels suggested that a close relationship may exist between tumor and endothelial cells, with cross-absorption of cellular antigens.

SUGGESTED READINGS

Arnn ET, Yam LT, Li CY: Systemic angioendotheliomatosis presenting with hemolytic anemia. *Am J Clin Pathol* 80:246–251, 1983.

Ferry JA, Harris NL, Picker LJ, et al: Intravascular lymphomatosis (malignant angioendotheliomatosis): A B-cell neoplasm expressing surface homing receptors. *Mod Pathol* 1:444–452, 1988.

Fulling KH, Gerssell DJ: Neoplastic angioendotheliomatosis: Histologic, immunohistochemical, and ultrastructural findings in two cases. *Cancer* 51:1107–1118, 1983.

Seo IS, Li CY: "Malignant angioendotheliomatosis" revisited: B-cell intravascular lymphomatosis. *J Histochem Cytochem* 38:1044, 1990.

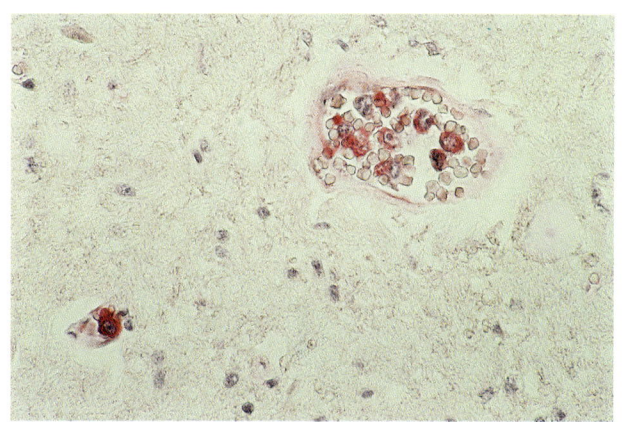

CASE 11-2. Another section of the brain showed positive staining (reddish granular staining) of factor VIII antigen in the cytoplasm of the neoplastic cells (immunoalkaline phosphatase stain for factor VIII antigen using naphthol AS phosphate and fast red violet LB salt, ×400). This finding is suggestive of an endothelial origin of the tumor cells.

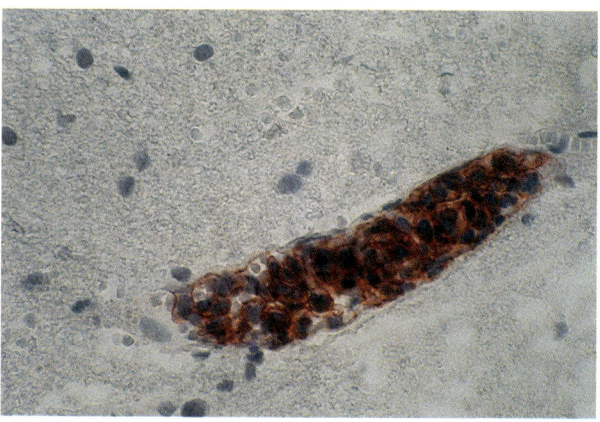

CASE 11-4. Another section of the brain showed positive immunostaining (brownish red granular staining) of CD20 in the cytoplasm of both intravascular tumor cells and vascular endothelial cells (indirect immunoperoxidase stain for CD20 using monoclonal antibody L26, ×400).

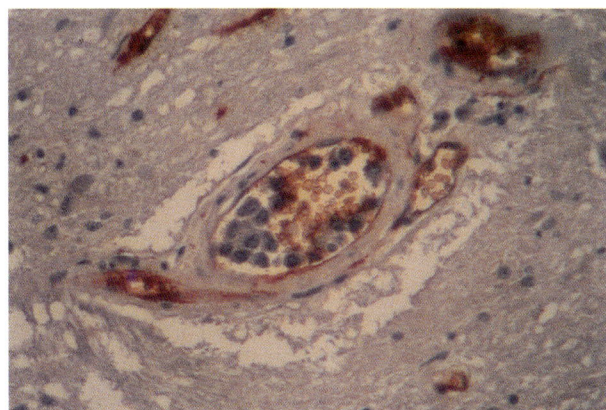

CASE 11-3. Another section of the brain showed positive immunostaining (brownish red granular staining) of Ulex europaeus 1 lectan (UEA-1) in the cytoplasm of vascular endothelial cells but negative staining in the intravascular tumor cells (peroxidase-antiperoxidase [PAP] immunoperoxidase stain for UEA-1, ×400).

CASE 12 Pre-T-Cell Acute Lymphoblastic Leukemia

A 54-year-old woman was initially seen because of recent onset of shortness of breath and a nonproductive cough. A chest roentgenogram showed a large mediastinal mass. Blood examination revealed a marked increase of WBCs (250.0×10^9/L) with 90% blasts.

Comments. This case illustrates the characteristic clinical presentation and morphologic and immunocytochemical features of pre-T-cell acute lymphoblastic leukemia.

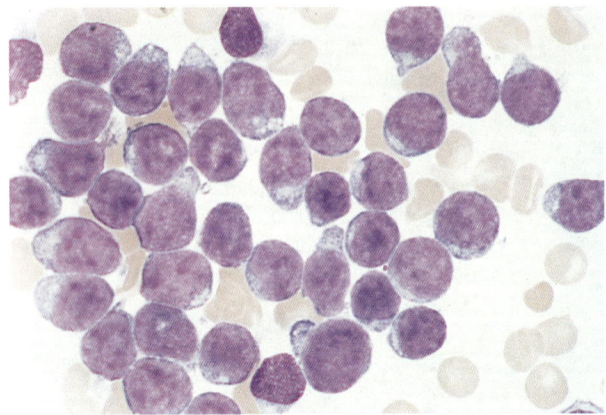

CASE 12-1. A marrow smear showed extensive replacement of marrow by blasts with L1 morphology (Wright's stain, ×1000). Blasts stained negatively with peroxidase, CD19, CD20, and CD22.

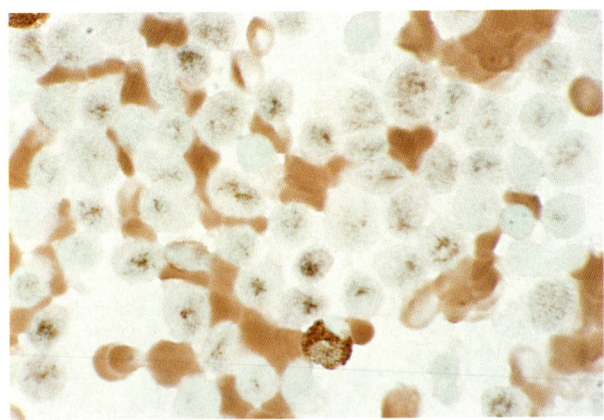

CASE 12-2. A marrow smear showed positive immunostaining of TdT (brownish granular staining) in the nuclei of the leukemic blasts (PAP immunoperoxidase stain for TdT, ×1000).

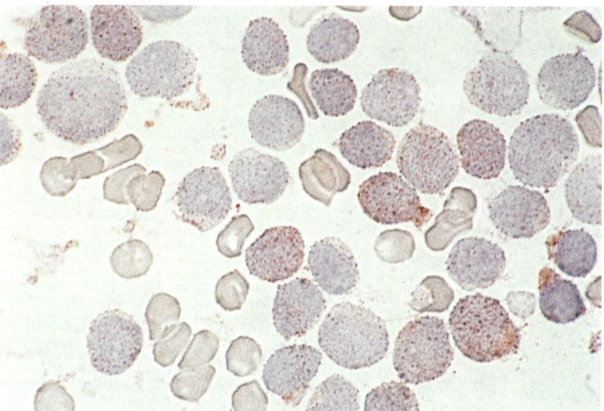

CASE 12-3. A marrow smear showed weakly positive immunostaining (brownish red granular staining) of CD10 on the surface of leukemic blasts (indirect immunoperoxidase stain for CD10, ×1000).

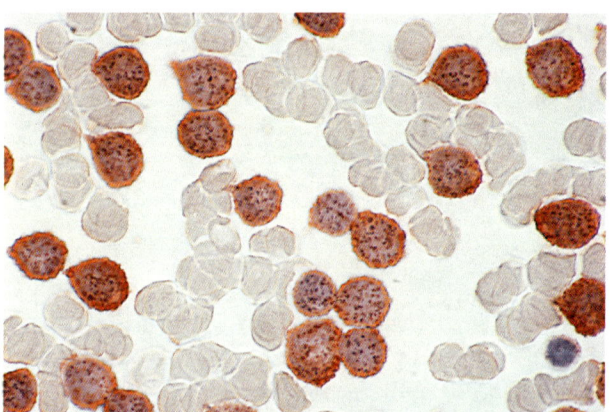

CASE 12-4. A blood smear showed strong positive immunostaining (brownish red granular staining) of CD7 on the surface of leukemic blasts (indirect immunoperoxidase stain for CD7 using monoclonal antibody Leu-9, ×1000).

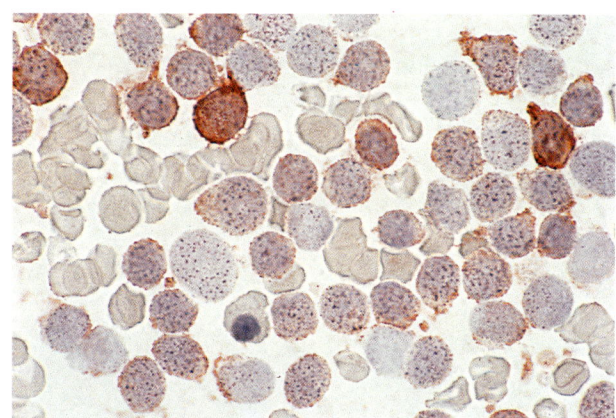

CASE 12-5. A marrow smear showed positive immunostaining (brownish red granular staining) of CD5 on the surface of leukemic blasts (indirect immunoperoxidase stain for CD5 using monoclonal antibody Leu-1, ×1000). Leukemic blasts were negative for CD2 by immunostaining.

CASE 13 Common Acute Lymphoblastic Leukemia

A 2½-year-old boy had had fever of 5 days' duration. Six months prior to this febrile episode, he had suffered from a febrile illness associated with severe neutropenia and marrow hypoplasia. Physical examination revealed redness of the pharynx with exudate. Blood examination yielded the following data: RBC 4.09×10^{12}/L ($4.09 \times 10^6/\mu$L); hemoglobin 112.0 g/L (11.2 g/dL); platelets 260.0×10^9/L ($260.0 \times 10^3/\mu$L); and WBC 5.6×10^9/L ($5.6 \times 10^3/\mu$L) with 20% neutrophils, 73% lymphocytes, 4% monocytes, and 2% eosinophils.

Comments. This case illustrates the characteristic cytochemical and immunocytochemical features of common ALL.

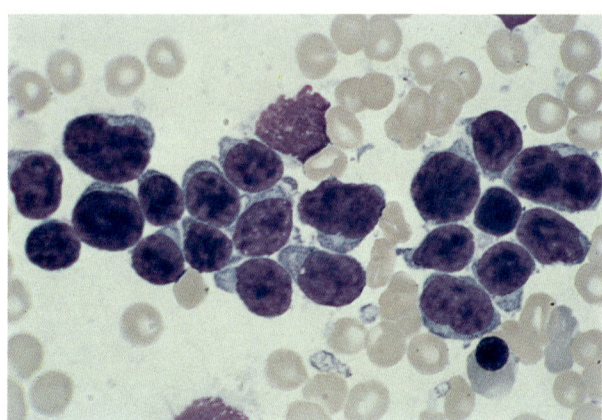

CASE 13-1. A marrow smear showed a hypercellular marrow with extensive replacement of the marrow by blasts (Wright stain, ×1000). This finding established the diagnosis of acute leukemia. The blasts stained negatively for peroxidase, nonspecific esterase, acid phosphatase, and T-cell surface antigens.

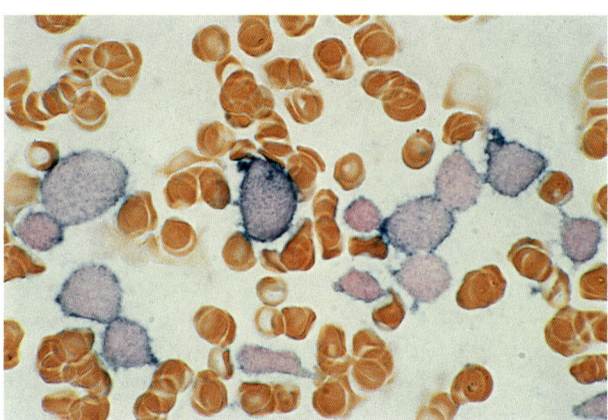

CASE 13-3. Another marrow smear showed positive staining (bluish granular staining) of HLA-DR antigens on the surface of most of the leukemic blasts (immunoalklaine phosphatase stain for HLA-DR antigen, ×1000).

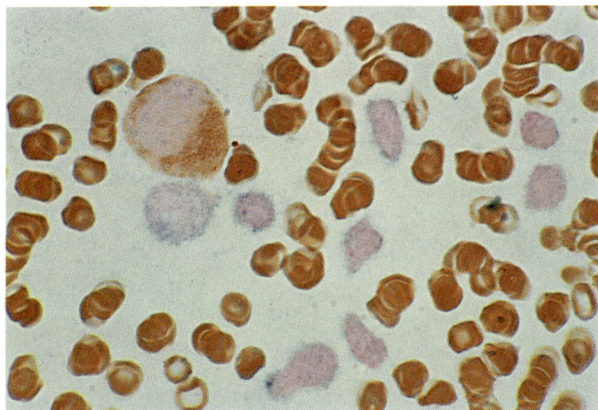

CASE 13-2. Another marrow smear showed positive staining (bluish granular staining on the cell surface) of common ALL surface antigens (CALLA, CD10) on most of the leukemic blasts (immunoalkaline phosphatase stain for CALLA and peroxidase stain, ×1000). An immature granulocyte positive for peroxidase (brownish granular cytoplasmic staining) was visible at the left upper corner of the field.

CASE 14 B-Cell Acute Lymphoblastic Leukemia (L3)

A 64-year-old man had had a 5-month history of a mildly progressive malaise. During the 3 weeks preceding his hospital admission, he experienced worsening symptoms: 9.1 kg weight loss, night sweats, some fever, a nonproductive cough, and exertional dyspnea. Physical examination at the time of admission revealed a shotty 1.0 cm node over the right side of his neck, hepatomegaly down to 2.0 cm below the right costal margin, and splenomegaly down to 2.0 cm below the left costal margin. Blood examination yielded the following data: RBC 4.17×10^{12}/L (4.17×10^6/μL); hemoglobin 116.0 g/L (11.6 g/dL); hematocrit 0.344 (34.4%); platelets 21.0×10^9/L (21.0×10^3/μL); and WBC 8.4×10^9/L (8.4×10^3/μL) with 27.5% neutrophils, 60.5% lymphocytes, 4.5% monocytes, 1% eosinophils, 0.5% basophils, 3% metamyelocytes, 2% myelocytes, and 1% plasma cells. Five days after admission, the WBC count increased to 10.6×10^9/L (10.6×10^3/μL) and contained 30% blasts.

Comments. This case illustrates the morphologic, cytochemical, and immunocytochemical features of L3 acute lymphoblastic leukemia that are characteristic of B-ALL.

Chromosome analysis of the bone marrow specimen in this case revealed a 46,XY karyotype with a translocation involving chromosomes 8 and 14 in all cells. This chromosomal abnormality has been consistently seen in L3 ALL (B-ALL) and Burkitt's lymphomas. Patients with t(8;14) ALL respond poorly to conventional therapy and have the shortest survival rates.

This patient died of persistent leukemia 2½ months after the diagnosis despite intensive chemotherapy, including systemic cyclophosphamide, doxorubicin hydrochloride, vincristine, and prednisone, as well as intrathecal cytarabine hydrochloride for the CNS disease.

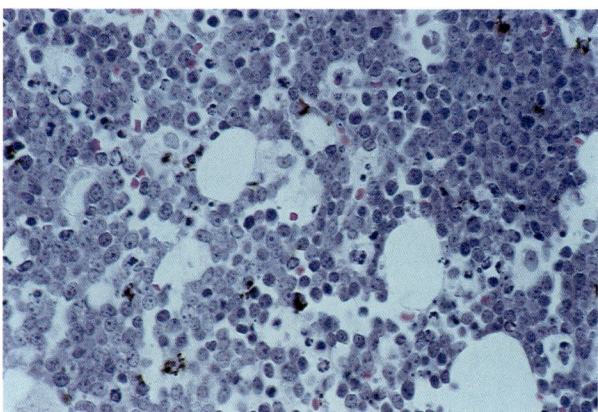

CASE 14-2. A marrow biopsy section showed a histopathologic feature similar to that of Burkitt's lymphoma (H&E stain, ×400). The leukemic blasts appeared uniform in size. The presence of scattered phagocytic histiocytes resulted in a starry-sky appearance.

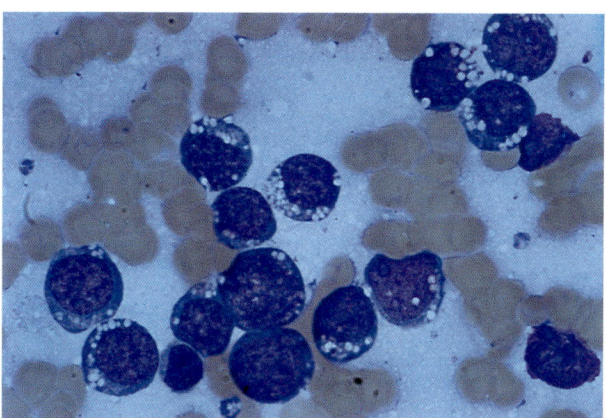

CASE 14-1. A marrow smear showed extensive replacement of the marrow by uniform, primitive lymphoid cells with vacuolated basophilic cytoplasm identical to the description of cells of the L3 type of ALL in the FAB classification (Wright's stain, ×1000). The blasts stained negatively with peroxidase and nonspecific esterase.

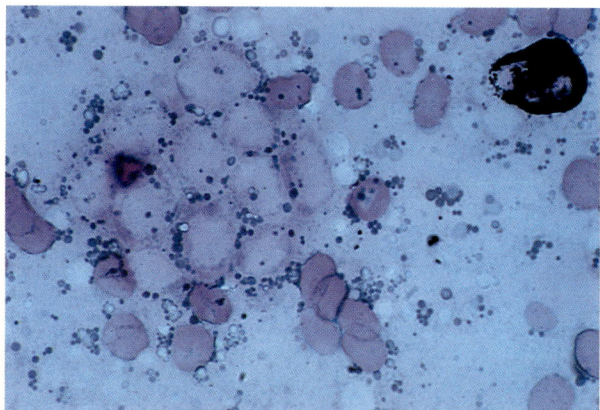

CASE 14-3. Another marrow smear showed light Sudan black B staining in the vacuoles of the leukemic blasts (Sudan black B stain, ×1000). This finding was in contrast to the intense cytoplasmic staining in a granulocyte in the right upper corner of the field. The leukemic blasts stained positively with CD20 and CD19 and stained negatively with TdT and CD10 by immunostaining.

CASE 15 Small Noncleaved Cell Lymphoma—Leukemic Phase (L3)

A 25-year-old man was initially seen because of acute abdominal pain. A laparotomy and resection of 12 cm of the distal ileum were performed because of a free perforation secondary to a small-bowel lymphoma. Staging laparotomy 1 month later established the diagnosis of small, noncleaved cell lymphoma (diffuse undifferentiated lymphoma, non-Burkitt's type) involving the para-aortic nodes.

Comments. Both B-ALL and small, noncleaved cell lymphomas (Burkitt's and non-Burkitt's types) are considered to be closely related diseases. Neoplastic cells of both diseases have similar morphologic features, immunologic phenotype, and karyotypic abnormalities.

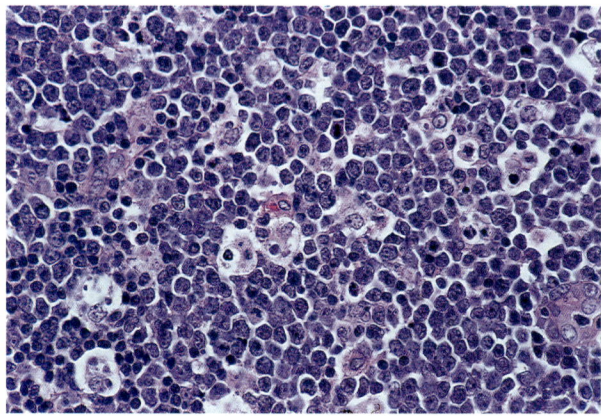

CASE 15-1. A section of a para-aortic lymph node showed small, noncleaved cell lymphoma with a starry-sky appearance due to scattered phagocytic histiocytes with clear cytoplasm (H&E stain, ×400).

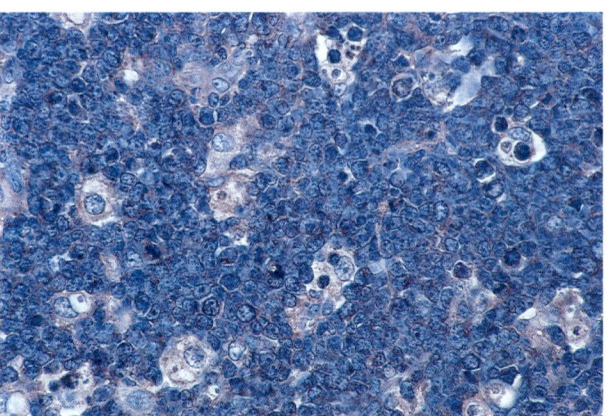

CASE 15-2. Another section of the para-aortic lymph node showed positive λ light chain staining in the cytoplasm of most of the lymphoma cells (immunoperoxidase stain for λ light chains, ×400). Positive staining is indicated by the brownish red staining of one pole of each cell. Staining for κ light chains was negative.
The patient was treated with 40 Gy of radiation to the para-aortic and pelvic lymph nodes. These lymph nodes showed no objective evidence of active disease at the conclusion of therapy. The patient returned 2 weeks later with a huge abdominal mass and bulky peripheral adenopathy. Blood examination yielded the following data: hemoglobin 139.0 g/L (13.0 g/dL); platelets 42.0×10^9/L ($42.0 \times 10^3/\mu$L); and WBC 20.5×10^9/L ($20.5 \times 10^3/\mu$L) with 18% circulating blasts.

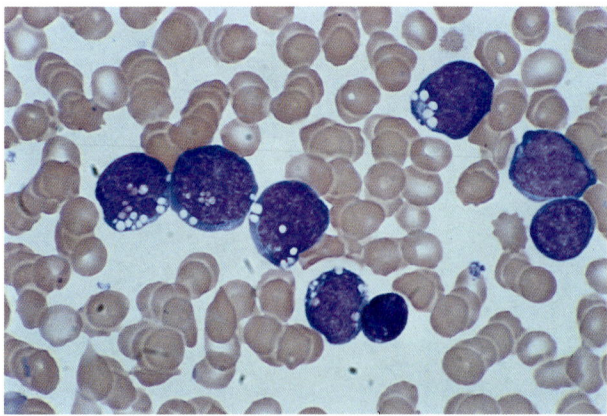

CASE 15-3. A marrow smear showed extensive replacement of the marrow by blasts with morphologic characteristics of the L3 type of ALL in the FAB classification, similar to those found in Case 14, Case 14-1. (Wright's stain, ×1000). Leukemic blasts stained negatively with TdT, CD10, and CD7 and positive with CD19 and CD20 by immunocytochemical stains.

CASE 16 Neuroblastoma

A 23-month-old girl had had a 2-week history of lethargy and irritability. Malignant cells were found on a recent bone marrow examination. Physical examination revealed several firm nodules over the posterior parietal skull and left periorbital edema. A skull roentgenogram showed marked separation of the sutures. A CT scan of the head disclosed a large left parietal mass extending from the cranium to the parietal cortex. Blood examination yielded the following data: RBC 4.62×10^{12}/L (4.62×10^{6}/µL); hemoglobin 122.0 g/L (12.2 g/dL); hematocrit 0.36 (36%); platelets 490.0×10^{9}/L (490.0×10^{3}/µL); and WBCs 12.4×10^{9}/L (12.4×10^{3}/µL) with 56.5% neutrophils, 28.5% lymphocytes, 12.5% monocytes, and 2.5% eosinophils. Levels of urinary vanillylmandelic acid and homovanillic acid were markedly elevated.

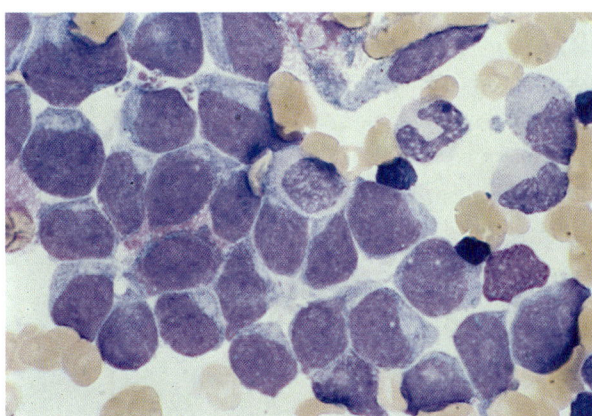

CASE 16-1. A marrow smear showed partial replacement of the marrow by blast-like cells (Wright's stain, ×1000). These cells stained negatively with peroxidase, nonspecific esterase, chloroacetate esterase, Sudan black, and PAS stains.

Comments. Morphologically, neuroblastoma cells may be difficult to differentiate from blasts of acute leukemia, particularly the lymphoblasts. This case illustrates some of the cytochemical characteristics of neuroblastoma cells. Neuroblastoma cells are usually positive for monoamine oxidase stain, and all other leukemic blasts are negative for monoamine oxidase. Monoamine oxidase stain is helpful in the differential diagnosis and positive identification of neuroblastoma cells.

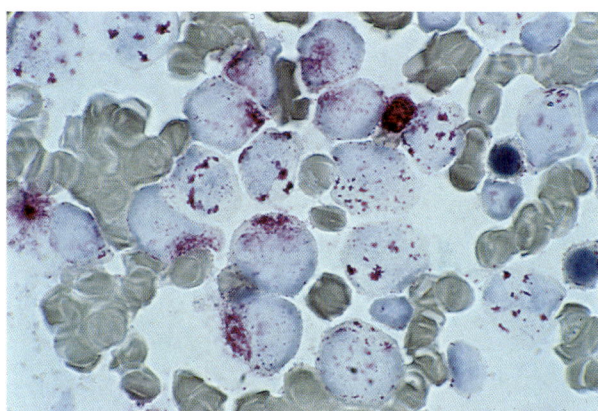

CASE 16-2. Another marrow smear showed moderate focal acid phosphatase staining (brownish red granular staining) in the Golgi area of some of the tumor cells (acid phosphatase stain, ×1000).

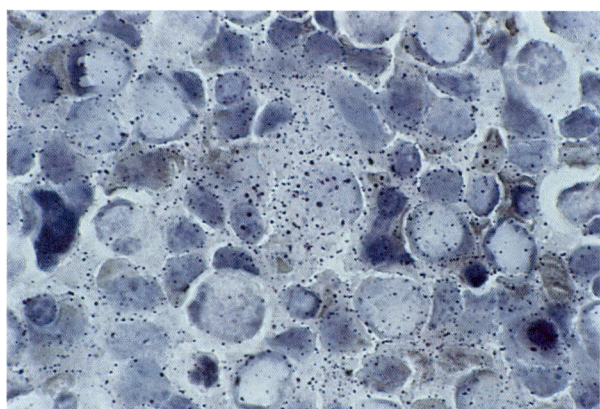

CASE 16-3. Another marrow smear showed positive monoamine oxidase staining (purple granular staining) in the cytoplasm of many tumor cells (monoamine oxidase stain, ×1000). This finding was consistent with the diagnosis of neuroblastoma. A biopsy specimen of the skull lesion also confirmed the diagnosis of neuroblastoma.

CASE 17 Ewing's Sarcoma

A 25-year-old man developed significant thrombocytopenia after 4 months of chemotherapy with vincristine, cyclophosphamide, and actinomycin for Ewing's sarcoma of his left fibula. His platelet count was $36.0 \times 10^9/L$ ($36.0 \times 10^3/\mu L$).

Comments. Ewing's sarcoma is one of the small round cell tumors with some morphologic similarity to acute leukemia or large-cell lymphoma. This case illustrates the characteristic morphologic and cytochemical features of Ewing's sarcoma that are helpful in making the differential diagnosis.

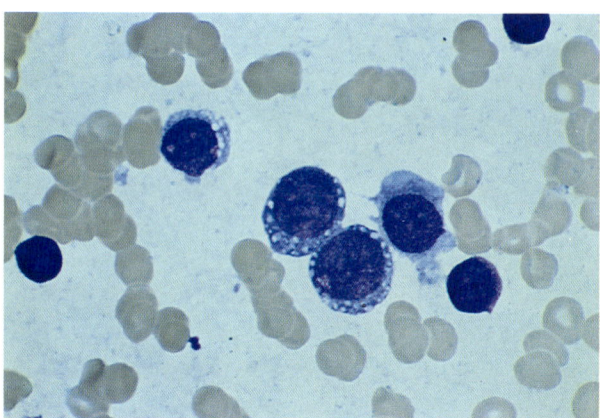

CASE 17-1. A marrow smear showed extensive replacement of the marrow by blast-like malignant cells with vacuolated basophilic cytoplasm, simulating L3-ALL (Wright's stain, ×1000). These cells stained negatively with monamine oxidase.

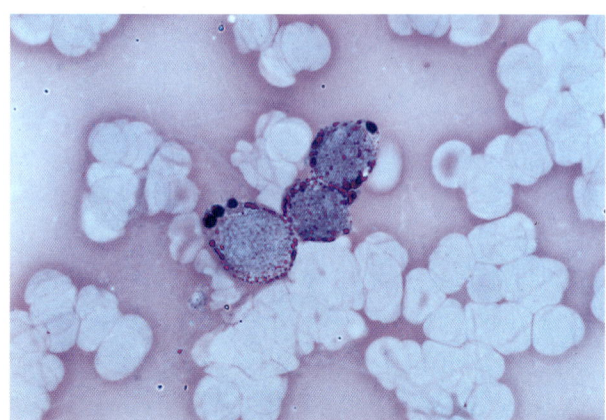

CASE 17-3. Another marrow smear showed strong PAS positivity (red granular cytoplasmic staining) in the tumor cells (PAS stain, ×1000). This finding confirmed the diagnosis of Ewing's sarcoma with marrow involvement.

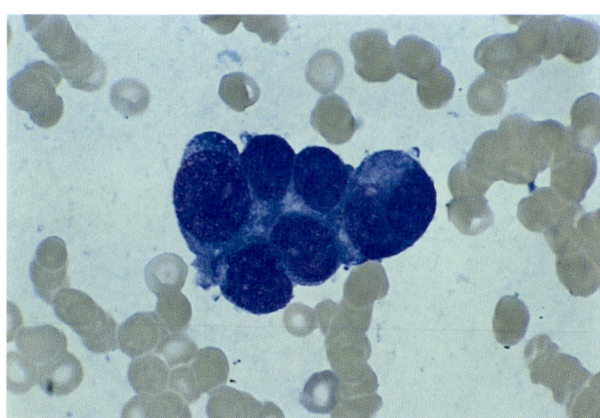

CASE 17-2. Another field of the same marrow smear as in Case 17-1. showed occasional malignant cells in clumps. This clumping is helpful in distinguishing nonhematopoietic neoplasms, in which the cells may form clumps, from hematopoietic neoplasms (such as lymphoma or leukemia), in which the cells do not form clumps (Wright's stain, ×1000).

CASE 18 Rhabdomyosarcoma

A 41-year-old man had had recurring sinus congestion for 3 months. More recently, he developed thoracic back pain after jumping out of bed to answer the telephone. Ten days ago, he developed persistent right epistaxis and right thigh hematoma and was found to be thrombocytopenic. Physical examination revealed a large ecchymotic area involving the right flank, right hip, and right thigh, extending across the lower back to the left hip, and ecchymoses on the sole of the right foot. A roentgenogram and CT scans of the head revealed a large soft tissue mass expanding to the right ethmoid sinus with associated bony destruction and extension into the right maxillary antrum, right nasal cavity, right spheroid sinus, and right supraorbital ethmoid. Blood examination yielded the following data: RBC 3.24×10^{12}/L (3.24×10^6/µL); hemoglobin 95.0 g/L (9.5 g/dL); hematocrit 0.288 (28.8%); mean corpuscular volume 88.8 fL (88.8 µm^3); reticulocytes 0.016 (1.6%); erythrocyte sedimentation rate 5.0 mm/hr; platelets 41.0×10^9/L (41.0×10^3/µL); and WBC 9.2×10^9/L (9.2×10^3/µL) with 52% neutrophils, 30% lymphocytes, 4% monocytes, 2.5% eosinophils, 1.5% basophils, 5% metamyelocytes, 2% myelocytes, 2% promyelocytes, 1% blasts, and 32% nucleated RBCs. Fibrinogen was 0.79 g/L (79.0 mg/dL); fibrin split product >40.0 µg/mL; lactate dehydrogenase 1770.0 U/L; aspartate aminotransferase 360.0 U/L; total bilirubin 37.2 µmol/L (2.2 mg/dL); and direct bilirubin 8.5 µmol/L (0.5 mg/dL).

Comments. This is a case of rhabdomyosarcoma with an unusual clinical presentation and morphologic features that may mimic malignant histiocytosis. The immunohistochemical characteristics, as demonstrated in this case, are helpful in establishing the diagnosis and in distinguishing it from other round cell tumors.

The patient was initially treated with heparin, transfusion of red blood cells, fresh frozen plasma, and cryoprecipitate for control of bleeding, followed by chemotherapy with doxorubicin hydrochloride, cyclophosphamide, etoposide, prednisone, and methotrexate, and he showed improvement. He was subsequently changed to a program that included cyclophosphamide, doxorubicin hydrochloride, and vincristine (CAV).

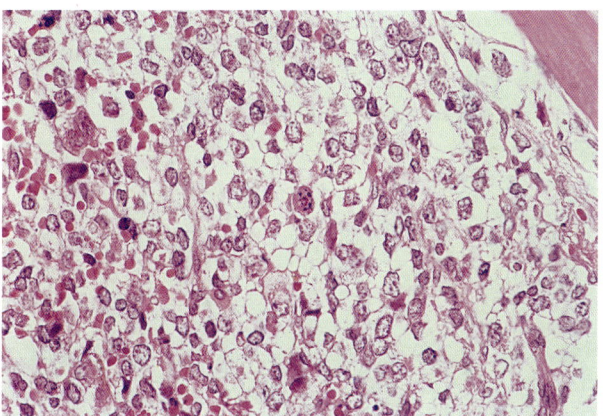

CASE 18-2. A marrow biopsy section showed extensive replacement of marrow by round cells with clear cytoplasm (H&E stain, ×400).

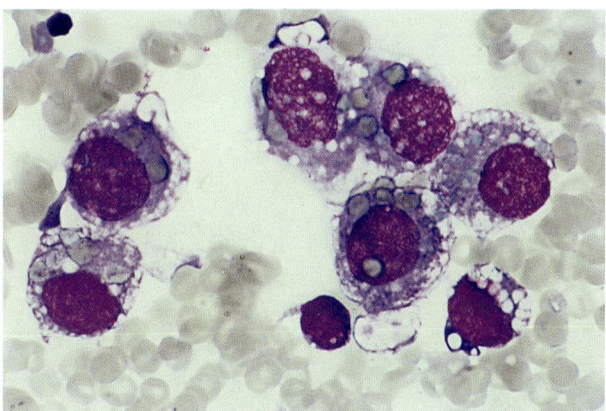

CASE 18-1. A marrow smear showed many large, malignant cells with erythrophagocytosis suggestive of malignant histiocytosis (Wright's stain, ×1000). The tumor cells were negative for keratin, CD14, CD2, and α-naphthyl butyrate esterase but weakly positive for α-naphthyl acetate esterase.

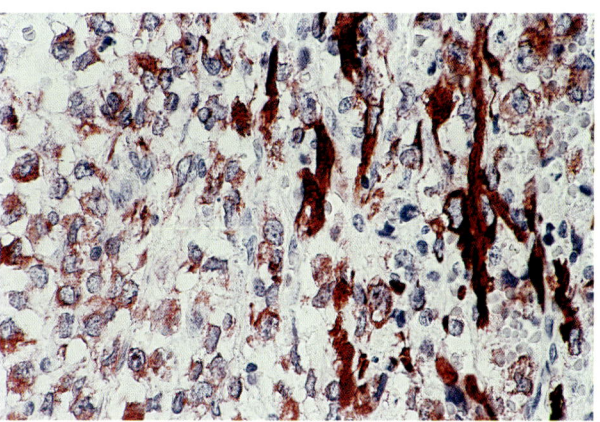

CASE 18-3. A marrow biopsy section showed positive immunostaining (brownish red granular staining) of desmin in the cytoplasm of the tumor cells, especially in the large, elongated cells (indirect immunoperoxidase stain for desmin, ×400).

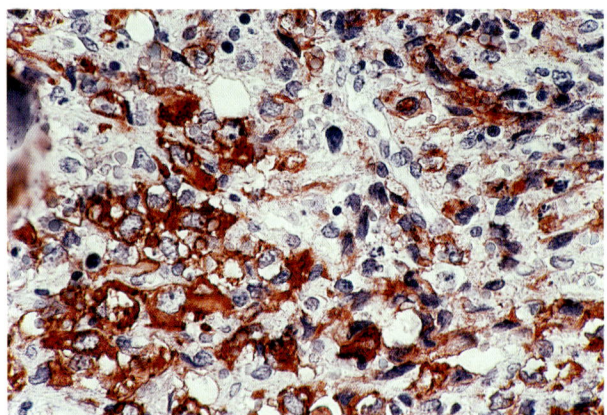

CASE 18-4. A marrow biopsy section showed positive immunostaining (brownish red granular staining) of muscle actin in the cytoplasm of tumor cells (indirect immunoperoxidase stain for muscle actin, ×400). These findings confirmed the diagnosis of rhabdomyosarcoma with extensive marrow replacement.

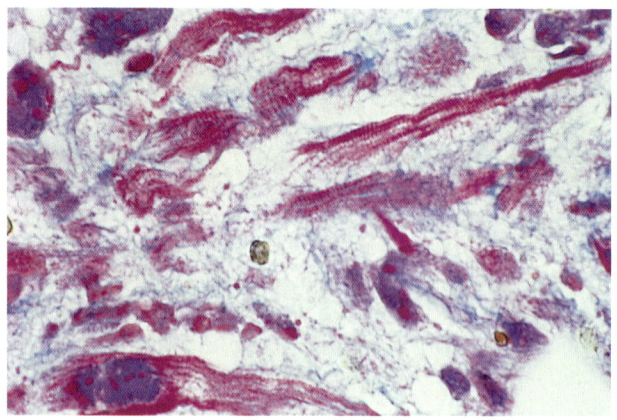

CASE 18-5. Another marrow biopsy section from the same patient 3 months after chemotherapy showed morphologically recognizable muscular differentiation with cross-striation, which further confirmed the diagnosis of rhabdomyosarcoma (trichrome stain, ×1000).

CASE 19 B-Cell Chronic Lymphocytic Leukemia

An asymptomatic 60-year-old man was known to have had mild absolute lymphocytosis for 7 years. During that time, his WBC count had increased from 12.0×10^9/L ($12.0 \times 10^3/\mu$L) to 17.3×10^9/L ($17.3 \times 10^3/\mu$L). Blood examination yielded the following data: RBC 4.55×10^{12}/L ($4.55 \times 10^6/\mu$L); hemoglobin 135.0 g/L (13.5 g/dL); hematocrit 0.383 (38.3%); platelets 229.0×10^9/L ($229.0 \times 10^3/\mu$L); and WBC 17.3×10^9/L ($17.3 \times 10^3/\mu$L) with 71.5% lymphocytes, 1% monocytes, 26.5% neutrophils, and 1% basophils. Conventional immunologic surface marker studies revealed 48% SIg-positive lymphocytes and 26% E-rosette-forming lymphocytes in the peripheral blood.

Comments. This case illustrates the characteristic morphologic, cytochemical, and immunologic features of common B-CLL. Occasional cytoplasmic inclusion may be seen in some cases of B-CLL, as shown in Cases 19-3 and 19-4.

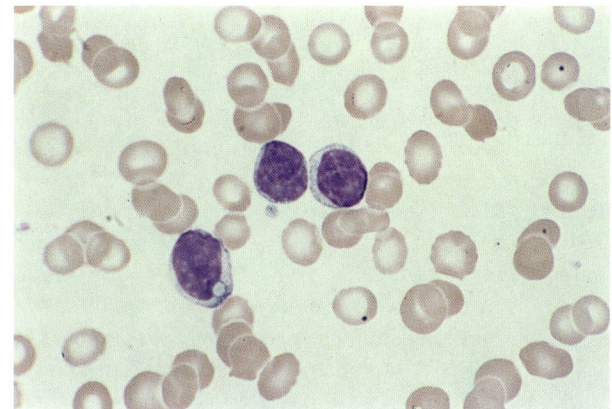

CASE 19-3. A blood smear from another patient with CLL showed a globular cytoplasmic inclusion in one of the lymphocytes (Wright's stain, ×1000). This globular inclusion is usually seen in the leukemic cells of B-CLL with monoclonal κ surface immunoglobulin.

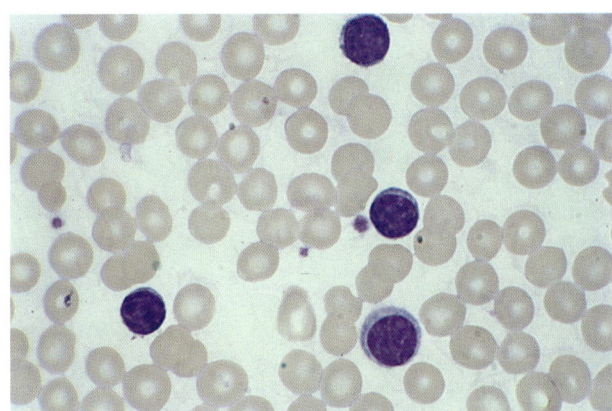

CASE 19-1. A blood smear showed a predominance of mature, small lymphocytes (Wright's stain ×1000). Most of the lymphocytes were negative for α-naphthyl acetate esterase stain and E-rosette formation.

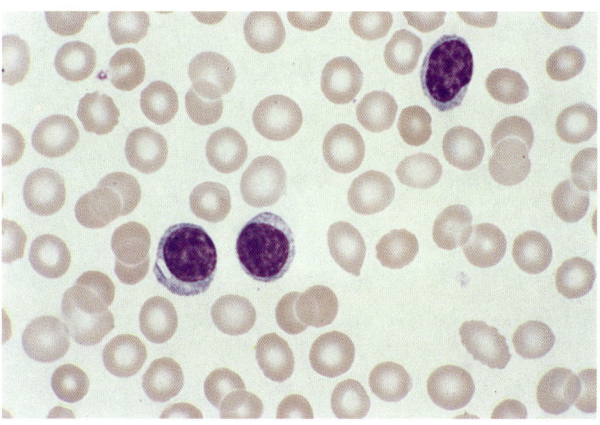

CASE 19-4. A blood smear from another patient with CLL showed immunoglobulin crystals in the cytoplasm of one of the lymphocytes (Wright's stain, ×1000). This type of cytoplasmic inclusion is usually seen in the leukemic cells of B-CLL with monoclonal λ immunoglobulin.

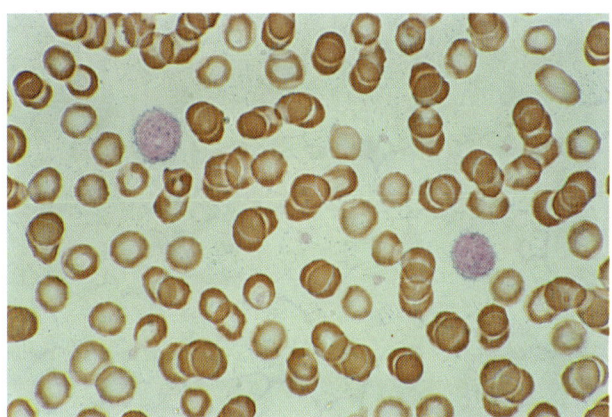

CASE 19-2. Another blood smear showed the positive bluish granular staining of HLA-DR antigens on the surface of most of the lymphocytes (immunoalkaline phosphatase stain using monoclonal antibody specific for HLA-DR antigen and fast blue BBN as the color reagent, ×1000). Staining for T-cell surface antigen was negative.

CASE 20 B Small Cleaved Cell Leukemia

A 70-year-old man had a 6-month history of fatigue, weight loss, and progressive adenopathy. Physical examination revealed prominent generalized peripheral adenopathy ranging from 1 to 5 cm in size and marked splenomegaly, with the spleen tip 5 cm below the left costal margin. A chest roentgenogram showed prominence of the left pulmonary artery, hilar adenopathy, and atelectasis in the right middle lobe. Blood examination revealed the following data: RBC $3.54 \times 10^{12}/L$ ($3.45 \times 10^{6}/\mu L$); hemoglobin 113.0 g/L (11.3 g/dL); hematocrit 0.32 (32%); reticulocytes 0.017 (1.7%); erythrocyte sedimentation rate 127.0 mm/hr; platelets $104.0 \times 10^{9}/L$ ($104.0 \times 10^{3}/\mu L$); and WBC $179.0 \times 10^{9}/L$ ($179.0 \times 10^{3}/\mu L$) with 4% neutrophils, 77.5% lymphocytes, 16% atypical lymphocytes, 1.5% monocytes, and 1% metamyelocytes. Serum protein electrophoresis revealed an increased total protein of 8.69 g/L and an increased γ globulin of 3.2 g/L with a prominent monoclonal spike. Serum immunoelectrophoresis demonstrated a monoclonal IgM λ protein.

Comments. This case illustrates the characteristic morphologic, immunologic, and immunocytochemical features of B small cleaved cell leukemia. In comparison with common B-CLL, positive staining for the pan-B marker CD20 is much stronger, and that for the surface immunoglobulin is also much stronger, with a tendency to capping.

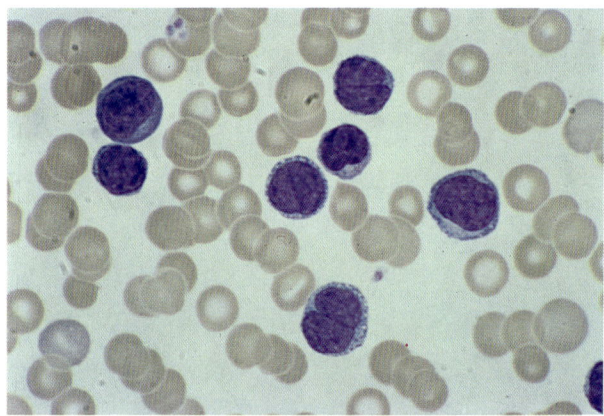

CASE 20-1. A blood smear showed moderate variation in the size of lymphocytes and the presence of many small cleaved cells (Wright's stain, ×1000).

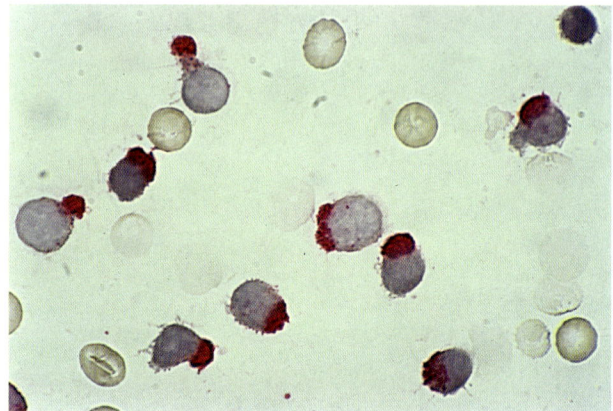

CASE 20-2. Another smear of washed blood cell showed strong immunostaining (bright red granular staining) of λ immunoglobulin with capping (at one pole of cells) on the surface of most of the leukemic cells (direct immunoalkaline phosphatase stain for λ light chain surface immunoglobulin, ×1000). Immunostaining for κ immunoglobulin was negative. This finding confirmed the λ monoclonal B-cell lineage of the leukemic cells.

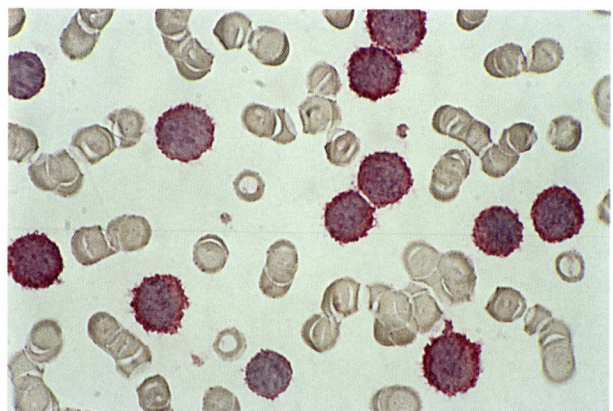

CASE 20-3. A blood smear showed strong positive immunostaining (bright red granular staining) of HLA-DR antigen on the surface of the leukemic lymphocytes (alkaline phosphatase–antialkaline phosphatase [APAAP] immunoalkaline phosphatase stain for HLA-DR antigen, ×1000).

B Small Cleaved Cell Leukemia

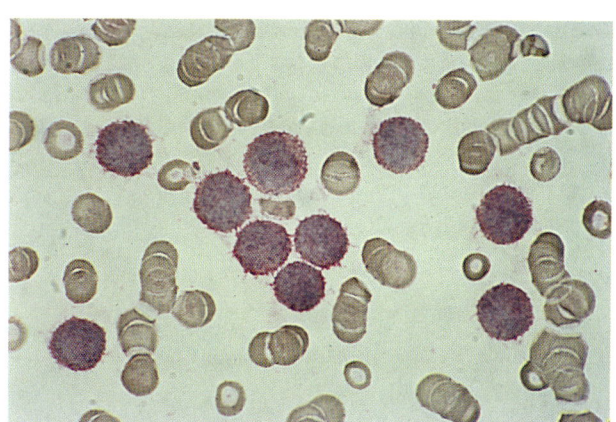

CASE 20-4. Another blood smear showed strong positive immunostaining (bright red granular staining) of CD20 on the surface of the leukemic lymphocytes (APAAP immunoalkaline phosphatase stain for CD20 using monoclonal antibody B1, ×1000). Immunostaininig of CD5 was negative.

CASE 21 Plasma Cell Leukemia

A 51-year-old woman was referred for evaluation of bruising. The condition had been diagnosed at her local hospital 18 months prior to this referral as chronic lymphocytic leukemia. At that time she had anemia, thrombocytopenia, and hepatosplenomegaly. She was treated with six courses of cytoxan, vincristine, and prednisone (CVP), which induced a remission. Six months later, she required a series of admissions for fatigue. Physical examination revealed numerous ecchymoses on the extremities. The liver was enlarged to 4 cm below the right costal margin, and the spleen was enlarged to 6 cm below the left costal margin. Roentgenographic examination revealed lytic lesions of the skull, left arm, femur, and pelvis. Blood examination yielded the following data: RBC $3.43 \times 10^{12}/L$ ($3.43 \times 10^6/\mu L$); hemoglobin 111.0 g/L (11.1 g/dL); hematocrit 0.31 (31%); platelets $29.0 \times 10^9/L$ ($29.0 \times 10^3/\mu L$); and WBC $82.0 \times 10^9/L$ ($82.0 \times 10^3/\mu L$) with 5.5% neutrophils, 1% monocytes, 1% basophils, 0.5% metamyelocytes, and 92% atypical mononuclear cells. Immunoelectrophoretic studies revealed monoclonal IgGλ protein in serum and urine. Urinalysis revealed heavy proteinuria (8.1 g/24 hr urine) with Bence-Jones protein.

Comments. This case illustrates the morphologic and immunocytochemical characteristics of plasma cell leukemia. The plasma cell, because of its terminal differentiation of B cells, tends to lose most of the B-cell markers (including CD19, CD20, HLA-DR, and SIg), except for cytoplasmic immunoglobulin.

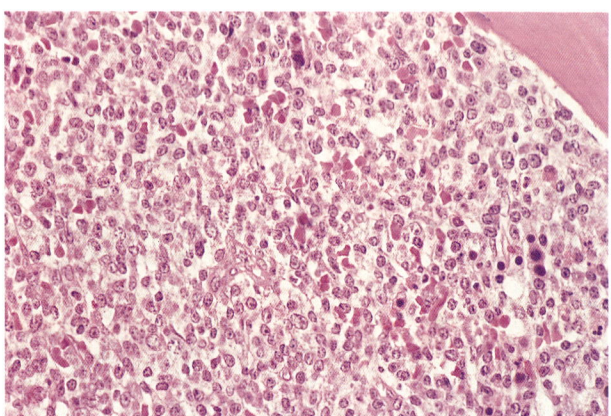

CASE 21-2. A marrow biopsy section showed extensive replacement of bone marrow by small plasmacytoid cells (H&E stain, ×400). Immunostaining of κ immunoglobulin was negative.

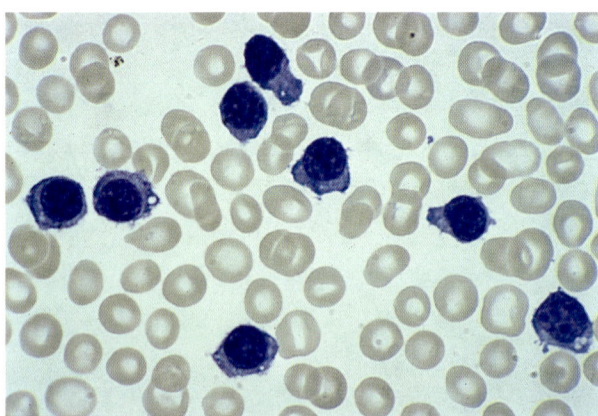

CASE 21-1. A blood smear showed a predominance of small plasmacytoid cells with intense basophilic cytoplasm and slightly eccentric nuclei (Wright's stain, ×1000). These leukemic cells were negative for CD3, CD5, CD20, and HLA-DR.

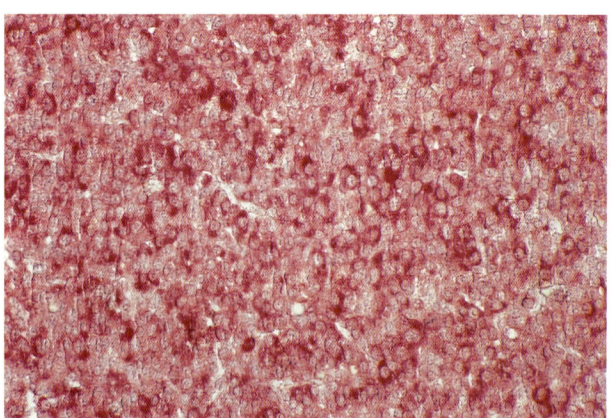

CASE 21-3. Another marrow biopsy section showed strong positive immunostaining (red granular staining) of λ immunoglobulin in the cytoplasm of atypical plasmacytoid cells, indicating the λ monoclonal plasma cell lineage of leukemic cells and confirming the diagnosis of plasma cell leukemia (indirect immunoalkaline phosphatase stain for λ light chain immunoglobulin, ×400).

CASE 22 — Persistent Polyclonal B Lymphocytosis

A 47-year-old woman, who was a smoker, was incidentally found to have lymphocytosis 4 years previously during her annual physical checkup. She remained asymptomatic and her lymphocytosis remained stable, with absolute counts ranging from 8 to 9×10^9/L. Lymphocyte enumeration studies by flow cytometry revealed increased polyclonal B lymphocytes with a normal T helper:suppressor ratio of 2.7. She had a normal hemoglobin level of 151 g/L (15.1 g/dL) and a platelet count of 168.0×10^9/L (168.0×10^3/μL). Her HLA-DR typing was A3, A32, B47, B61, DR5, and DR7. Viral serology for Epstein-Barr virus revealed a viral capsid antigen (VCA) IgG titer of 1:160 and negativity for IgM, indicating past exposure to Epstein-Barr virus.

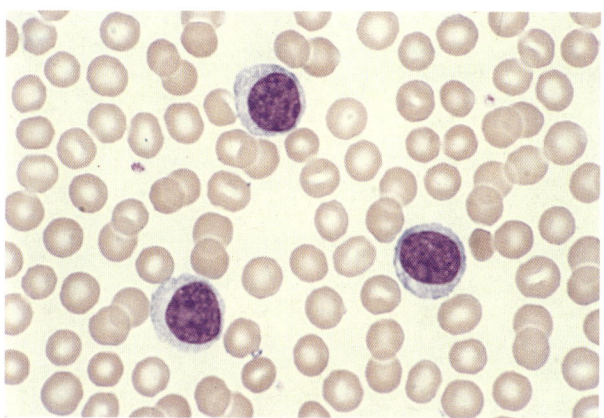

CASE 22-1. A blood smear showed an increase in the number of atypical lymphocytes, which were slightly larger than normal small lymphocytes (Wright's stain, ×1000).

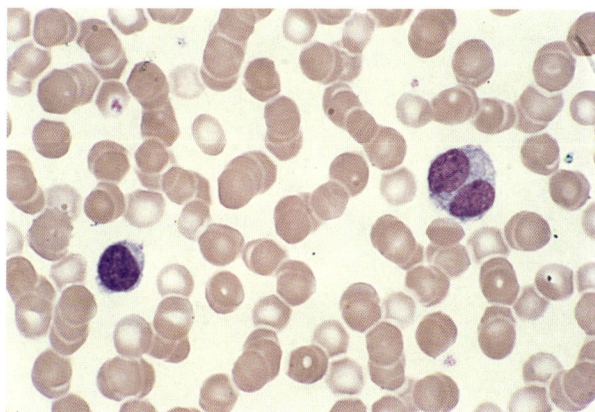

CASE 22-2. Another area of the same blood smear showed atypical binucleated lymphocytes (Wright's stain, ×1000). Immunostaining of CD3 was negative on these lymphocytes.

Comments. This case illustrates the characteristic clinical presentation and morphologic, immunocytochemical, and in situ hybridization features of persistent polyclonal B lymphocytosis. This entity is considered a benign disease and is frequently associated with female smokers with the HLA-DR7 phenotype.

SUGGESTED READINGS

Chow KC, Nacilla JQ, Witzig TE, et al: Is persistent polyclonal B lymphocytosis caused by Epstein-Barr virus? A study with polymerase chain reaction and in situ hybridization. Am J Hematol 41:270–275, 1992.

Gordon DS, Jones BM, Browning SW, et al: Persistent polyclonal lymphocytosis of B lymphocytes. N Engl J Med 307:232–236, 1982.

Troussard X, Valensi F, Debert C, et al: Persistent polyclonal lymphocytosis with binucleated B lymphocytes: A genetic predisposition. Br J Haematol 88:275–280, 1994.

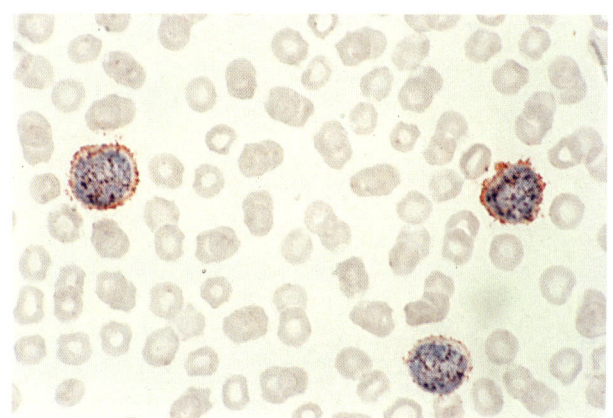

CASE 22-3. Another blood smear showed positive immunostaining (brownish red granular staining) of CD20 on the surface of most of the atypical lymphocytes (indirect immunoperoxidase stain for CD20 using monoclonal antibody B1, ×1000).

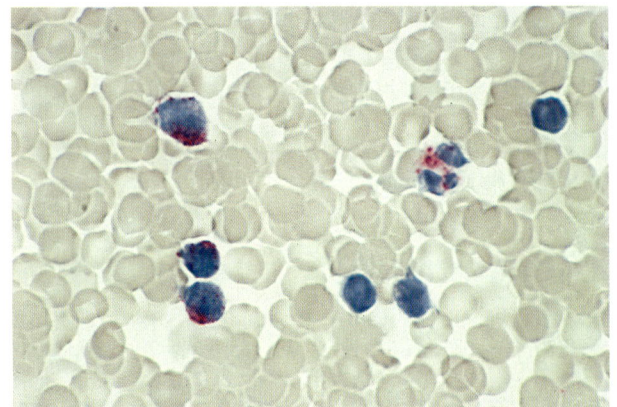

CASE 22-4. A smear of washed blood cells showed positive immunostaining (bright red granular staining) of κ immunoglobulin on the surface of three atypical lymphocytes (with capping) on the left side of this field (direct immunoalklaine phosphatase stain for κ light chain immunoglobulin, ×1000). The immunostaining of λ immunoglobulin showed a similar result. Enumeration of positive cells resulted in 47% of lymphocytes positive for κ and 44% positive for λ, which indicated a polyclonal B lymphocytosis.

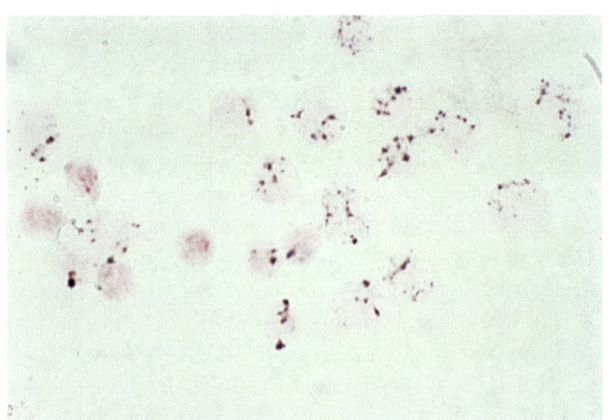

CASE 22-5. A smear of lymphocyte preparation showed positive in situ hybridization of the Epstein-Barr virus genome (dot-like dark brownish staining) in the nuclei of most of the atypical lymphocytes (in situ hybridization for Epstein-Barr virus using peroxidase-conjugated Epstein-Barr virus oligonucleotides, ×1000). This finding indicates that persistent polyclonal B lymphocytosis is strongly associated with Epstein-Barr virus.

CASE 23 Helper T-Cell Chronic Lymphocytic Leukemia

A 61-year-old man was found to have absolute lymphocytosis during an evaluation of leg edema that had been present for 4 months. Physical examination revealed generalized lymphadenopathy of 1 to 2 cm and splenomegaly down to 7 cm below the left costal margin. Blood examination yielded the following data: RBC 3.04×10^{12}/L (3.04×10^{6}/μL); hemoglobin 105.0 g/L (10.5 g/dL); hematocrit 0.28 (28.0%); platelets 97.0×10^{9}/L (97.0×10^{3}/μL); and WBC 66.4×10^{9}/L (66.4×10^{3}/μL) with 92% lymphocytes.

Comments. T-CLLs have been recognized more recently. These cases illustrate the cytochemical, immunologic, and immunocytochemical characteristics of the helper T-cell subtype of T-CLL, characteristics similar to those of normal helper/inducer T lymphocytes. Although nuclear irregularity is not present in normal lymphocytes, it is commonly present in the lymphocytes of cord blood and newborn babies. The immunocytochemical characteristics of T-CLL, however, are quite different from those in common B-CLL, as illustrated in Case 19.

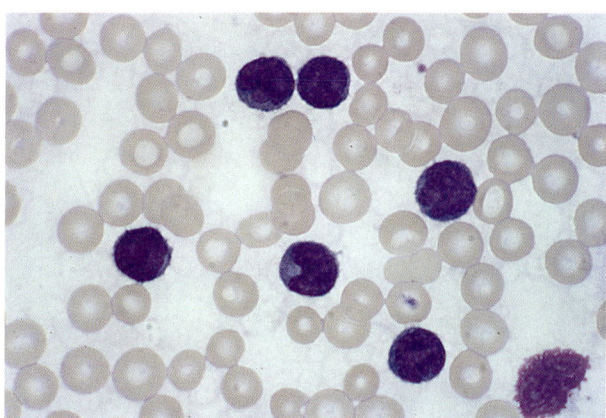

CASE 23-1. A blood smear showed marked lymphocytosis with a predominance of atypical small lymphocytes with irregular, convoluted nuclei (Wright's stain, ×1000).

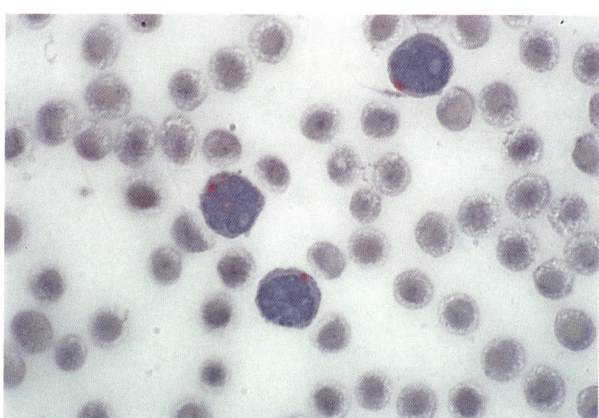

CASE 23-3. Another blood smear showed weak focal acid phosphatase activity (reddish granular staining) in the cytoplasm of the leukemic cells (acid phosphatase stain, ×1000).

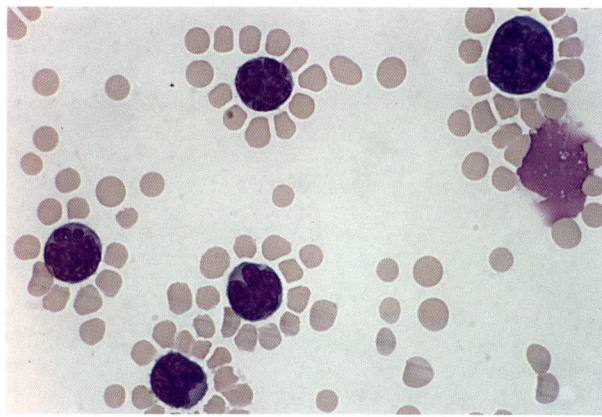

CASE 23-2. E-rosettes formed on most of the atypical leukemic cells (E-rosette preparation with Wright's stain, ×1000). This finding confirmed the suspicion of T-CLL.

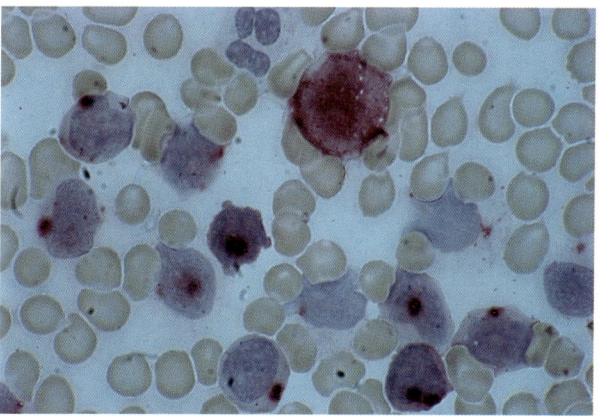

CASE 23-4. Another blood smear showed focal globular α-naphthyl acetate esterase activity (brownish red staining) in the cytoplasm of the leukemic cells similar to that found in normal helper/inducer T cells (α-naphthyl acetate esterase stain, ×1000). This finding is in contrast to the diffuse cytoplasmic staining found in the monocyte at the middle upper portion of the field. The leukemic cells also stained positively for CD5 and CD4 but negatively for CD8 and HLA-DR, further confirming the helper T-cell lineage of the leukemic cells.

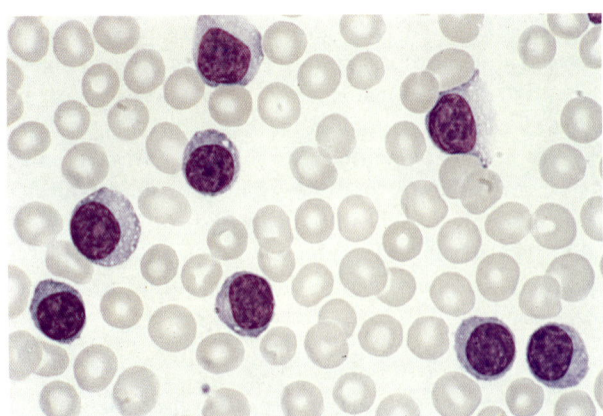

CASE 23-5. A blood smear from another case of helper T-cell CLL showed marked lymphocytosis with a predominance of small lymphocytes with round nuclei (Wright's stain, ×1000). Although most cases of helper T-cell CLL tend to show atypical nuclear irregularity, occasional cases may be morphologically indistinguishable from common B-CLL, as in this case.

CASE 24 Suppressor T-Cell Chronic Lymphocytic Leukemia

An asymptomatic 36-year-old man was known to have splenomegaly and persistent lymphocytosis. He underwent splenectomy 1½ years ago. The spleen weighted 500 g, and a splenic section showed scattered small perivascular lymphocytic aggregates suggestive of lymphoproliferative disorder. During the past 1½ years, his WBC count ranged from 12.0 to 13.0×10^9/L (12.0 to $13.0 \times 10^3/\mu$L) with 90% lymphocytes.

Comments. This case illustrates the morphologic and immunocytochemical characteristics of the suppressor T-cell subtype of T-CLL, which has features of the suppressor/cytotoxic T lymphocytes.

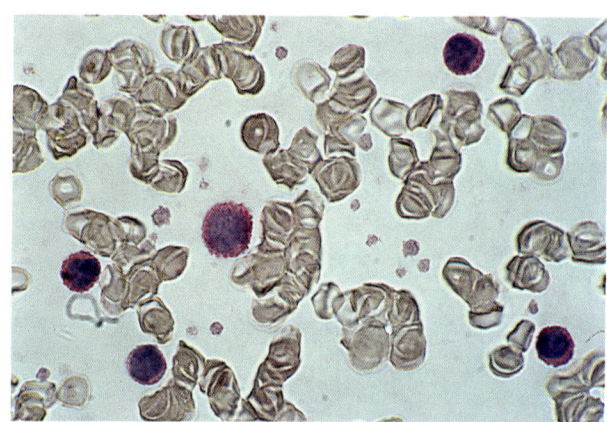

CASE 24-2. Another blood smear showed strong positive staining (reddish granular staining) of suppressor T-cell antigens on the surface of most of the lymphocytes (immunoalkaline phosphatase stain using CD8 monoclonal antibody specific for suppressor T-cell antigens, ×1000).

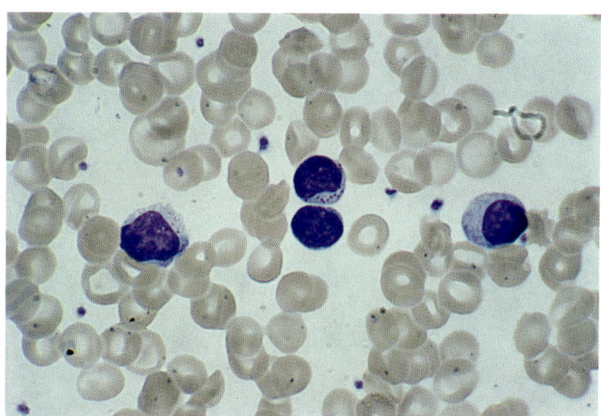

CASE 24-1. A blood smear showed marked lymphocytosis. Most of the lymphocytes had abundant cytoplasm that contained azurophilic granules similar to those found in normal suppressor/cytotoxic T cells (Wright's stain, ×1000). These lymphocytes were negative for HLA-DR antigens and CD4 but weakly positive for CD3.

CASE 25 Chronic Myelocytic Leukemia

A 53-year-old man was initially seen because of a 1-month history of aching and stiffness of the proximal portions of his arms and legs. Physical examination revealed petechiae scattered over the legs, especially on the dorsum of both feet. Examination of his extremities revealed a slow gait with minimal activity of the joints and decreased range of motion, especially of the shoulders and hips. A 1 cm left anterior cervical node was present, and two confluent left inguinal 1 cm nodes were palpated. No hepatosplenomegaly was present. Blood examination yielded the following data: RBC 3.70×10^{12}/L (3.70×10^6/μL); hemoglobin 95.0 g/L (9.5 g/dL); hematocrit 0.30 (30.0%); platelets 113.0×10^9/L (113×10^3/μL); and WBC 85.0×10^9/L (85.0×10^3/μL) with 83.5% neutrophils, 6% lymphocytes, 3.5% monocytes, 2% eosinophils, 1.5% metamyelocytes, 2.5% myelocytes, 0.5% progranulocytes, and 0.5% blasts. Bone marrow examination revealed a hypercellular marrow with marked granulocytic hyperplasia and slight left-shifted maturation. Cytogenetic analysis was not performed owing to insufficient numbers of mitotic figures.

Comments. Leukemoid reactions with unusually large numbers of leukocytes and immature cells in the blood may occur in association with a variety of infections, intoxications, malignant diseases, and even severe hemorrhage or sudden hemolysis. This blood picture is similar to that of CML. The LAP stain is helpful in differentiating CML (low LAP score) from a leukemoid reaction (high LAP score).

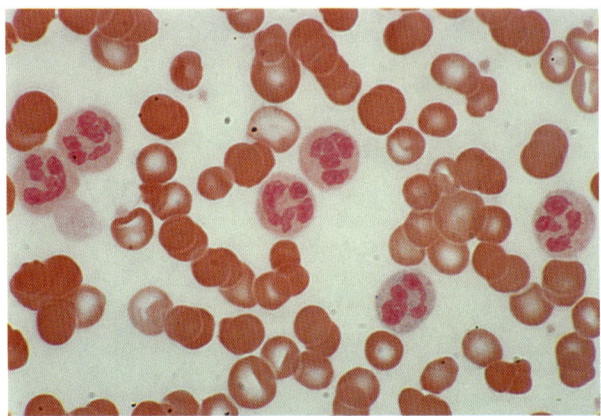

CASE 25-2. Another blood smear showed very low alkaline phosphatase activity in the neutrophils (alkaline phosphatase stain using naphthol AS phosphate and fast blue BBN, ×1000). This finding was consistent with chronic granulocytic leukemia. The leukocyte alkaline phosphatase (LAP) score was 5 (see Part 2, Section 5.22, for information on scoring).

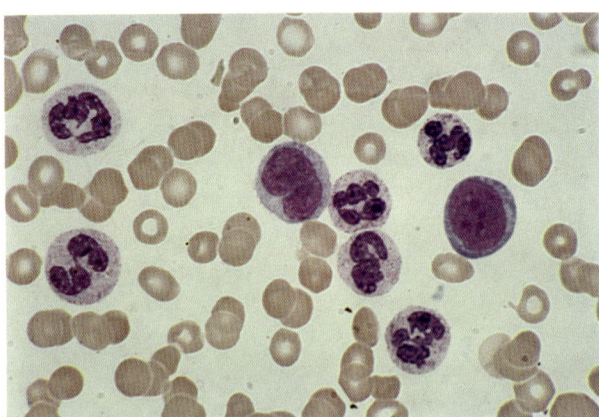

CASE 25-1. A blood smear showed marked neutrophilia with slight left-shifted maturation (Wright's stain, ×1000).

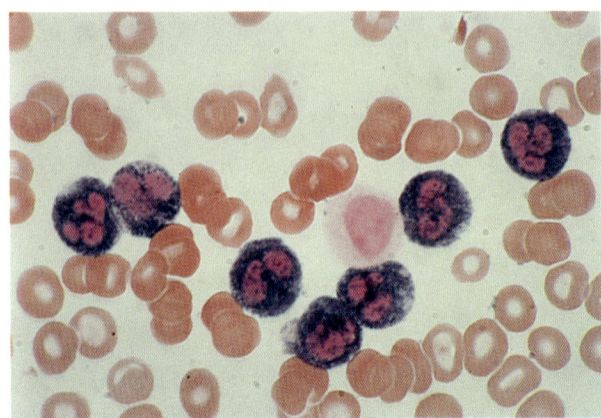

CASE 25-3. This blood smear, from a patient with a leukemoid reaction, was used as a positive control. It showed strong alkaline phosphatase activity (bluish granular staining) in the cytoplasm of the neutrophils (alkaline phosphatase stain using naphthol AS phosphate and fast blue BBN, ×1000). The LAP score was 231.

CASE 26 Chronic Myelomonocytic Leukemia in Transition to M4

A 75-year-old man was seen because of shortness of breath, increasing confusion, and weight loss. He had been asymptomatic 4 months earlier, when initial laboratory examination revealed the following data: WBC 70.0×10^9/L ($70.0 \times 10^3/\mu$L) with 59% neutrophils, 26% monocytes, 13% lymphocytes, 1% metamyelocytes, and 1% eosinophils; hemoglobin 113.0 g/L (11.3 g/dL); platelets 263.0×10^9/L ($263.0 \times 10^3/\mu$L), and normal results of bone marrow cytogenetic studies. He was treated with hydroxyurea at that time. Physical examination revealed signs of right lower lung pneumonia and mild splenomegaly. Blood examination yielded the following data: hemoglobin 72.0 g/L (7.2 g/dL); platelets 93.0×10^9/L ($93.0 \times 10^3/\mu$L); and WBC 332.0×10^9/L ($332.0 \times 10^3/\mu$L) with 75% blasts.

Comments. This case illustrates the characteristic morphologic, cytochemical, and immunocytochemical features of chronic and acute myelomonocytic leukemias. Combined α-naphthyl butyrate and chloroacetate esterase stains are the most useful in identifying both monocytic and granulocytic components on the same smear.

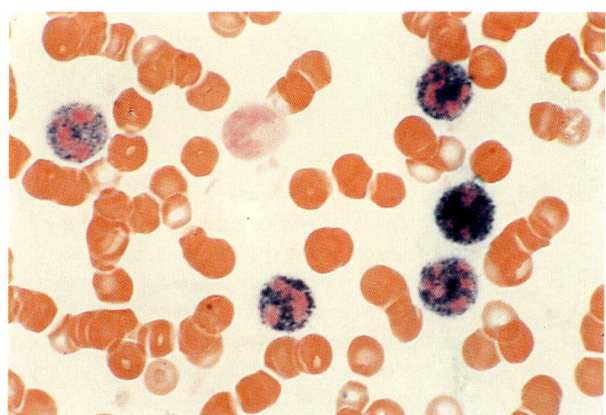

CASE 26.2. Another blood smear showed positive alkaline phosphatase staining (bluish granular staining) in the cytoplasm of most of the neutrophils (alkaline phosphatase stain using naphthol AS phosphate and fast blue BBN, ×1000). The LAP score was 159. This finding makes the diagnosis of chronic myelocytic leukemia very unlikely.

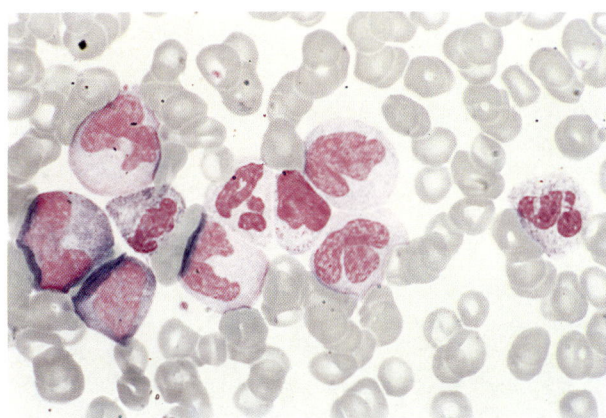

CASE 26-1. Initial blood smear showed marked leukocytosis with left-shifted granulocytic maturation and monocytosis (Wright's stain, ×1000). The major differential diagnoses include chronic myelocytic leukemia, leukemoid reaction, and chronic myelomonocytic leukemia.

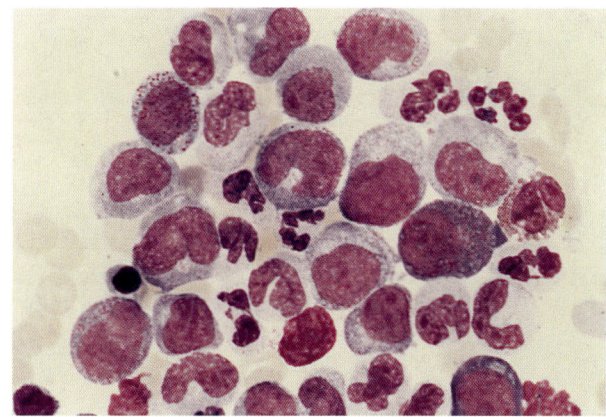

CASE 26-3. Initial marrow smear showed marked granulocytic hyperplasia with slight left-shifted maturation (Wright's stain, ×1000).

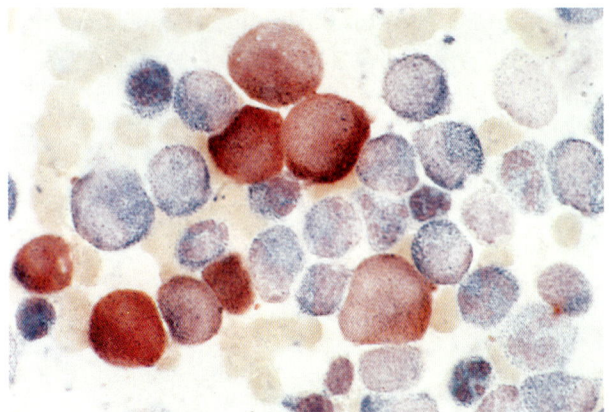

CASE 26-4. Another marrow smear showed positive α-naphthyl butyrate esterase staining (brownish red cytoplasmic staining) in more than 20% of nucleated cells and positive chloroacetate esterase staining (bluish granular staining) in the cytoplasm of the rest of the cells (combined α-naphthyl butyrate esterase and chloroacetate esterase stains, ×1000). This finding indicates proliferation of both monocytic and granulocytic cell types and is consistent with the diagnosis of chronic myelomonocytic leukemia.

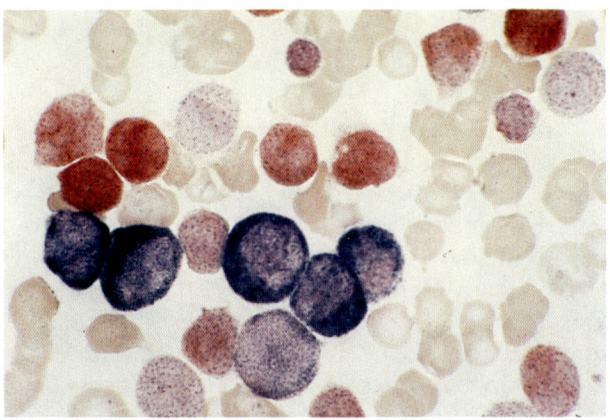

CASE 26-6. Another blood smear again showed positive α-naphthyl butyrate esterase staining (brownish red cytoplasmic staining) in more than 20% of leukemic cells and positive chloroacetate esterase staining (bluish granular staining) in the cytoplasm of some immature cells (combined α-naphthyl butyrate esterase and chloroacetate esterase stains, ×1000). This finding is consistent with the diagnosis of acute myelomonocytic leukemia (M4).

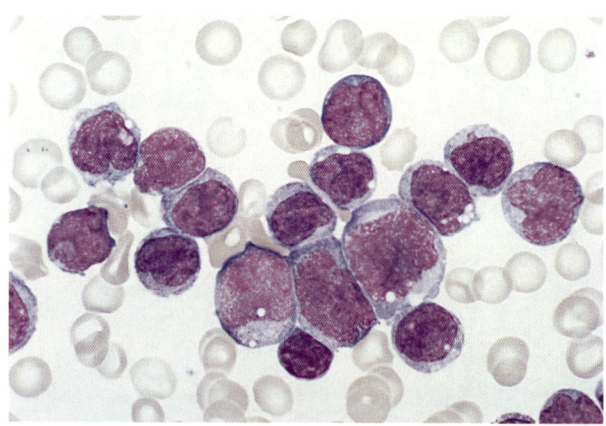

CASE 26-5. A subsequent blood smear showed a marked increase in blasts consistent with transformation into acute leukemia (Wright's stain, ×1000).

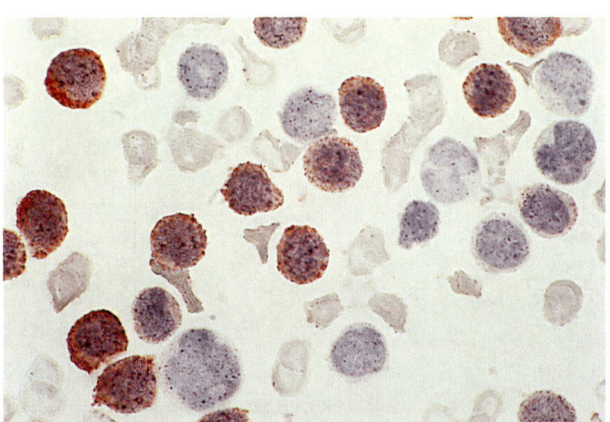

CASE 26-7. Another blood smear showed positive immunostaining (brownish red granular staining) of CD14 on the surface of monocytic components of the leukemic cells (indirect immunoperoxidase stain for CD14 using monoclonal antibody Leu-M3, ×1000). Immunostaining for CD11b and CD11c was also positive in many immature leukemic cells.

CASE 27 Chronic Basophilic Leukemia with Erythroblastic Transformation

A 65-year-old man presented with a 2-year history of fatigue, mild fever, night sweats, epigastric pain, and "red skin." Physical examination revealed prominent facial flushing and splenomegaly extending 7 cm below the left costal margin. Blood examination yielded the following data: RBC $2.17 \times 10^{12}/L$ ($2.17 \times 10^{6}/\mu L$); hemoglobin 68.0 g/L (6.8 g/dL); hematocrit 0.23 (23%); platelets $98.0 \times 10^{9}/L$ ($98.0 \times 10^{3}/\mu L$); and WBC $54.0 \times 10^{9}/L$ ($54.0 \times 10^{3}/\mu L$) with 24.5% neutrophils, 7.5% lymphocytes, 1.5% eosinophils, 62% basophils, 0.5% metamyelocytes, 2% myelocytes, 2% blasts, and 2% nucleated RBCs. The blood histamine level was 591.0 µg/100 mL (normal, 3.0–9.0). Cytogenetic study of the bone marrow showed the following karyotype: $7 = 46,XY/1 = 45,XY,-7/1 = 44,-4,-7$. Gastroduodenoscopy revealed the presence of a 1 cm gastric ulcer.

Comments. This case illustrates the characteristic morphologic and cytochemical features of chronic basophilic leukemia. Blastic transformation of chronic myeloproliferative disorders or myelodysplastic syndromes can be of any cell type.

The patient was treated for chronic basophilic leukemia with prednisone and hydroxyurea, which resulted in a remarkable decrease in his hyperhistaminic symptoms. He remained in remission for 2 years, when fatigue, fever, splenomegaly, and basophilia recurred.

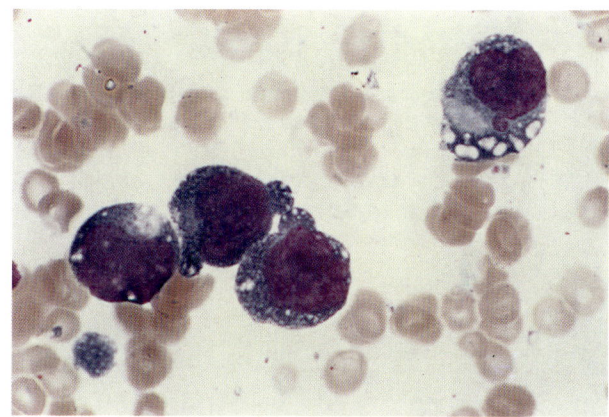

CASE 27-3. A subsequent marrow smear showed extensive replacement of the marrow by large, primitive blasts with intense basophilic cytoplasm (Wright's stain, ×1000). The blasts were negative for peroxidase and toluidine blue stains and positive with PAS.

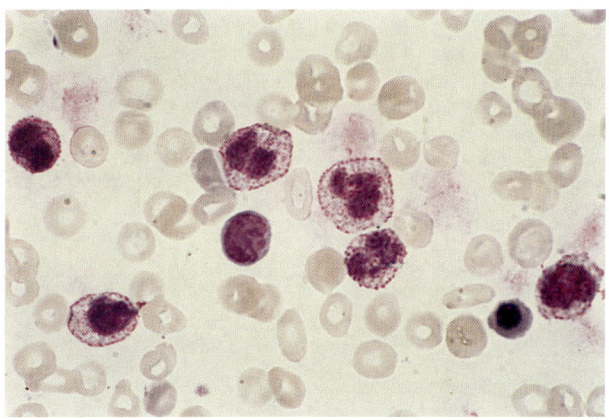

CASE 27-1. A blood smear showed marked basophilia (Wright's stain, ×1000).

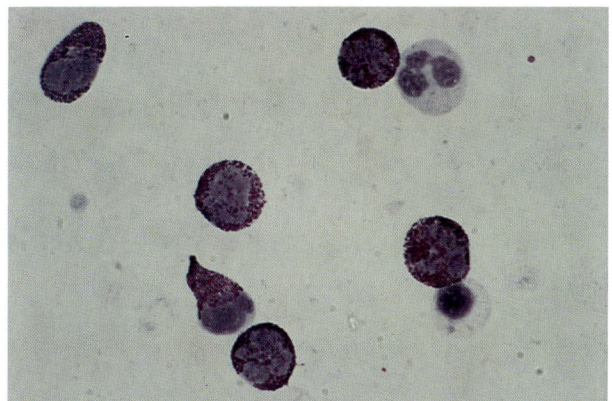

CASE 27-2. Another blood smear showed well-preserved metachromatic granules in the cytoplasm of basophils (toluidine blue stain, ×1000). A neutrophil at the right upper corner of the field stained negatively. The basophils were negative for peroxidase, chloroacetate esterase, and aminocaproate esterase.

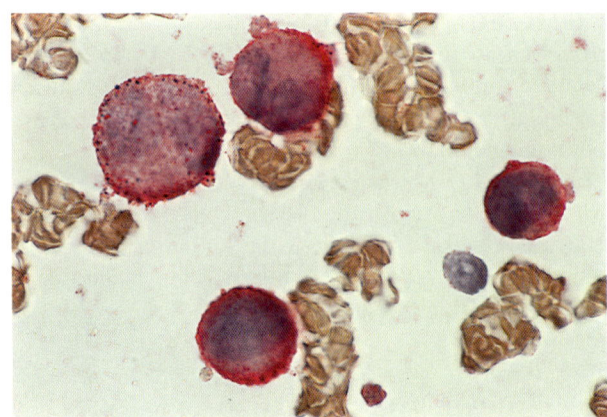

CASE 27-4. Another marrow smear showed strong positive immunostaining (bright red granular staining) of early erythroid antigen on the surface and cytoplasm of leukemic blasts, establishing the diagnosis of erythroblastic transformation of chronic basophilic leukemia (APAAP immunoalkaline phosphatase stain for early erythroid antigen using monoclonal antibody RC 82.4, ×1000).

CASE 28 Hairy Cell Leukemia—Blood and Marrow

A 47-year-old man had a 3-year history of increasing fatigue and weakness with night sweats. In addition, splenomegaly, pancytopenia, and increased fibrosis of the bone marrow were present. He had been treated with androgen, folic acid, and high-dose prednisone but had experienced no improvement. He had received approximately 50 units of blood in the past 8 months. Splenectomy for an enlarged spleen (2870 g) resulted in normalization of the WBC and platelet counts and stabilization of the hemoglobin level at approximately 110.0 g/L (11.0 g/dL) without transfusion.

Comments. This case illustrates the clinical presentation and characteristic morphologic and cytochemical features of hairy cell leukemia (leukemic reticuloendotheliosis) involving the blood and bone marrow. TRAP staining of the peripheral blood or a buffy coat smear is helpful in identifying small numbers of leukemic cells present to establish the diagnosis.

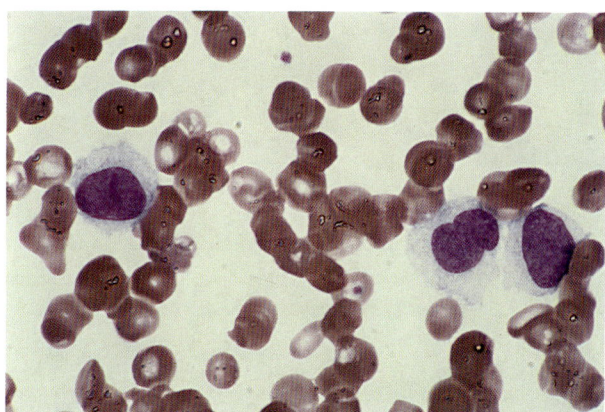

CASE 28-1. A blood smear showed the "hairy cells"—mononuclear cells with indented nuclei, a fine chromatin pattern, and faint, filamentous cytoplasmic projections (Wright's stain, ×1000).

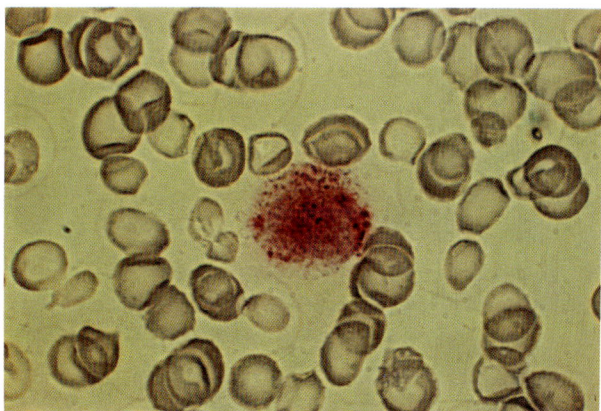

CASE 28-2. Another blood smear showed strong tartrate-resistant acid phosphatase (TRAP) activity (brownish red granular staining) in the cytoplasm of the mononuclear cells (TRAP stain, ×1000).

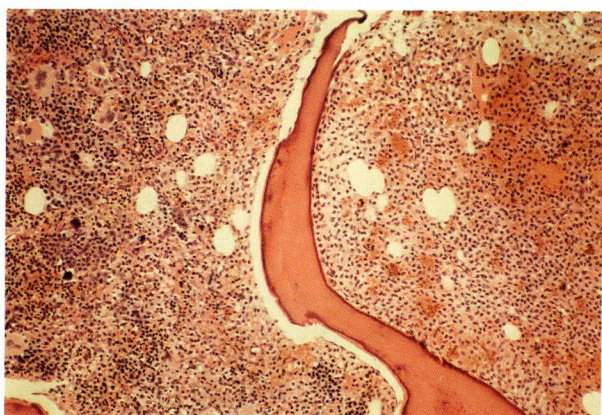

CASE 28-3. A marrow biopsy section showed the characteristic monomorphic loose mononuclear cell infiltration on the right side of the field and the more compact pleomorphic residual normal marrow cells on the left side (H&E stain, ×160).

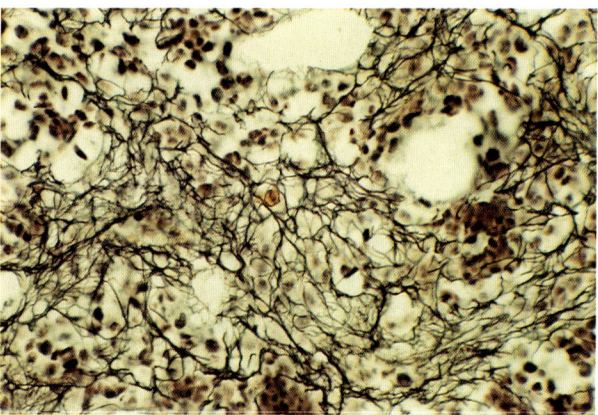

CASE 28-4. Another marrow biopsy section showed a fine reticulin network surrounding the mononuclear cell infiltrates (reticulin stain, ×400).

CASE 29 Hairy Cell Leukemia—Spleen and Liver

A 42-year-old woman had a 6-month history of anemia that had been unresponsive to iron therapy. Physical examination revealed moderate splenomegaly down to 4 cm below the left costal margin. Blood examination yielded the following data: RBC 2.99×10^{12}/L ($2.99 \times 10^{6}/\mu$L); hemoglobin 85.0 g/L (8.5 g/dL); hematocrit 0.268 (26.8%); reticulocytes 0.02 (2%); platelets 50.0×10^{9}/L ($50.0 \times 10^{3}/\mu$L); and WBC 1.4×10^{9}/L ($1.4 \times 10^{3}/\mu$L) with 63% neutrophils, 36% lymphocytes, and 1% monocytes. A bone marrow biopsy specimen revealed extensive replacement of the marrow by loose mononuclear cell infiltrates that were associated with reticulin fibrosis. Splenectomy for an enlarged spleen (540 g) resulted in normalization of platelet and WBC counts.

Comments. This case illustrates the sites of hairy cell infiltration in the spleen and liver. The extensive infiltration of the cords of Billroth form an additional barrier and tend to trap the circulating blood cells excessively when they pass through the spleen. This may explain the extraordinarily beneficial effect of splenectomy on patients with this disease.

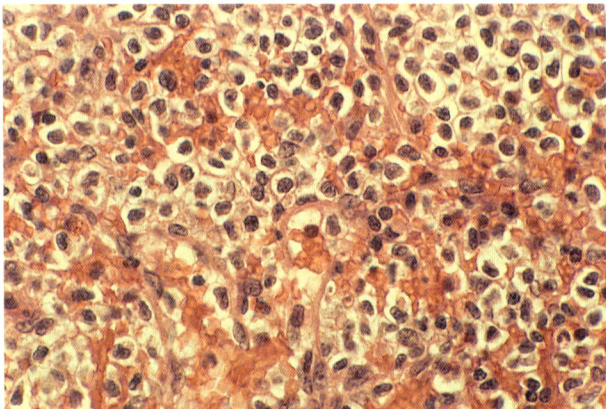

CASE 29-3. A splenic section showed extensive infiltration of the red pulp by hairy cells, the monomorphic mononuclear cells with clear cytoplasm (H&E stain, ×400).

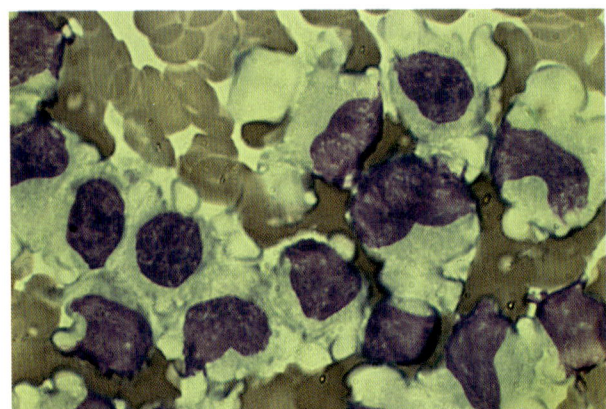

CASE 29-1. A splenic touch imprint showed aggregates of mononuclear cells with abundant cytoplasm (Wright-Giemsa stain, ×1000).

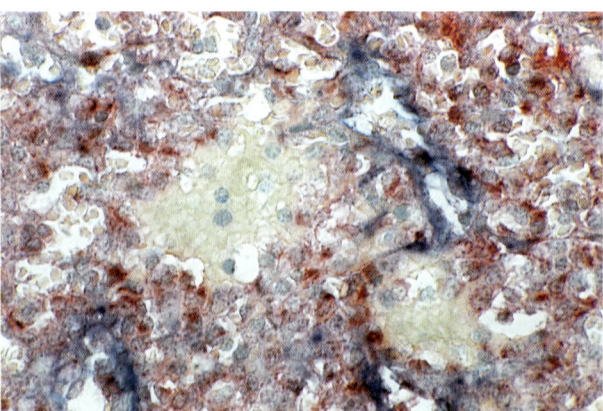

CASE 29-4. A cryostat section of the spleen showed expansion of the cord owing to hairy cell infiltration and trapping of RBCs, with pseudosinus formation (combined naphthol AS acetate esterase and TRAP stains, ×400). Hairy cells were stained reddish by TRAP stain, and the sinus lining cells were stained bluish by naphthol AS acetate esterase stain.

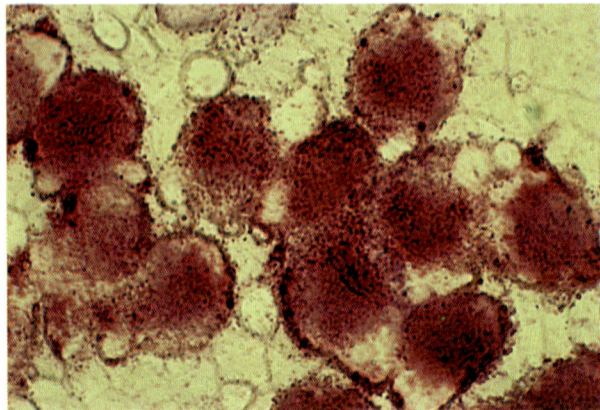

CASE 29-2. Another splenic touch imprint showed intense TRAP activity (brownish red granular staining) in the cytoplasm of the mononuclear cells (TRAP stain, ×1000). This finding confirmed the diagnosis of hairy cell leukemia.

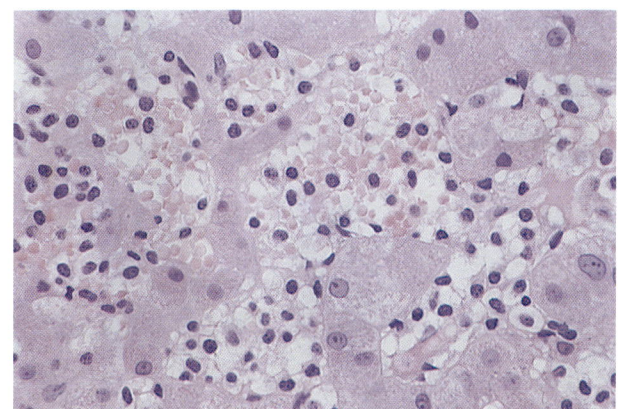

CASE 29-5. A plastic section of the liver biopsy specimen showed diffuse sinusoidal infiltration by monomorphic mononuclear cells with abundant clear cytoplasm (H&E stain, ×400).

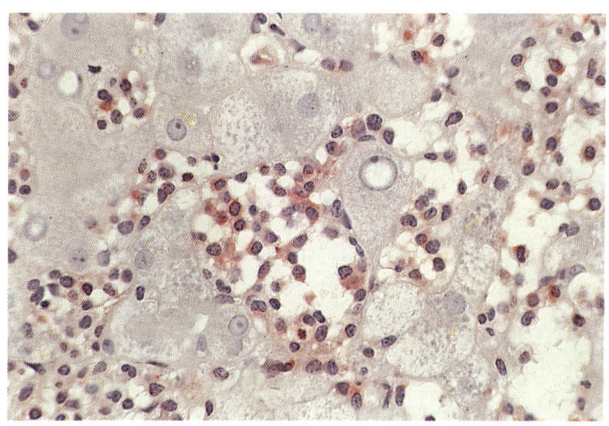

CASE 29-6. Another plastic section of the liver biopsy specimen showed strong positive staining (reddish cytoplasmic staining) with TRAP (TRAP stain, ×400). This finding confirmed the hairy cell infiltration of the liver.

CASE 30 Systemic Mast Cell Disease—Marrow

A 38-year-old woman had a long history of flushing, recurrent headaches, and gastrointestinal tract symptoms consistent with reflux esophagitis. Increasing bony sclerosis was visible on roentgenographic examinations during the past 8 years. Dermographism was noted during the physical examination. Roentgenographic examination of the abdomen with tomograms demonstrated splenomegaly and a patchy, sclerotic density of the visualized bones. Blood examination yielded the following data: RBC 4.8×10^{12}/L ($4.8 \times 10^{6}/\mu$L); hemoglobin 145.0 g/L (14.5 g/dL); hematocrit 0.408 (40.8%); platelets 324.0×10^{9}/L ($324.0 \times 10^{3}/\mu$L); and WBC 13.8×10^{9}/L ($13.8 \times 10^{3}/\mu$L) with 67% neutrophils, 21.5% lymphocytes, 3.5% monocytes, 6% eosinophils, and 2% basophils. Her serum histamine level was elevated.

Comments. Aminocaproate esterase is a specific enzyme marker for the mast cells. The histochemical stain, for aminocaproate esterase, is helpful in confirming the diagnosis of mast cell disease, particularly in the study of marrow lesions when other stains failed to demonstrate the characteristic metachromatic substances in the mast cell granules. However, special processing of the specimen is necessary to preserve enzyme activity.

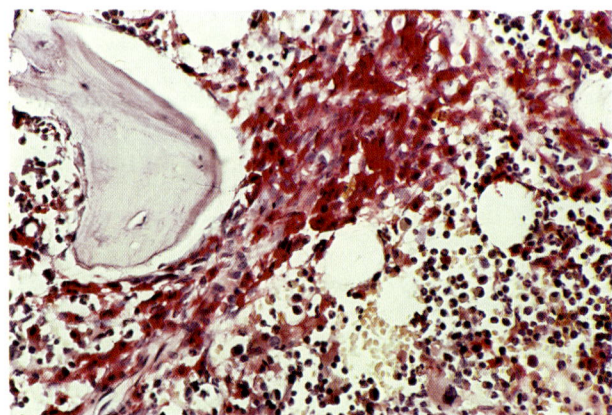

CASE 30-3. A cryostat section of the marrow biopsy specimen showed a characteristic perivascular mast cell lesion with intense reddish cytoplasmic staining for aminocaproate esterase activity, which is the specific enzyme marker for mast cells (aminocaproate esterase stain on a cryostat section of cold formalin-fixed, EDTA-decalcified marrow biopsy specimen, ×400).

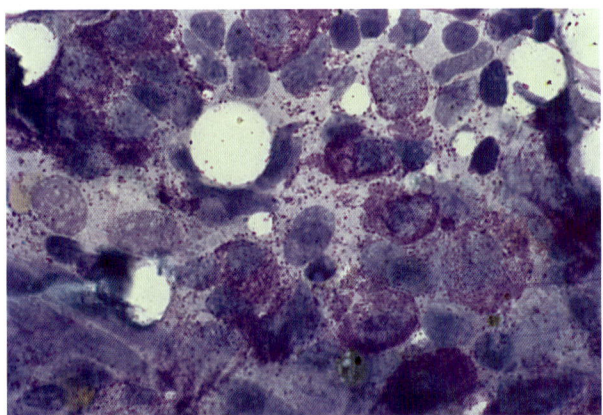

CASE 30-1. A marrow smear showed aggregates of mast cells (Wright's stain, ×1000).

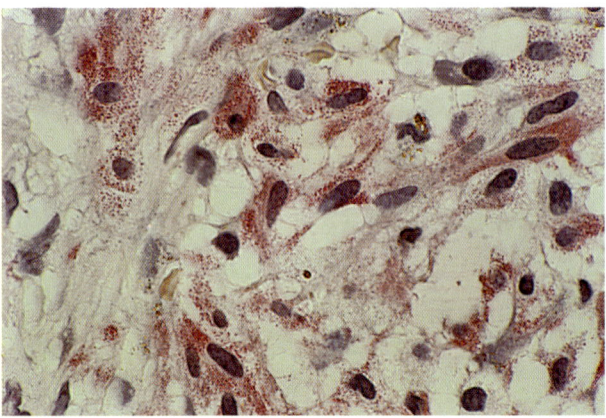

CASE 30-4. A plastic section of the marrow biopsy specimen showed a paratrabecular mast cell lesion with intense reddish granular cytoplasmic staining for aminocaproate esterase activity and with well-preserved cellular morphology (aminocaproate esterase stain on a marrow biopsy specimen embedded in glycol methacrylate at a low temperature, ×1000).

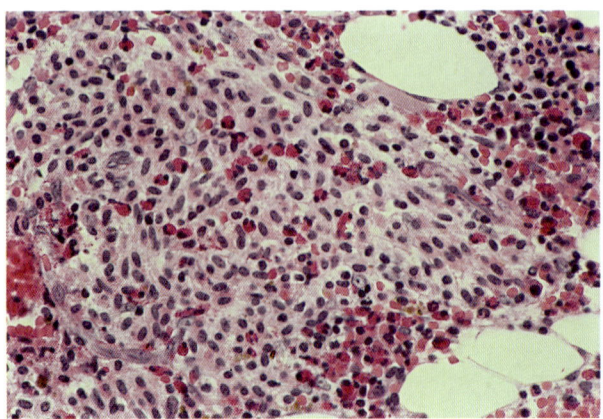

CASE 30-2. A paraffin section of the marrow biopsy specimen showed a cluster of monomorphic mononuclear cells intermixed with eosinophils (H&E stain, ×400). A toluidine blue stain was equivocal for metachromatic granules.

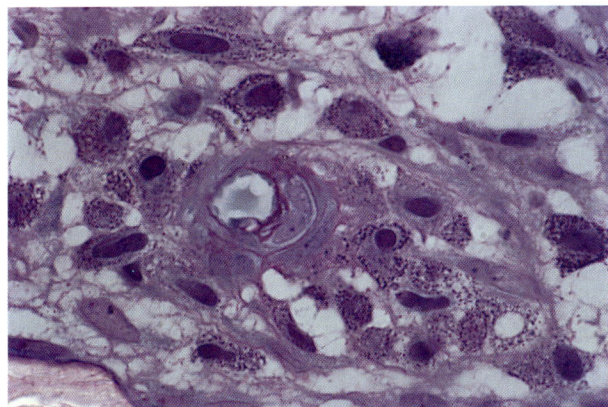

CASE 30-5. Another plastic section of the marrow biopsy specimen showed a perivascular infiltration of mast cells with cytoplasmic basophilic granules (Giemsa stain, ×1000).

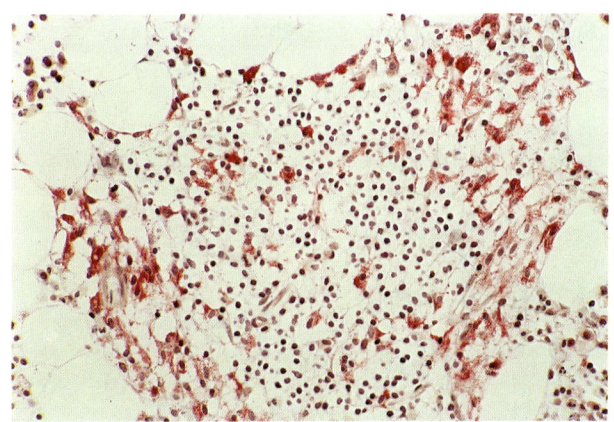

CASE 30-6. Another plastic section of a bone marrow biopsy section from other patient with systemic mast cell disease showed a perifollicular infiltration of mast cells with intense reddish granular cytoplasmic staining for aminocaproate esterase activity (aminocaproate esterase stain, ×250).

CASE 31 Mast Cell Leukemia

A 52-year-old woman had a 2-year history of duodenal ulcer and a 6-month history of intermittent diarrhea, fever, hot flashes, and weight loss. Physical examination revealed splenomegaly extending to 9 cm below the left costal margin. Blood examination yielded the following data: RBC 2.79×10^{12}/L (2.79×10^6/μL); hemoglobin 95.0 g/L (9.5 g/dL); hematocrit 0.291 (29.1%); mean corpuscular volume 104.4 fL (104.4 μm^3); platelets 82.0×10^9/L (82.0×10^3/μL); and WBC 6.5×10^9/L (6.5×10^3/μL) with 54.5% neutrophils, 30.5% lymphocytes, 2.5% monocytes, 0.5% eosinophils, 0.5% metamyelocytes, 0.5% myelocytes, 0.5% blasts, 1.5% nucleated RBCs, and 10.5% unidentified cells. The LAP score was 175.

Comments. This case illustrates the characteristic clinical presentation and morphologic and cytochemical features of mast cell leukemia. In comparison to systemic mast cell disease, the infiltration pattern in the bone marrow, spleen, liver, and lymph nodes in mast cell leukemia is more diffuse (similar to other types of leukemic infiltration). Clinically, mast cell leukemia is also much more aggressive than systemic mast cell disease.

Subsequently, this patient underwent vagotomy, pyloroplasty, and patch repair surgery for a perforated duodenal ulcer 2 weeks after splenectomy. She had a progressively downhill course with increasing ascites, hepatomegaly, increasing liver enzyme levels, increasing circulating mast cells, and disseminated intravascular coagulation. Cytogenetic study of circulating leukemic cells showed the following karyotype: 46,XX,dir ins (10;16)(q2?2;q13q22). Treatment with hydroxyurea, vincristine, and methylprednisolone sodium succinate was unsuccessful. She died 2 months later.

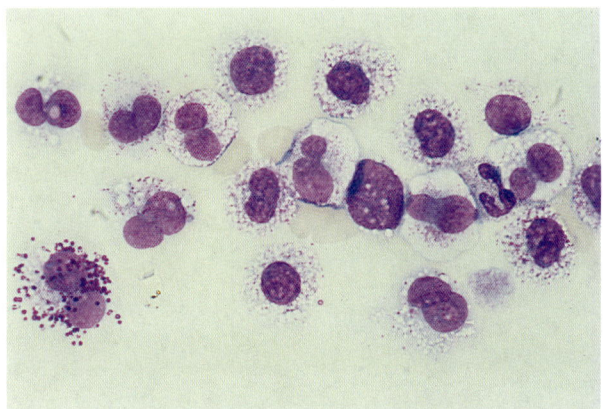

CASE 31-1. A feather edge of a blood smear showed many atypical degranulated cells with elongated and indented nuclei (Wright's stain, ×625).

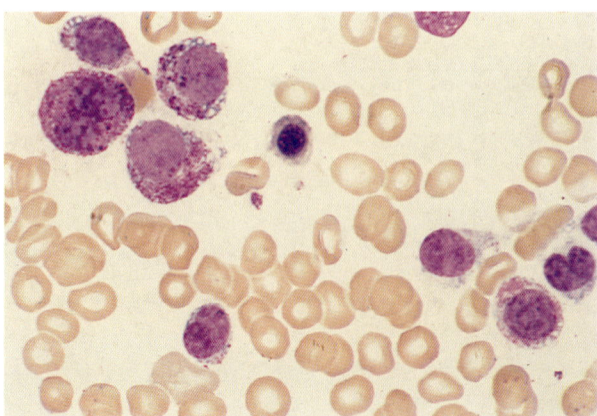

CASE 31-2. A marrow smear showed extensive replacement of the bone marrow by atypical mononuclear cells with various numbers of basophilic granules in the cytoplasm (Wright's stain, ×1000). These atypical mononuclear cells were negative for peroxidase.

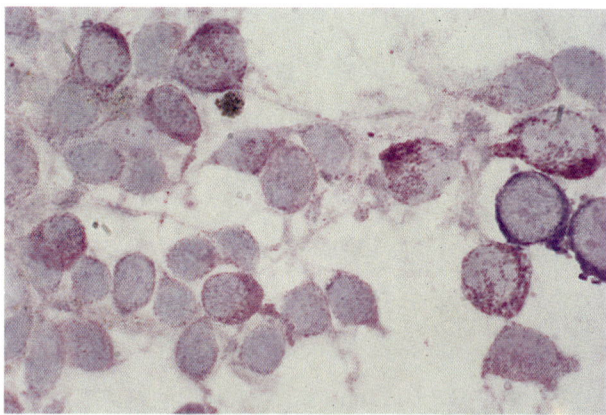

CASE 31-3. Another marrow smear showed metachromatic granules in the cytoplasm in atypical cells (toluidine blue stain, ×1000).

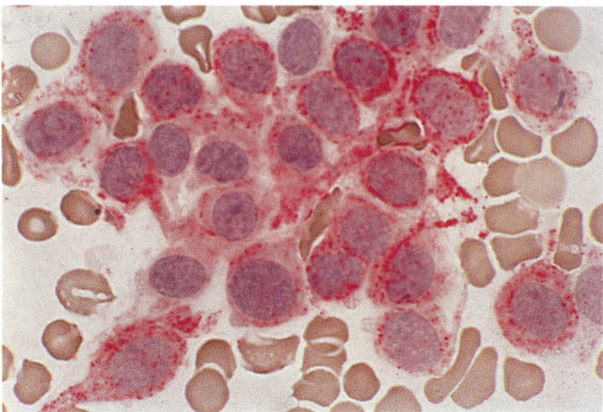

CASE 31-4. Another marrow smear showed positive chloroacetate esterase staining (bright red granular staining) in the cytoplasm of atypical cells (chloroacetate esterase stain, ×1000).

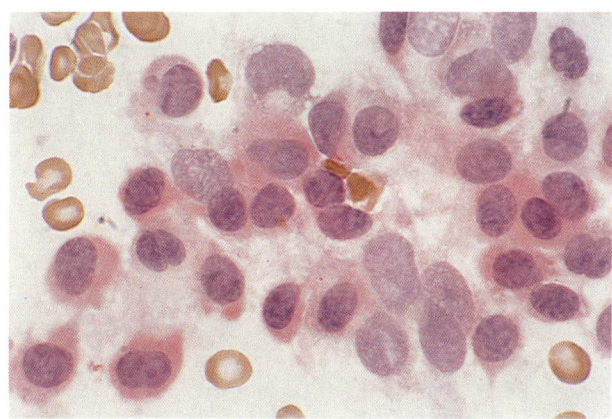

CASE 31-5. Another marrow smear showed positive aminocaproate esterase staining (pink granular staining) in the cytoplasm of the atypical cells (aminocaproate esterase stain, ×1000). These findings indicate the mast cell lineage of atypical cells and confirm the diagnosis of mast cell leukemia.

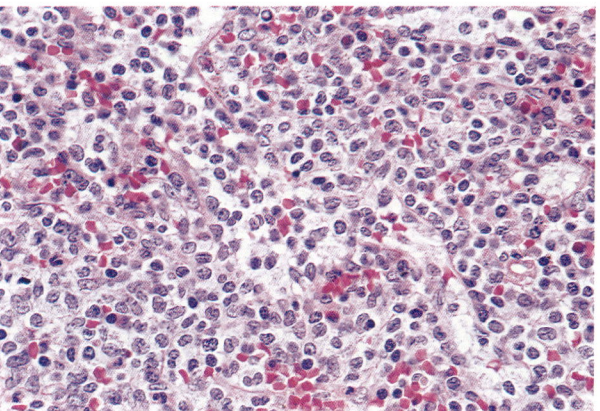

CASE 31-7. The splenic section showed diffuse red pulp infiltration in addition to the trabecular and perifollicular infiltration seen in systemic mast cell disease (H&E stain, ×400).

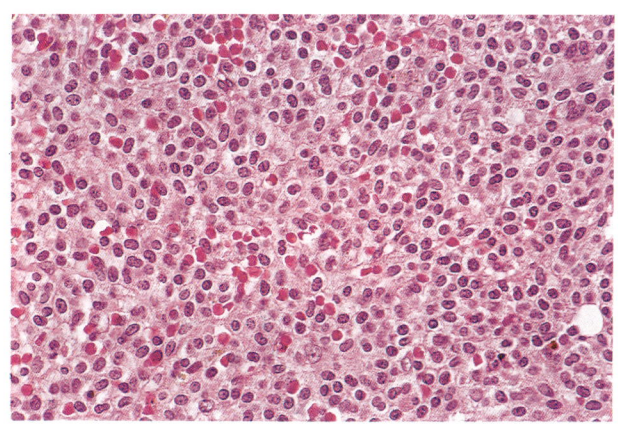

CASE 31-6. A marrow biopsy section showed diffuse replacement of marrow by mononuclear cells with abundant cytoplasm, similar to hairy cell leukemia (H&E stain, ×400). The patient underwent splenectomy, with some symptomatic improvement.

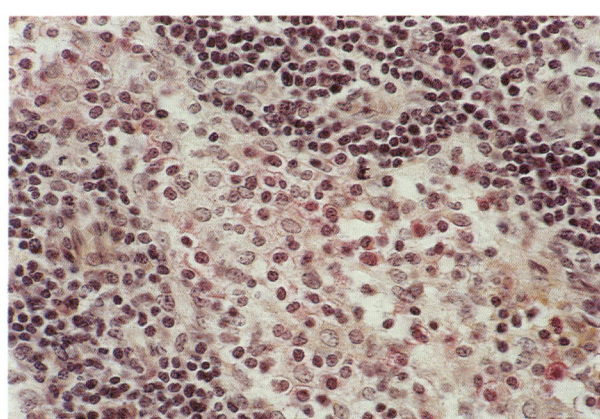

CASE 31-8. The lymph node section showed positive chloroacetate esterase staining (pink granular staining) in the cytoplasm of leukemic cells involving the sinuses (chloroacetate esterase stain, ×400).

CASE 32 Hodgkin's Disease—Nodular Sclerosing Type

A 31-year-old woman had a 2-week history of night sweats, including chills and rigors during the first few days, as well as a persistent low-grade fever. Physical examination revealed a grade 2 to 6 midsystolic murmur and a palpable spleen tip. A roentgenogram and a CT scan of the chest showed focal areas of consolidation of the right lower lobe and left upper lobe of the lungs, as well as mediastinal adenopathy. A CT scan of the abdomen showed an enlarged spleen without evidence of retroperitoneal adenopathy. Blood examination yielded the following data: RBC 2.34×10^{12}/L (2.34×10^6/μL); hemoglobin 65.0 g/L (6.5 g/dL); hematocrit 0.194 (19.4%); mean corpuscular volume 82.9 fL (82.9 μm^3); erythrocyte sedimentation rate 112.0 mm/hr; platelets 159.0×10^9/L (159.0×10^3/μL); and WBC 3.4×10^9/L (3.4×10^3/μL) with 63% neutrophils, 20% lymphocytes, 9% monocytes, 7% eosinophils, and 1% basophils. Serum alkaline phosphatase was 446.0 U/L; lactate dehydrogenase 269.0 U/L; and haptoglobin 5.17 g/L (517.0 mg/dL).

Comments. This case illustrates the characteristic clinical presentation and morphologic and immunohistochemical features of Reed-Sternbeg cells in nodular sclerosing and mixed-cell Hodgkin's disease.

Subsequent left cervical lymph node biopsy in this case further confirmed the diagnosis of nodular sclerosing Hodgkin's disease, stage 4b. The patient was treated with a hybrid regimen, including mechlorethamine hydrochloride, vincristine sulfate, procarbazine hydrochloride, prednisone, doxorubicin hydrochloride, bleomycin sulfate, and vinblastine sulfate. Her intermittent fever abated prior to her dismissal from the hospital. She remained well at last follow-up 15 months after the diagnosis.

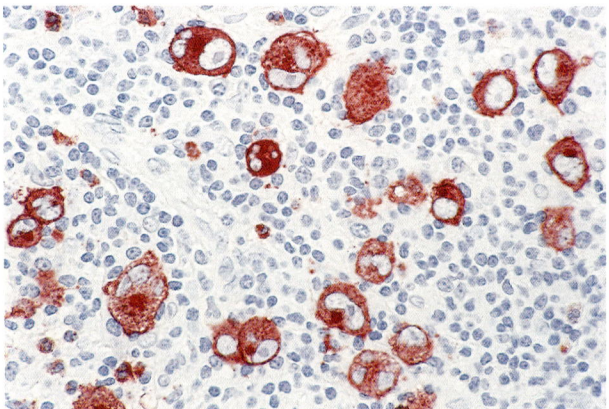

CASE 32-2. Another marrow biopsy section showed strong immunostaining (brownish red granular staining) of CD15 on the surface and cytoplasm of all large, atypical cells, including Reed-Sternberg cells (labeled streptavidin-biotin immunoperoxidase stain for CD15 using monoclonal antibody Leu-M1, ×400). The clear membrane staining with a dot-like paranuclear positivity is characteristic of Hodgkin's cells.

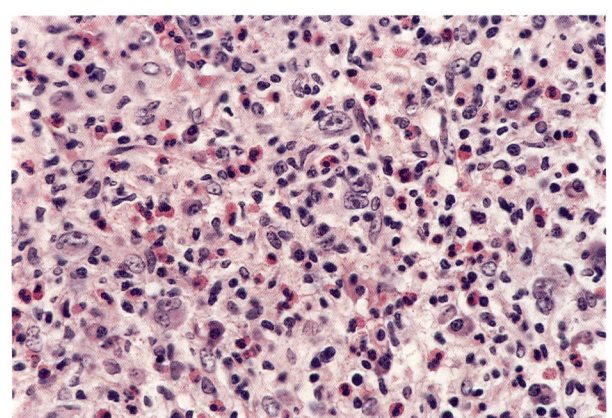

CASE 32-1. A marrow biopsy section showed plemorphic lymphoid infiltrates with eosinophilia and Reed-Sternberg cells consistent with Hodgkin's disease (H&E stain, ×400).

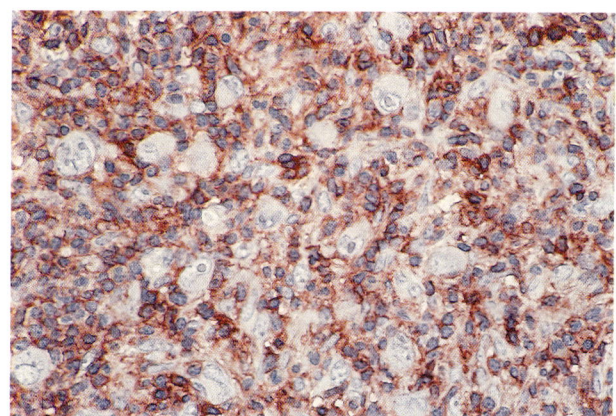

CASE 32-3. Another marrow biopsy section showed positive immunostaining (brownish red granular staining) of CD45 on the surface of background small lymphocytes but negative staining of the large, atypical cells (labeled strepatvidin-biotin immunoperoxidase stain for CD45 using monoclonal antibody LCA, ×400). Immunostaining using monoclonal antibody OPD4 showed a staining pattern similar to that of CD45. The immunostaining for CD20 was negative.

CASE 33 Malignant Lymphoma—Lymphoblastic Type

A 30-year-old man was initially seen because of generalized lymphadenopathy of 1 month's duration. Physical examination revealed massive generalized lymphadenopathy (up to 4 cm in diameter) over the cervical, axillary, and inguinal regions. Blood examination yielded the following data: RBC 5.7×10^{12}/L (5.7×10^{6}/μL); hemoglobin 162.0 g/L (16.2 g/dL); hematocrit 0.468 (46.8%); platelets 102.0×10^{9}/L (102.0×10^{3}/μL); and WBC 24.2×10^{9}/L (24.2×10^{3}/μL) with 6% neutrophils, 79.5% lymphocytes, 2% eosinophils, 0.5% basophils, and 12% atypical lymphocytes.

Comments. This case illustrates the characteristic morphologic and cytochemical features of lymphoblastic lymphoma. The characteristic focal aid phosphatase staining pattern in this disease is helpful in distinguishing lymphoblastic lymphoma from small noncleaved cell lymphoma, which may show similar morphology on an H&E-stained section. The immunostaining of TdT and CD7 is also helpful in highlighting marrow involvement by lymphoblastic lymphoma, as illustrated in Cases 33-4, 33-5, and 33-6.

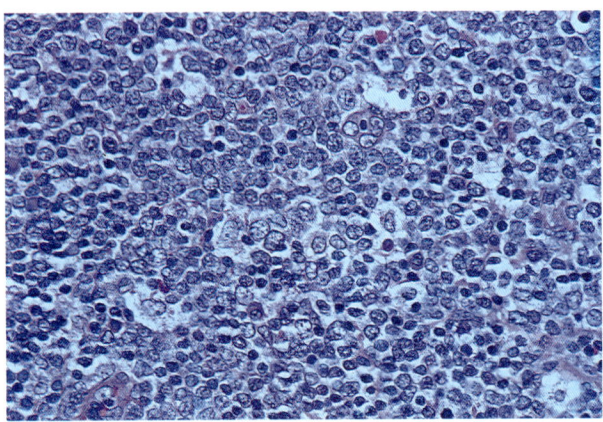

CASE 33-1. A section of a cervical lymph node showed diffuse replacement of the node by medium-sized lymphoid cells with round nuclei and scanty cytoplasm (H&E stain, ×400). The nuclei had blast-like features with finely stippled, delicate chromatin and inconspicuous nucleoli. A starry-sky pattern of interspersed macrophages was present. This feature is consistent with lymphoblastic lymphoma, which is a neoplasm of T or pre-T lymphoblasts. The methyl green–pyronine stain showed very weak staining in these cells.

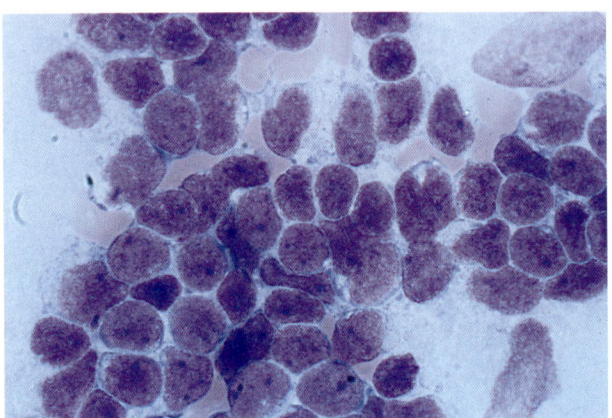

CASE 33-2. The morphology of the lymphoma cells on this touch imprint of the lymph node was indistinguishable from the morphology of the lymphoblasts of ALL, except for that of the L3 type (FAB classification) (Giemsa stain, ×1000).

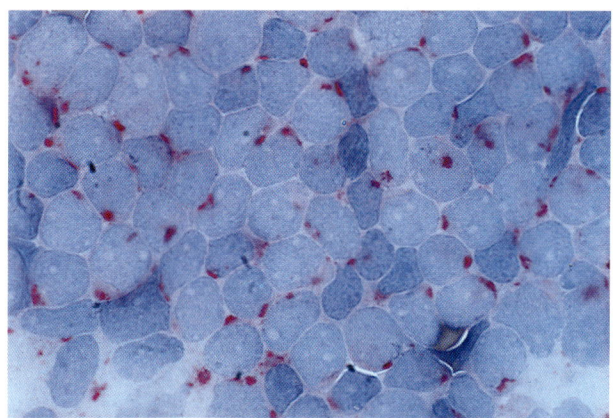

CASE 33-3. Another touch imprint of the lymph node showed the characteristic focal acid phosphatase pattern (reddish staining) in the Golgi area of T or pre-T lymphoblasts (acid phosphatase, ×1000). This finding confirmed the diagnosis of lymphoblastic lymphoma.

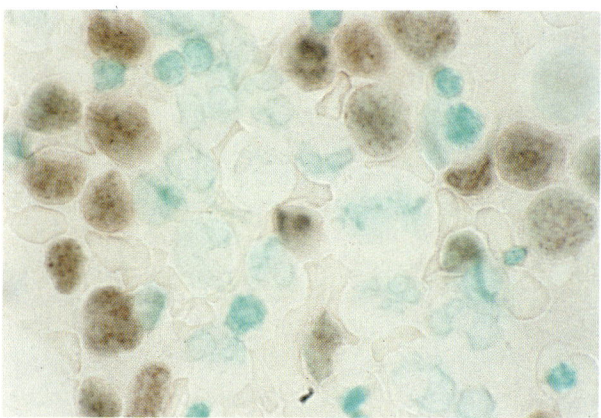

CASE 33-5. A marrow smear showed positive immunostaining of TdT (brownish granular staining) in the nuclei of lymphoblasts, indicating the increased number of lymphoblasts and confirming the early marrow involvement by lymphoblastic lymphoma (labeled streptavidin-biotin immunoperoxidase stain for TdT, ×1000).

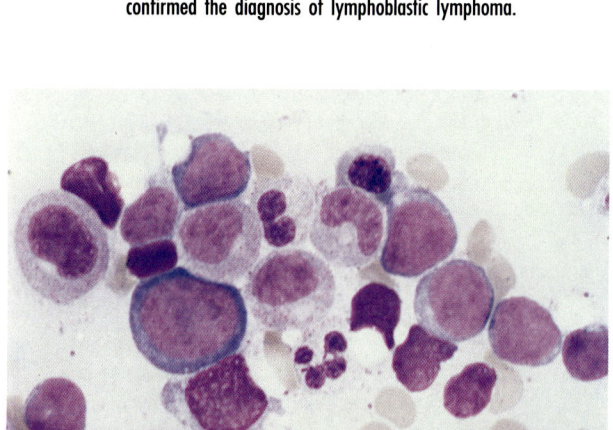

CASE 33-4. A marrow smear from another patient with lymphoblastic lymphoma showed a small aggregate of lymphoblasts on the right side of the field suggestive of early involvement by lymphoblastic lymphoma (Wright's stain, ×1000).

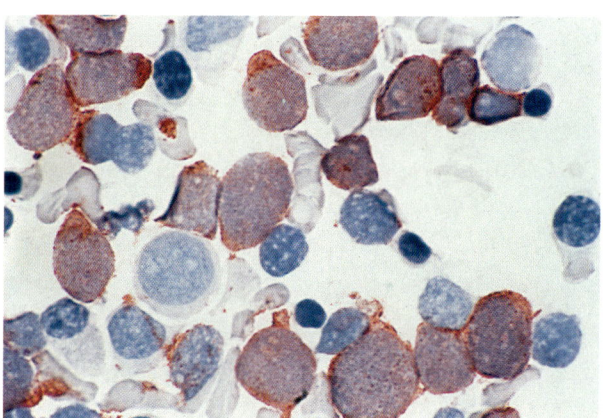

CASE 33-6. A marrow smear showed positive immunostaining of CD7 (brownish red granular staining) on the surface of lymphoblasts. This is another immunocytochemical characteristic of the lymphoma cells of lymphoblastic lymphoma and can also be used to highlight the lymphoma cells in the marrow (labeled streptavidin-biotin immunoperoxidase stain for CD7 using monoclonal antibody Leu-9, ×1000).

CASE 34 Burkitt's Lymphoma

A 3-year-old boy was initially seen because of a 2-week history of painless enlargement of the jaw. Physical examination revealed bilateral swelling of the jaw and an ill-defined, firm mass that seemed to involve the mandible bilaterally, with extension into the buccal mucosa and submandibular tissue. Distortion of the mandibular molars and swelling of the gingivae were also present. Blood examination yielded the following data: RBC 4.27×10^{12}/L (4.27×10^6/μL); hemoglobin 120.0 g/L (12.0 g/dL); hematocrit 0.34 (34.0%); platelets 334.0×10^9/L (334.0×10^3/μL); and WBC 6.6×10^9/L (6.6×10^3/μL) with 44.5% neutrophils, 44.5% lymphocytes, 3.5% monocytes, 6% eosinophils, 1% basophils, and 0.5% atypical lymphocytes. The lactic dehydrogenase level was 1359 U/L.

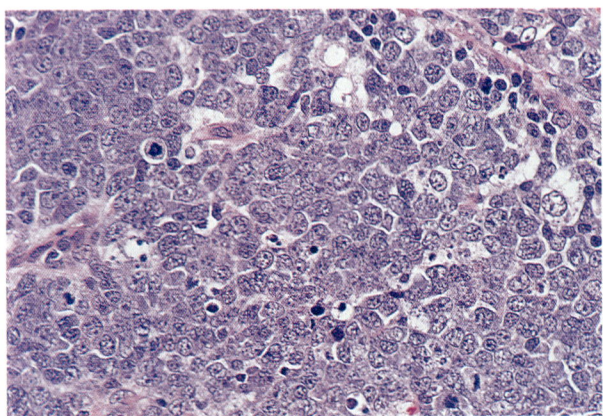

CASE 34-1. A section of the right submandibular biopsy specimen showed the characteristic features of Burkitt's lymphoma, a neoplasm of B lymphoblasts (small, noncleaved, follicular center cells) (H&E stain, ×400).

Comments. This case illustrates the morphologic and immunohistochemical characteristics of Burkitt's lymphoma.

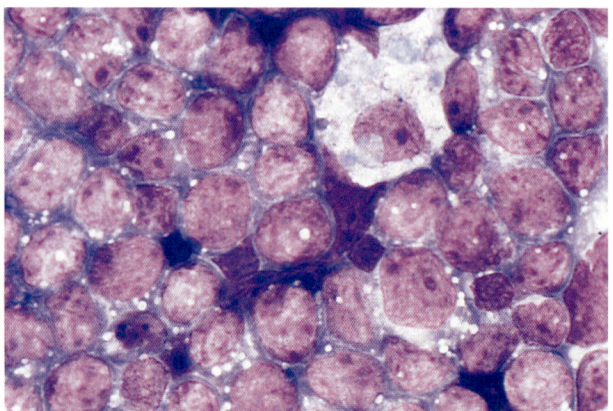

CASE 34-2. A touch imprint preparation from the same biopsy specimen showed morphologic similarity to the lymphoblasts of L3-ALL (FAB classification) or B-ALL (Giemsa stain, ×1000). A macrophage with abundant clear cytoplasm is seen in the right upper quadrant of this field.

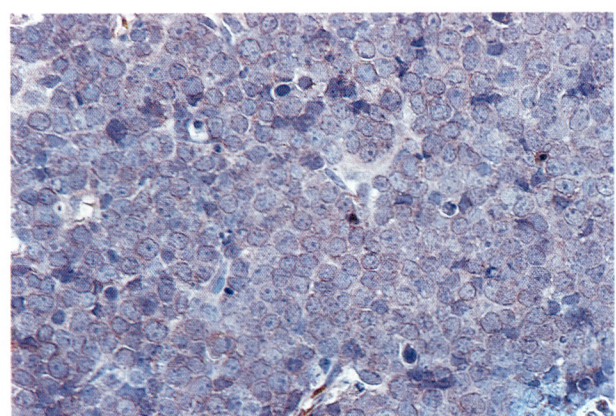

CASE 34-3. Another section of the same biopsy specimen showed positive λ light chain staining (brownish red staining) in the cytoplasm of the lymphoma cells (immunoperoxidase stain for λ light chains, ×400). Kappa light chain staining was negative, indicating monoclonal B-cell proliferation consistent with the diagnosis of Burkitt's lymphoma.

CASE 35 Diffuse Large-Cell Lymphoma—Follicular Center Cell Type

A 58-year-old man was initially seen because of swelling in the left side of the neck, which had been present for 8 months. The swelling was unresponsive to antibiotic treatment. Physical examination revealed a firm, fixed 5 × 6 cm left infra-auricular mass. Blood cell counts were all within normal limits.

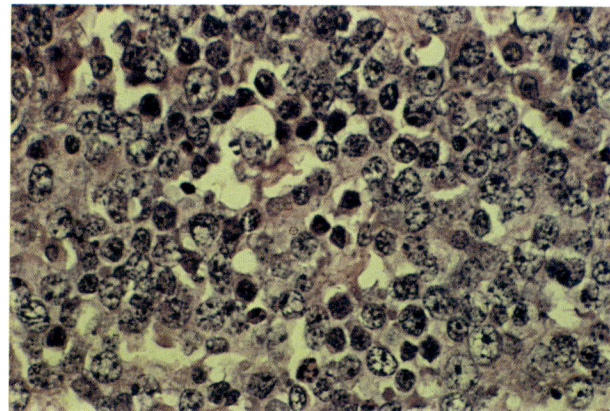

CASE 35-1. A paraffin section of a left cervical lymph node showed features of diffuse large-cell lymphoma, predominantly composed of large noncleaved cells, each with a round nucleus slightly larger than the nucleus of the phagocytes (H&E stain, ×640). Nuclear chromatin was finely distributed, and one to three small nucleoli were present near the nuclear membrane. On cryostat sections, the lymphoma cells showed weak diffuse acid phosphatase activity. Lymphoma cells were negative for α-naphthyl butyrate esterase, lysozyme, and κ light chains staining.

Comments. This case illustrates the characteristic morphologic, histochemical, and immunohistochemical features of the most common type of diffuse large-cell lymphoma—the follicular center cell type (also known as *diffuse large noncleaved follicular center cell lymphoma* and *diffuse histiocytic lymphoma of Rappaport*).

This patient was treated with radiation therapy to both areas of the neck, followed by combination chemotherapy of mechlorethamine hydrochloride, vincristine sulfate, procarbazine, and prednisone (MOPP). He was well as of the seventh year of follow-up.

He eventually died of pulmonary thromboembolism 10 years after the diagnosis of malignant lymphoma. At autopsy, malignant mesothelioma with extensive peritoneal involvement and massive ascites was noted, but no residual lymphoma was identified.

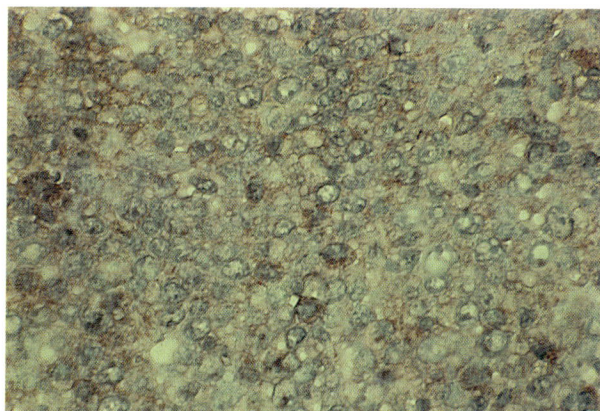

CASE 35-2. A paraffin section of the same node showed positive staining (brownish red granular staining) for λ light chains in the cytoplasm of most of the lymphoma cells (immunoperoxidase stain for λ light chains, ×640). This finding confirmed the B-cell nature of the lymphoma.

CASE 36 Diffuse Large-Cell Lymphoma—B-Cell Immunoblastic Lymphoma

A 33-year-old woman had persistent back pain of 1 month's duration and had lost 2.3 kg. Physical examination revealed left cervical adenopathy and a palpable mass in the right upper quadrant of the abdomen. A CT scan of the abdomen revealed huge abdominal confluent masses. Most of these masses were located in the retroperitoneum, but they also occupied the upper abdomen and epigastrium. Blood examination yielded the following data: RBC 4.15×10^{12}/L (4.15×10^6/μL); hemoglobin 121.0 g/L (12.1 g/dL); hematocrit 0.341 (34.1%); platelets 373.0×10^9/L (373.0×10^3/μL); and WBC 5.3×10^9/L (5.3×10^3/μL) with 75.4% neutrophils, 13.8% lymphocytes, 7% monocytes, 2.4% eosinophils, and 0.5% basophils.

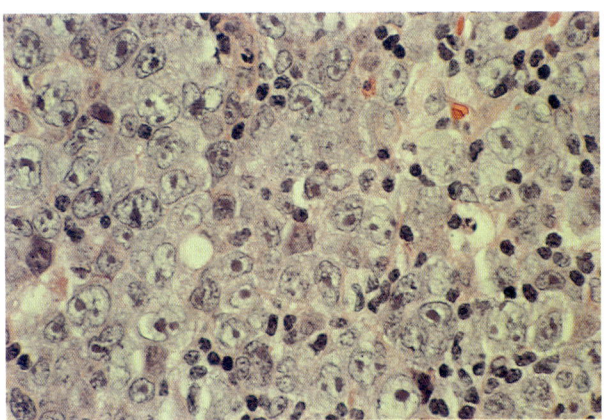

CASE 36-1. A section of a left cervical lymph node showed diffuse large-cell lymphoma with features of immunoblastic lymphoma (H&E stain, ×400). The cells were slightly larger than large noncleaved follicular center cells. A large, prominent central nucleolus was present in many of the large cells.

Comments. This case illustrates the characteristic morphologic and immunohistochemical features of B-cell immunoblastic lymphoma. B-cell immunoblastic lymphomas are generally much more aggressive than the B-cell neoplasms of the follicular center cell type.

This patient survived for less than 4 months despite administration of systemic combination therapy consisting of cyclophosphamide, vincristine sulfate, prednisone, and doxorubicin hydrochloride (COPA), plus radiation to the abdomen.

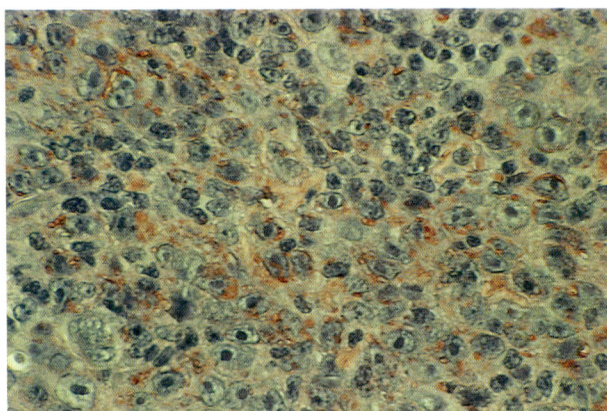

CASE 36-2. Another section of the same node showed positive staining (brownish red granular staining) for κ light chains in the cytoplasm of the lymphoma cells (immunoperoxidase stain for κ light chains, ×400). This finding confirmed the diagnosis of B-cell immunoblastic lymphoma. Staining for λ light chains was negative.

CASE 37 Diffuse Large-Cell Lymphoma—T-Cell Type

A 19-year-old woman was initially seen because of a 1-month history of fever, lymphadenopathy, and pleuritic pain on the left side of the chest. Physical examination revealed enlarged nodes over the cervical, left axillary, and right inguinal areas, but no hepatosplenomegaly was found. A chest roentgenogram showed bilateral interstitial infiltrates, and an excretory urogram demonstrated an obstruction of the left ureter at the level of L3. Blood examination yielded the following data: RBC 3.69×10^{12}/L (3.69×10^6/μL); hemoglobin 112.0 g/L (11.2 g/dL); hematocrit 0.329 (32.9%); platelets 374.0×10^9/L (374.0×10^3/μL); and WBC 19.6×10^9/L (19.6×10^3/μL) with 90% neutrophils, 5.5% lymphocytes, 4% monocytes, and 0.5% metamyelocytes. Results of a Monospot test were negative.

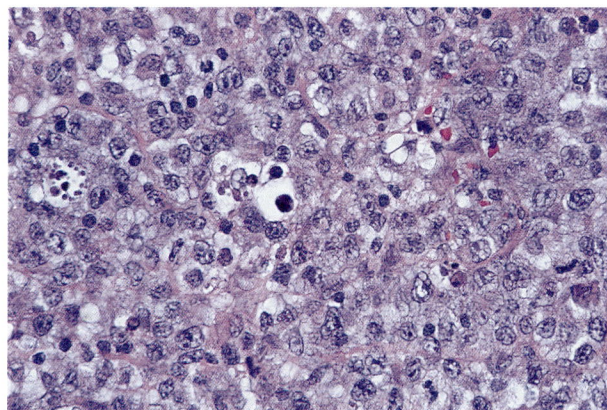

CASE 37-1. A section of a right inguinal lymph node showed diffuse replacement of the node by large lymphoid cells with abundant cytoplasm and variable nuclear morphology (H&E stain, ×400). This finding is consistent with diffuse large-cell lymphoma.

Comments. Diffuse large-cell lymphoma of the T-cell type may show wide varieties in morphology, and morphologic distinction between the B-cell type and the histiocytic type may be difficult. Acid phosphatase stain on a touch imprint preparation is probably the easiest way to demonstrate the characteristic intense focal staining pattern of T-lymphoma cells, which is similar to the transformed T cells of phytohemagglutinin culture.

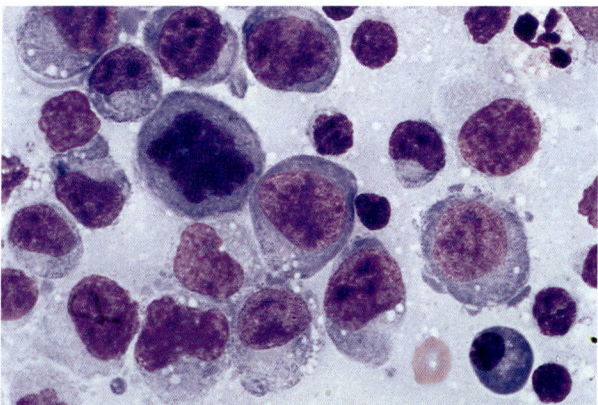

CASE 37-2. A touch imprint preparation of the same node showed wide variation in cell size and morphologic features similar to those of normal T cells transformed in culture by phytohemagglutinin (Giemsa stain, ×1000). These cells do not have nonspecific esterase activity.

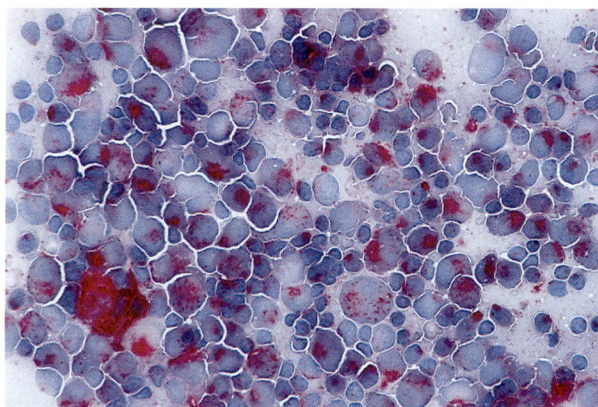

CASE 37-3. Another touch imprint preparation of the same node showed intense focal acid phosphatase activity (reddish staining) in the Golgi areas of most of the lymphoma cells (acid phosphatase stain, ×400). This finding confirmed the T-cell type of diffuse large-cell lymphoma.

CASE 38 Diffuse Large-Cell Lymphoma—T-Cell Immunoblastic Lymphoma

A 53-year-old man had noticed cervical and axillary adenopathy of 10 days' duration. This was preceded by a 9.1 kg weight loss in 1 year and a 3-week history of night sweats. Physical examination revealed 1 to 3 cm lymphadenopathy over both the cervical and axillary regions. Blood examination yielded the following data: RBC 4.85×10^{12}/L (4.85×10^{6}/µL); hemoglobin 136.0 g/L (13.6 g/dL); hematocrit 0.396 (39.6%); platelets 420.0×10^{9}/L (420.0×10^{3}/µL); and WBC 7.0×10^{9}/L (7.0×10^{3}/µL) with 83% neutrophils, 7% lymphocytes, and 10% monocytes. The chest roentgenogram showed bilateral mediastinal enlargement. Findings from a lymphangiogram were negative.

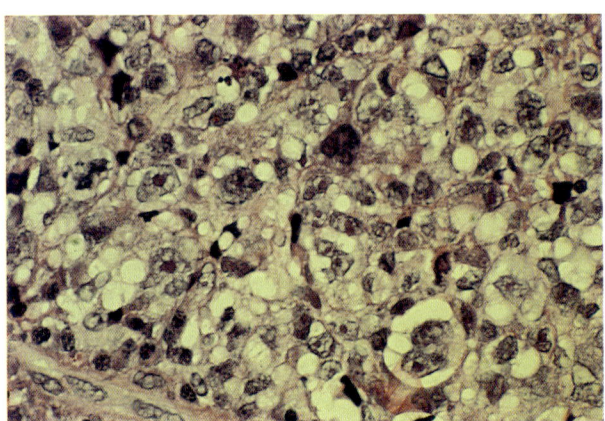

CASE 38-1. A paraffin section of a left axillary lymph node showed diffuse replacement of the node by lymphoid cells, with wide variation in cell size and nuclear morphology (H&E stain, ×400). Many of the large cells showed features of immuoblasts with a large, prominent central nucleolus. These lymphoma cells were negative for α-naphthyl butyrate esterase, excluding the possibility of a histiocytic neoplasm.

Comments. This case again illustrates the variation in the morphologic features of T-cell lymphomas. The T-cell nature of the lymphoma cells was further confirmed by the conventional E-rosette technique.

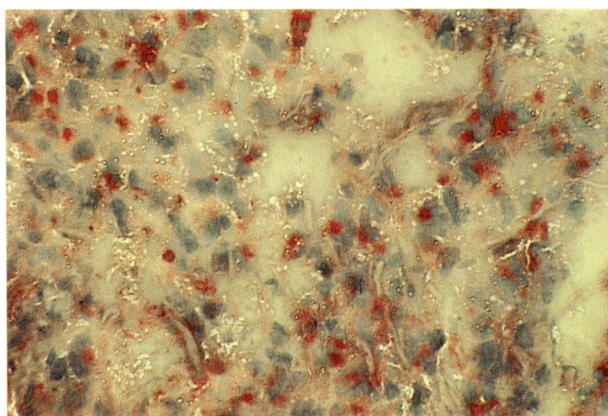

CASE 38-2. A cryostat section of the same node showed characteristic focal acid phosphatase activity (reddish staining) in the Golgi areas of the lymphoma cells (acid phosphatase stain, ×400). This finding confirmed the T-cell nature of the lymphoma cells.

CASE 39 Diffuse Large-Cell Lymphoma—Histiocytic Type

A 39-year-old man was initially seen because of a 2-month history of malaise, fever, headache, and nonproductive cough. These symptoms were associated with an 11.4 kg weight loss. Physical examination revealed small but definite adenopathy over the left cervical, right axillary, and bilateral inguinal regions. The abdomen appeared distended, with a diffuse periumbilical tenderness. The spleen had enlarged to three fingerbreadths below the left costal margin. Blood examination yielded the following data: RBC 4.2×10^{12}/L (4.2×10^{6}/μL); hemoglobin 96.0 g/L (9.6 g/dL); hematocrit 0.287 (28.7%); platelets 248.0×10^{9}/L (248.0×10^{3}/μL); and WBC 2.5×10^{9}/L (2.5×10^{3}/μL) with 81.5% neutrophils, 0.5% lymphocytes, 11% monocytes, and 1% basophils.

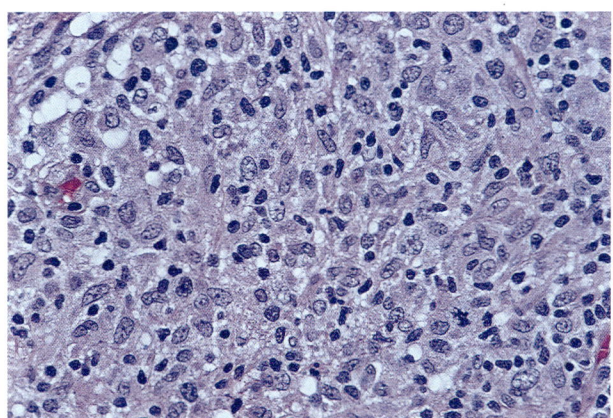

CASE 39-1. A paraffin section of a left supraclavicular lymph node showed diffuse replacement of the node by large cells with elongated nuclei and abundant cytoplasm (H&E stain, ×400). This finding was consistent with diffuse large-cell lymphoma.

Comments. This case illustrates the morphologic, histochemical, and immunohistochemical features of a fairly well-differentiated histiocytic lymphoma.

Although the patient was treated with a combination chemotherapy regimen of cyclophosphamide, vincristine sulfate, procarbazine, and prednisone (modified COPP), he died 6 months later because the histiocytic lymphoma was widely disseiminated and a perforation developed in the duodenum.

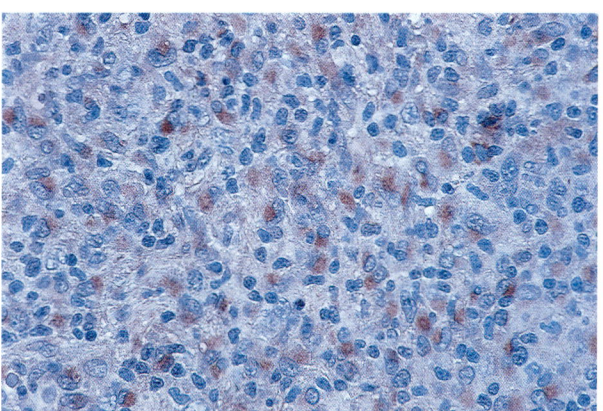

CASE 39-2. Another paraffin section of the same node showed positive staining (brownish red granular staining) for lysozyme in the cytoplasm of most cells (immunoperoxidase stain for lysozyme, ×400). This finding established the histiocytic nature of the neoplastic cells.

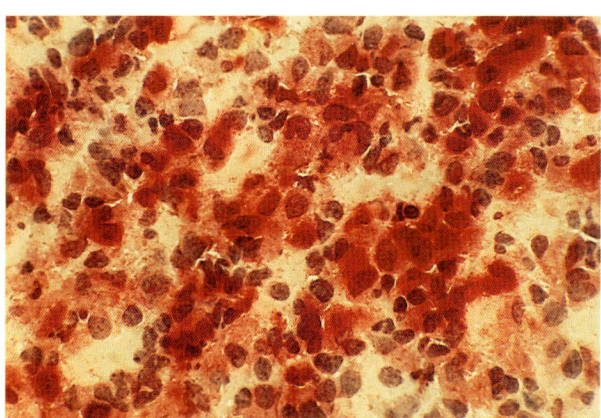

CASE 39-3. A cryostat section of the same node showed intense α-naphthyl butyrate esterase activity (brownish red staining) in the cytoplasm of all the cells (α-naphthyl butyrate esterase stain, ×400). This finding further confirmed the diagnosis of diffuse histiocytic lymphoma.

CASE 40   Large-Cell Lymphoma—B-Cell Type

A 29-year-old woman had a 6-month history of fever, night sweats, anorexia, and a 9.0 kg weight loss. She also experienced a dry cough associated with shortness of breath and occasional hemoptysis. She had several extensive examinations. Results of all cultures and serologic tests were negative. No evidence of neoplastic disease was noted on exploratory laparotomy, histologic examination of the spleen, liver biopsy, lymph node biopsy, and bone marrow biopsies. Physical examination revealed mild hepatomegaly and a 1.9 × 1.8 cm thyroid nodule. A fine needle aspiration of the thyroid mass suggested the possibility of Hürthle cell carcinoma. Blood examination yielded the following data: RBC 2.69×10^{12}/L (2.69×10^{6}/μL); hemoglobin 90.0 g/L (9.0 g/dL); hematocrit 0.25 (25.0%); erythrocyte sedimentation rate 33.0 mm/hr; platelets 81.0×10^{9}/L (81.0×10^{3}/μL); and WBC 15.3×10^{9}/L (15.3×10^{3}/μL) with 50.5% neutrophils, 29.5% lymphocytes, 3% monocytes, 11% nucleated RBCs, and 18% unidentified cells. The lactate dehydrogenase level was 1890 U/L. Flow cytometric analysis of blood lymphocytes revealed the following data: lymphocytes 3800/μL, B cells 76/μL, T cells 3427/μL, helper T cells 1732/μL, suppressor T cells 118/μL, and a helper:suppressor ratio of 1.47.

Comments. This is an unusual case of large-cell lymphoma primarily involving the bone marrow and pulmonary capillaries. Cytochemical and immunocytochemical stains were helpful in the differential diagnosis and in establishing the diagnosis of stage 4b large-cell lymphoma, B-cell type.

The patient was treated with a combination chemotherapy regimen of methotrexate with leucovorin rescue, doxorubicin, cyclophosphamide, vincristine, prednisone, and bleomycin. The spiking fever and dyspnea disappeared promptly, and she became ambulatory within a few days. Reexamination after 10 weeks of chemotherapy still showed bone marrow involvement. She was then switched to a combination chemotherapy regimen of cyclophosphamide, vincristine, prednisone, bleomycin, doxorubicin, and procarbazine. She underwent restaging 7 months after diagnosis, showed no evidence of disease, and was taken off all therapy.

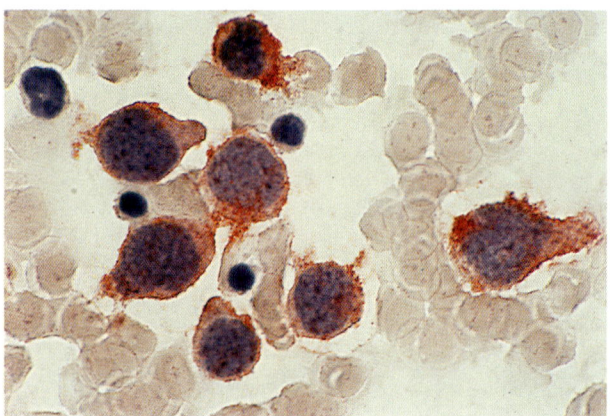

CASE 40-2. Another marrow smear showed strong positive immunostaining (brownish red granular staining) of CD22 on the surface of all large, immature cells (indirect immunoperoxidase stain for CD22 using monoclonal antibody Leu-14, ×1000). This finding established the diagnosis of large-cell lymphoma, B-cell type.

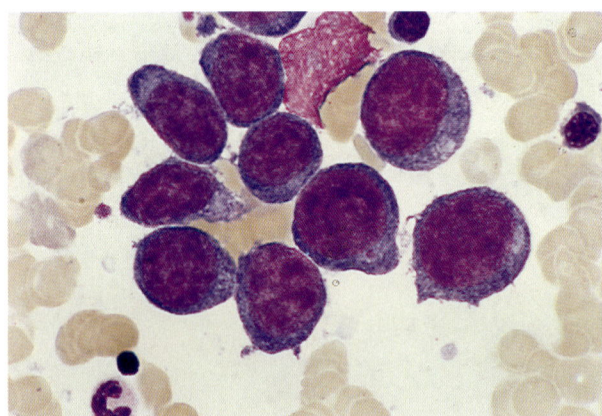

CASE 40-1. A marrow smear showed many large, immature cells with intense basophilic cytoplasm (Wright's stain, ×1000). The differential diagnosis included acute leukemia, malignant histiocytosis, and malignant lymphoma. These large, immature cells stained negative for peroxidase, α-napthyl buyrate esterase, α-naphthyl acetate esterase, hemoglobin, CD41A (glycoprotein IIb/IIIa complex), and CD5. These findings helped rule out the possibility of acute leukemia, malignant histiocytosis, and T-cell lymphoma.

Large-Cell Lymphoma—B-Cell Type

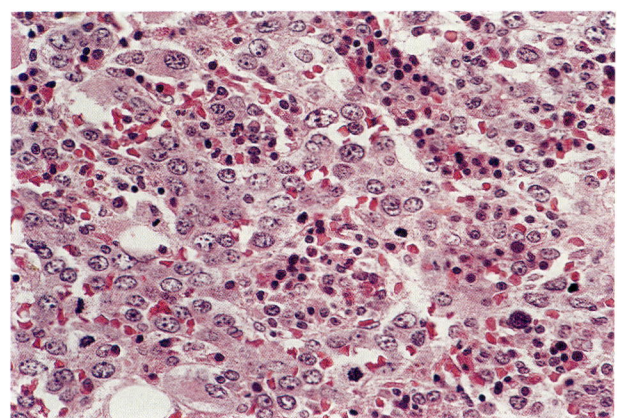

CASE 40-3. A marrow biopsy section showed interstitial and sinusoidal infiltration by large, immature cells, consistent with large-cell lymphoma with marrow involvement (H&E stain, ×400).

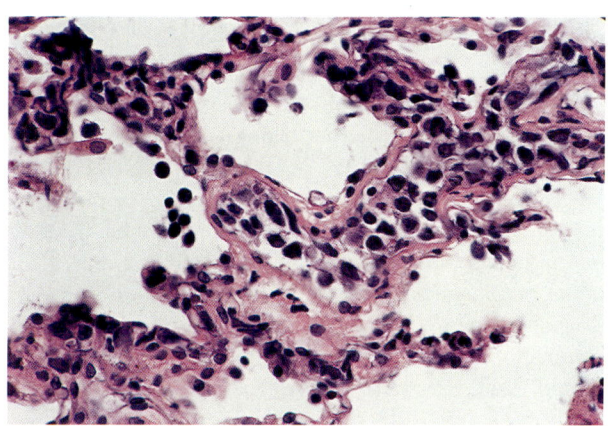

CASE 40-5. A transbronchial lung biopsy section showed numerous lymphoma cells in the capillaries of alveolar septi (H&E stain, ×400).

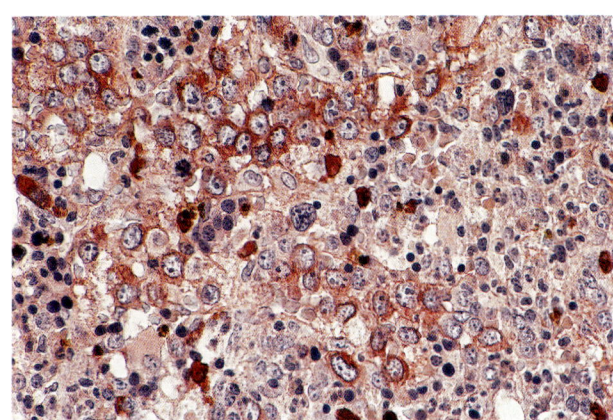

CASE 40-4. Another marrow biopsy section showed positive immunostaining (brownish red granular stain) of κ immunoglobulin in the cytoplasm of most large, immature cells (indirect immunoperoxidase stain for κ light chain immunoglobulin, ×400). Immunostaining of λ immunoglobulin was negative, confirming the monoclonal B-cell nature of the lymphoma cells.

CASE 41 — Small Cleaved Follicular Center Cell Lymphoma with Bone Marrow Involvement

A 63-year-old man had been taking combination chemotherapy for 1 year for diffuse, poorly differentiated lymphocytic lymphoma with abdominal pain. He underwent splenectomy (spleen weight (1580 g) 1 month earlier, and his abdominal discomfort abated. Histologic and immunologic studies of the splenic tissue established a diagnosis of small cleaved cell lymphoma of the B-cell type (IgM-κ). Physical examination revealed no palpable adenopathy. A CT scan showed mild to moderate retroperitoneal para-aortic lymphadenopathy. Blood examination yielded the following data: RBC 4.14×10^{12}/L ($4.14 \times 10^6/\mu L$); hemoglobin 127.0 g/L (12.7 g/dL); hematocrit 0.385 (38.5%); mean corpuscular volume 92.9 fL (92.9 μM^3); reticulocytes 0.017 (1.7%); erythrocyte sedimentation rate 31.0 mm/hr; platelets 413.0×10^9/L ($413.0 \times 10^3/\mu L$); and WBC 12.4×10^9/L ($12.4 \times 10^3/\mu L$) with 27% neutrophils, 55.5% lymphocytes, 5% monocytes, 11.5% eosinophils, and 1% basophils. The immunoglobulin gene rearrangement assay of blood showed no evidence of clonal rearrangement within either the μ heavy chain or the light chain locus.

Comments. This case illustrates the morphologic and immunohistochemical characteristics of bone marrow lesions in small cleaved follicular center cell lymphoma. These lesions are different from normal aggregates of small lymphocytes at the paratrabecular lesion, which usually consist of an equal mixture of T and B lymphocytes.

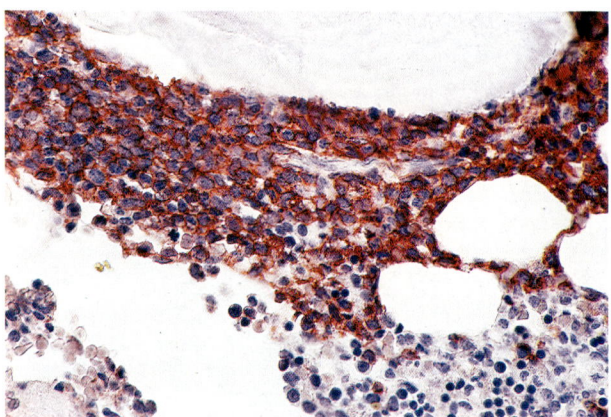

CASE 41-2. Another marrow biopsy section showed positive immunostaining (brownish red granular staining) of CD20 on the surface of all small cleaved lymphoma cells (indirect immunoperoxidase stain for CD20 using monoclonal antibody L26, ×400).

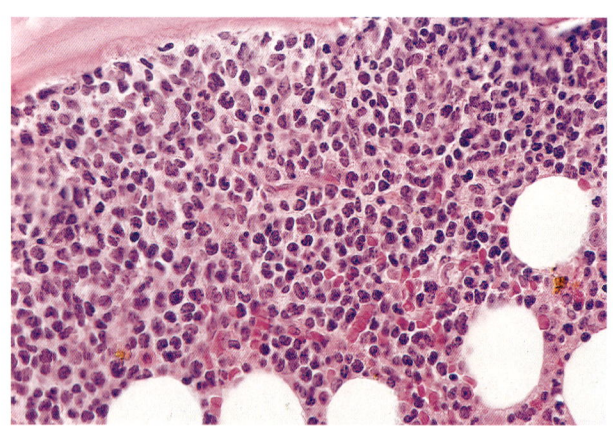

CASE 41-1. A marrow biopsy section showed an abnormal paratrabecular lymphoid lesion consisting mostly of small cleaved cells, characteristic of small cleaved follicular center cell lymphoma with marrow involvement (H&E stain, ×400).

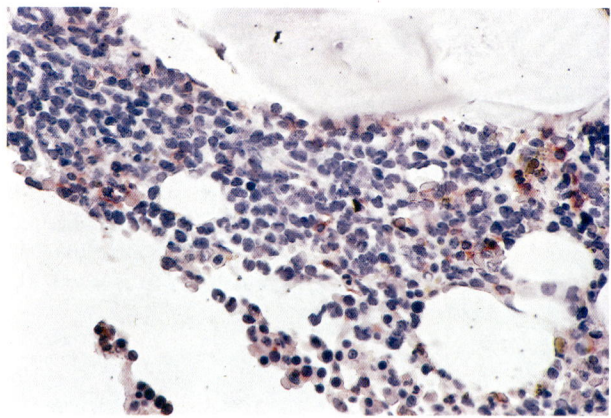

CASE 41-3. Another marrow biopsy section showed negative immunostaining of CD45RO on the lymphoma cells (indirect immunoperoxidase stain for CD45RO using monoclonal antibody UCHL-1, ×400). Only a few small lymphocytes were positive for CD45RO in the lesion.

CASE 42 Small Lymphocytic Lymphoma with Plasmacytoid Differentiation

A 58-year-old man had been taking chlorambucil for his lymphocytic lymphoma for the past 2½ years. Physical examination revealed a resolving paronychia of the right index finger. No palpable lymphadenopathy or hepatosplenomegaly was present. Blood examination yielded the following data: RBC 4.08×10^{12}/L (4.08×10^{6}/µL); hemoglobin 130.0 g/L (13.0 g/dL); hematocrit 0.381 (38.1%); mean corpuscular volume 93.3 fL (93.3 µM^3); reticulocytes 0.018 (1.8%); erythrocyte sedimentation rate 6.0 mm/hr; platelets 142.0×10^9/L (142.0×10^3/µL); and WBC 2.3×10^9/L (2.3×10^3/µL) with 64% neutrophils, 25% lymphocytes, 10% monocytes, and 1% basophils.

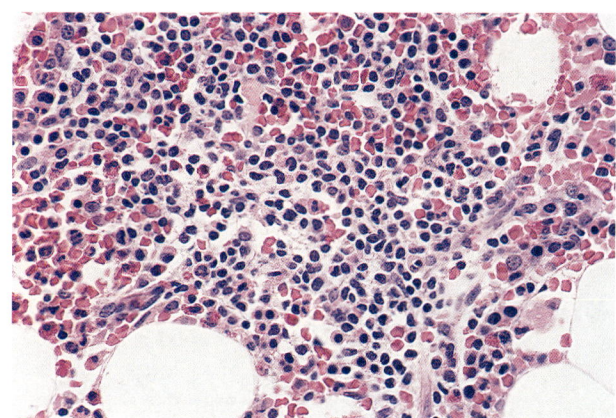

CASE 42-1. A marrow biopsy section showed a focal aggregate of small lymphocytes, which were considered quantitatively normal for the patient's age (H&E stain, ×400).

Comments. Immunohistochemical staining of κ and λ light chains is helpful in demonstrating the clonality of lymphoid lesions. In paraffin sections, however, many of the small lymphocytic lymphoma cells may be negative for both κ and λ light chains, except for small lymphocytic lymphoma with plasmacytoid differentiation.

Chlorambucil treatment was discontinued, and this patient remained well at the last follow-up 2½ years later.

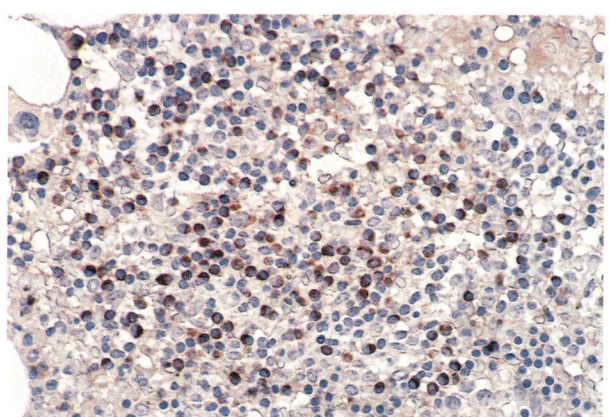

CASE 42-2. Another marrow biopsy section showed positive immunostaining (brownish red granular staining) of κ immunoglobulin in the cytoplasm of most of the small lymphocytes in the aggregate (indirect immunoperoxidase stain for κ light chains, ×400). Immunostaining of λ immunoglobulin was negative, indicating the presence of monoclonal B cells. This established the diagnosis of residual small lymphocytic lymphoma with plasmacytoid differentiation.

CASE 43 Small Lymphocytic Lymphoma—B-Cell Type with Marrow Involvement

A 73-year-old man had a 5-month history of transfusion-dependent anemia. He was treated with cyclophosphamide and prednisone for chronic lymphocytic leukemia without improvement. Physical examination revealed mucosal pallor and a small (0.4 cm) left posterior cervical node. Blood examination yielded the following data: RBC 3.17×10^{12}/L (3.17×10^{6}/µL); hemoglobin 96.0 g/L (9.6 g/dL); hematocrit 0.276 (27.6%); mean corpuscular volume 87.2 fL (87.2 µM^3); reticulocytes 0.0121 (1.21%); erythrocyte sedimentation rate 26.0 mm/hr; platelets 262.0×10^{9}/L (262.0×10^{3}/µL); and WBC 5.6×10^{9}/L (5.6×10^{3}/µL) with 27% neutrophils, 63% lymphocytes, 9% monocytes, and 1% basophils. Serum ferritin was 4775.0 µg/L (4775.0 ng/mL), and serum iron was 32.0 µmol/L (181 µg/dL) with 98% saturation. Serum vitamin B_{12} and folate levels were normal. Serum immunoelectrophoresis studies showed a monoclonal IgG-λ protein.

Comments. This case illustrates the immunohistochemical characteristics of a bone marrow lesion in small lymphocytic lymphoma of the B-cell type, which is different from a normal small lymphocytic aggregate of similar size (the latter usually consists of an equal mixture of T and B lymphocytes).

Follow-up examination of this patient 3 months later revealed an increase in leukocytes to 10,000/µL with a preponderance of mature lymphocytes consistent with chronic lymphocytic leukemia or the leukemic phase of B-cell small lymphocytic lymphoma.

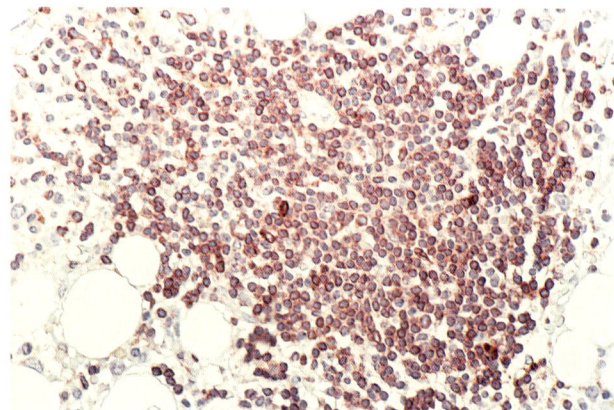

CASE 43-2. Another marrow biopsy section showed strong positive immunostaining (brownish red granular staining) of LN2 in the cytoplasm of most of the small lymphocytes in the aggregate. This finding indicated a disproportionate increase in small B lymphocytes, which supported the diagnosis of small lymphocytic lymphoma of the B-cell type with marrow involvement (labeled streptavidin-biotin immunoperoxidase stain for LN2, ×400). Immunoglobulin gene rearrangement studies also detected a minor B-cell clonal population, which further confirmed the diagnosis.

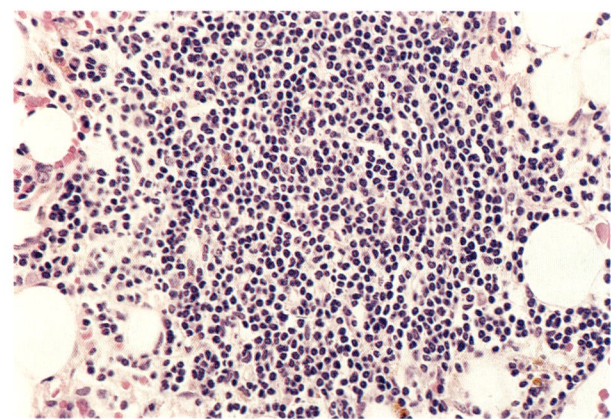

CASE 43-1. A marrow biopsy section showed a slight increase of small lymphocytes in aggregates (H&E stain, ×400). Immunohistochemical staining of κ and λ light chains was negative in the aggregate of small lymphocytes. Staining of CD20 was also very weak.

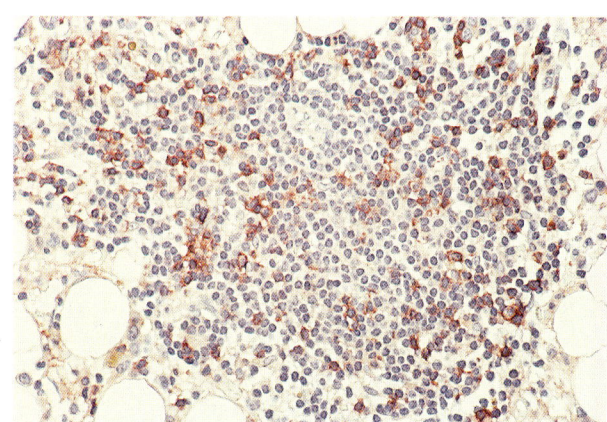

CASE 43-3. Another marrow biopsy section showed positive immunostaining (brownish red granular staining) of CD45RO on the surface of a few scattered small lymphocytes at the periphery of the aggregate (labeled streptavidin-biotin immunoperoxidase stain for CD45RO using monoclonal antibody UCHL-1, ×400).

CASE 44 Small Lymphocytic Lymphoma/Leukemia—Helper T-Cell Type with Marrow Involvement

A 47-year-old man was examined because of epigastric discomfort, a distended abdomen, lethargy, anorexia, sweats, and splenomegaly. Seven weeks ago, he was found to have lymphadenopathy, splenomegaly, and leukocytosis of 66,000/μL during a workup for his abdominal discomfort, early satiety, and sweats. An inguinal lymph node biopsy at that time revealed small lymphocytic lymphoma, and he was treated with chlorambucil and prednisone, with improvement. Positive physical findings included a temperature of 38°C, proptosis of the right eye, bilateral cervical and inguinal adenopathy, and a distended abdomen with marked splenomegaly (extending below the umbilicus). Blood examination yielded the following data: RBC 3.6×10^{12}/L (3.6×10^6/μL); hemoglobin 107.0 g/L (10.7 g/dL); hematocrit 0.318 (31.8%); mean corpuscular volume 88.3 fL (88.3 μM^3); platelets 26.0×10^9/L (26.0×10^3/μL); and WBC 61.6×10^9/L (61.6×10^3/μL) with 3% neutrophils, 82% lymphocytes, 13.5% atypical lymphocytes, and 1.5% eosinophils. T-cell receptor (TCR) assay showed evidence of a major clonal rearrangement with the β chain and γ chain of the TCR. Right axillary lymph node biopsy established a diagnosis of small lymphocytic lymphoma of the helper T-cell phenotype with lymphoma cells selectively positive for CD3, CD4, and CD5. Serum calcium was 2.67 mmol/L (10.7 mg/dL), and lactate dehydrogenase was 750.0 U/L.

Comments. This case illustrates the characteristic clinical presentation and morphologic and immunohistochemical features of small lymphocytic lymphoma/leukemia of the helper T-cell type. This is an aggressive disease compared to small lymphocytic lymphoma/leukemia of the B-cell type.

This patient died of respiratory failure 2 weeks later.

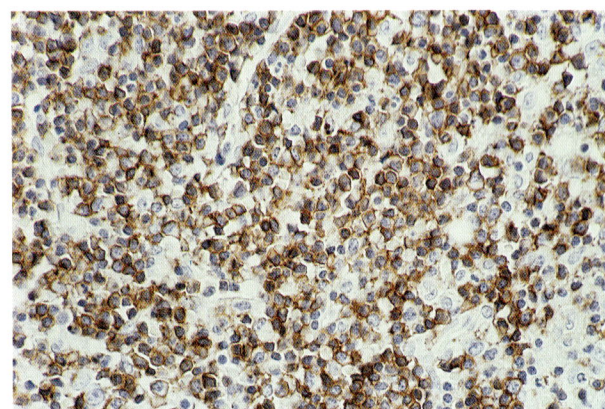

CASE 44-2. Another marrow biopsy section showed strong positive immunostaining (brownish granular staining) of OPD4 on the surface of most of the small lymphocytes, consistent with the helper T-cell phenotype of the lymphoma/leukemic cells (labeled streptavidin-biotin immunoperoxidase stain for OPD4, ×400). Immunostaining of LN2 on most of the small lymphocytes was negative.

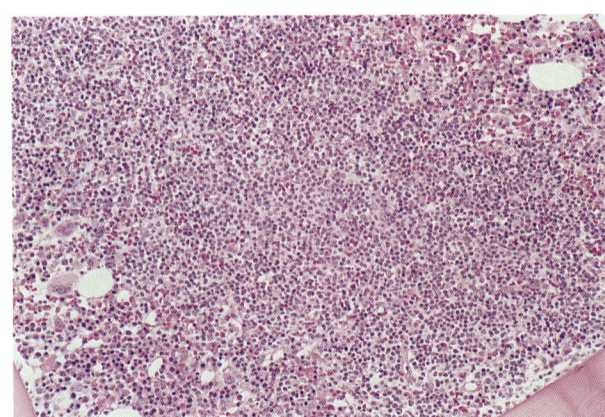

CASE 44-1. A marrow biopsy section showed extensive interstitial infiltration of marrow by small lymphocytes, consistent with either small lymphocytic lymphoma or chronic lymphocytic leukemia (H&E stain, ×160).

CASE 45 Lymphoproliferative Disorder of Granular Lymphocytes

A 67-year-old man had a 6-year history of neutropenia. Physical examination revealed no palpable lymphadenopathy or hepatosplenomegaly. Blood examination yielded the following data: RBC 4.74×10^{12}/L (4.74×10^6/μL); hemoglobin 136.0 g/L (13.6 g/dL); hematocrit 0.409 (40.9%); mean corpuscular volume 86.2 fL (86.2 μM^3); erythrocyte sedimentation rate 20.0 mm/hr; platelets 137.0×10^9/L (137.0×10^3/μL); and WBC 2.5×10^9/L (2.5×10^3/μL) with 2% neutrophils, 80.5% lymphocytes, 12.5% monocytes, 3% eosinophils, and 2% basophils. T- and B-cell quantitation by flow cytometry revealed the following data: lymphocytes 2000/μL, B cells (CD20) 60/μL (3%), T cells (CD2) 1900/μL (95%), helper T cells (CD4) 440/μL (22%), suppressor T cells (CD8) 1260/μL (63%), and a helper:suppressor ratio of 0.3.

Comments. This case illustrates the characteristic clinical presentation and morphologic and immunohistochemical features of a lymphoproliferative disorder of granular lymphocytes (suppressor T or NK phenotype). This is an indolent disease, but it may cause various types of cytopenia.

This patient was treated with a course of prednisone and low-dose cyclophosphamide, with improvement of his neutropenia. He remained asymptomatic at the last follow-up 3 years later.

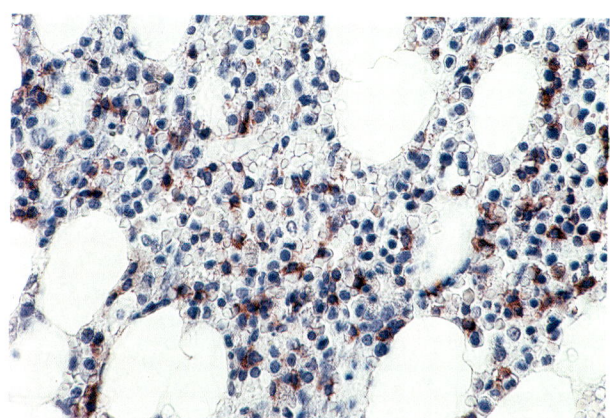

CASE 45-3. Another marrow biopsy section showed positive immunostaining (brownish red granular staining) of CD57 on the surface of many small lymphocytes, consistent with a lymphoproliferative disorder of the granular lymphocytes (indirect immunoperoxidase stain for CD57 using monoclonal antibody Leu-7, ×400).

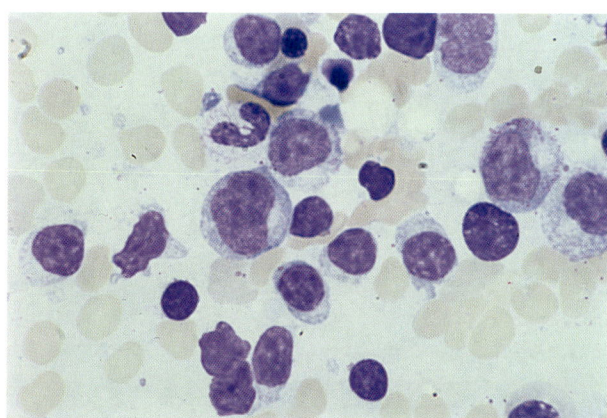

CASE 45-1. A marrow smear showed mild lymphocytosis with many granular lymphocytes and left-shifted granulopoiesis (Wright's stain, ×1000). A minor clonal T-cell population was detected by TCR gene rearrangement studies.

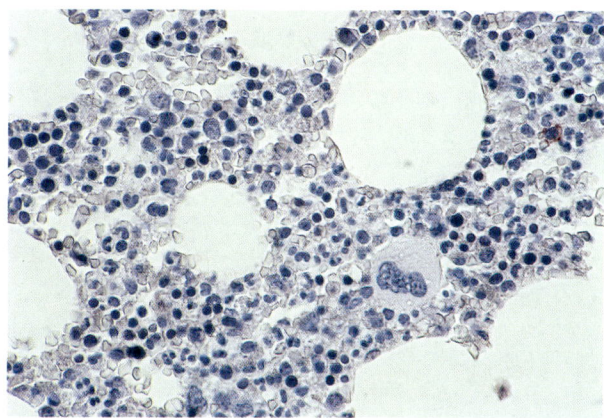

CASE 45-4. A normal marrow biopsy section, for comparison, showed positive immunostaining (brownish red granular staining) of CD57 on the surface of the rare small lymphocytes (indirect immunoperoxidase stain for CD57 using monoclonal antibody Leu-7, ×400).

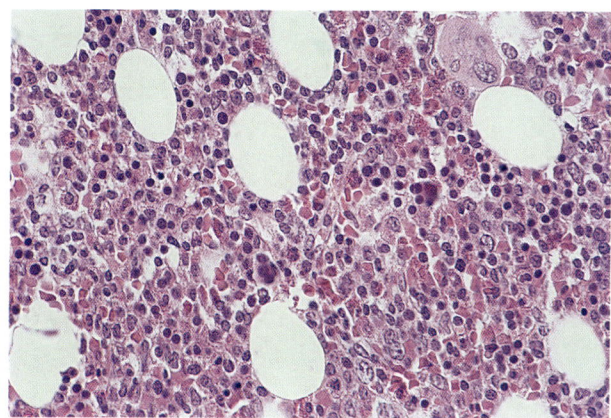

CASE 45-2. A marrow biopsy section showed left-shifted granulopoiesis without an appreciable increase in lymphoid cells (H&E stain, ×400).

CASE 46 Peripheral T-Cell Lymphoma with Multiorgan Failure

A 71-year-old man was transferred from another hospital with a 1-month history of hospitalization for fever, sweats, pancytopenia, progressive hepatic and renal dysfunction, and hypotension. Prior to this admission (2½ years ago), the patient was noted to have bilateral axillary and inguinal adenopathy. A lymph node biopsy specimen at that time showed atypical paracortical hyperplasia. A subsequent skin biopsy specimen showed lymphoid infiltrates. He was treated with five courses of combination chemotherapy consisting of cyclophosphamide, doxorubicin hydrochloride, vincristine sulfate, and prednisone (CHOP), with a good response. Physical examination on admission revealed jaundice, extensive petechiae, splenomegaly, and hypotension (blood pressure 60/0 mmHg). Blood examination yielded the following data: RBC 2.77×10^{12}/L (2.77×10^{6}/μL); hemoglobin 85.0 g/L (8.5 g/dL); hematocrit 0.235 (23.5%); mean corpuscular volume 85.0 fL (85.0 μM³); platelets 20.0×10^{9}/L (20.0×10^{3}/μL); and WBC 1.5×10^{9}/L (1.5×10^{3}/μL) with 71% neutropils, 26% lymphocytes, 1% monocytes, 1% eosinophils, 1% myelocytes, and 5% nucleated RBCs. Coagulation studies showed diffuse factor deficiency consistent with severe liver disease. Serum alkaline phosphatase was 1016 U/L, uric acid was 740 μmol/L (12.5 mg/dL), and creatinine was 510 μmol/L (5.8 mg/dL). Cytogenetic studies of the bone marrow revealed the following karyotype: 46-47,X,−Y,der(7)-t(7;?)(q3?2;?),der(19)t(19;?)(q13.1;?),+1-2mar [AA].

Comments. Peripheral T-cell lymphomas are a biologically heterogeneous group of lymphoproliferative disorders that evolve from a postthymic stage of T-lymphocyte maturation. A wide spectrum of clinical manifestations and morphologic features exist. Differentiating peripheral T-cell lymphoma from B-cell lymphoma and other hematologic neoplasms by clinical and morphologic features may sometimes be difficult, as illustrated in this case. The availability of monoclonal antibodies to detect mature T-cell antigens has improved the diagnosis of T-cell lymphoproliferative disorders.

This patient had rapid, progressive multiorgan failure despite intensive supportive treatment and died shortly after hospital admission. Postmortem examination confirmed the presence of disseminated lymphoma involving multiple organs.

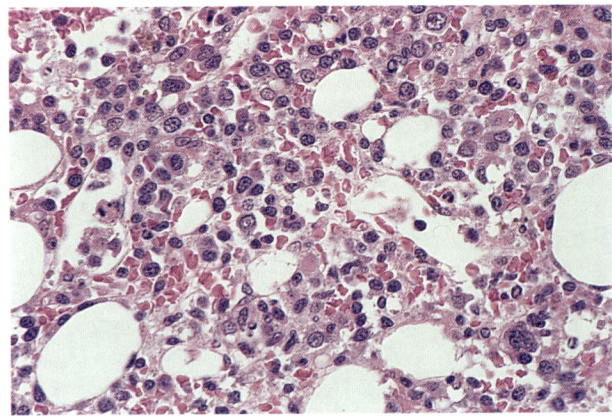

CASE 46-2. A marrow biopsy section showed extensive interstitial infiltration by medium-sized, atypical cells (H&E stain, ×400).

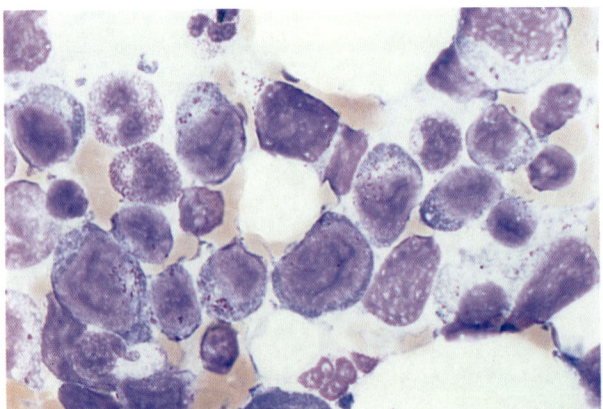

CASE 46-1. A marrow smear showed many atypical, immature cells with dense granules in the cytoplasm (Wright's stain, ×1000). Differential diagnosis included acute leukemias and T-cell lymphoma. The atypical cells stained negatively for peroxidase, toluidine blue, and TdT.

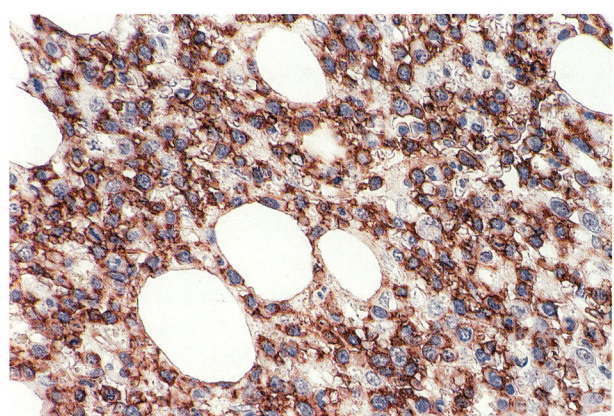

CASE 46-3. Another marrow biopsy section showed strong positive immunostaining (brownish red granular staining) of CD45RO on the surface of most of the atypical cells, establishing the diagnosis of T-cell lymphoma (indirect immunoperoxidase stain for CD45RO using monoclonal antibody UCHL-1, ×400). The immunostaining of CD2 was negative. The TCR gene rearrangement study also detected a major T-cell clonal population, which further confirmed the diagnosis of T-cell lymphoma.

CASE 47 Extranodal Peripheral T-Cell Lymphoma with Paraneoplastic Complications

A previously healthy 24-year-old man presented with a 1-month history of high fever, malaise, weight loss, jaundice, and hepatomegaly. Physical examination revealed jaundice, extensive ecchymoses, and gingival bleeding. No palpable lymphadenopathy or splenomegaly was present. A chest roentgenogram revealed bilateral small pleural effusions. Blood examination yielded the following data: RBC 3.12×10^{12}/L (3.12×10^6/µL); hemoglobin 90.0 g/L (9.0 g/dL); hematocrit 0.26 (26.0%); mean corpuscular volume 83.3 fL (83.3 µM³); reticulocytes 0.022 (2.2%); erythrocyte sedimentation rate 5.0 mm/hr; platelets 23.0×10^9/L (23.0×10^3/µL); and WBC 0.5×10^9/L (0.5×10^3/µL) with 57% neutrophils, 36% lymphocytes, and 7% monocytes. Coagulation studies showed prolonged thrombin and reptilase times, indicating either inhibition or abnormal fibrinogen. Serum alkaline phosphatase was 1782 U/L, aspartate aminotransferase 411 U/L, total bilirubin 222 µmol/L (13.0 mg/dL), direct bilirubin 173 µmol/L (10.1 mg/dL), creatinine 320.0 µmol/L (3.6 mg/dL), lactate dehydrogenase 1465 U/L, and creatinine kinase 19,650.0 U/L. Results of extensive serologic tests were all negative. The skin, muscle, and sural nerve biopsy results were nondiagnostic. The liver biopsy showed an atypical lymphoid infiltrate in the portal areas. Cytogenetic study of the bone marrow revealed the following karyotype: 16 = 41 − 44,X,−Y,+?4,−5,−12,−17,der(3)t(3;?)(p2?5;?),der-(4)t(4;?)(p3?1;?),del(6)(q?23q?27),der(8)t(Y;8)(q11;p23),?del(8)(q22?q24),der(9)t(9;?)(p2?2;?),+4 − 6mar/3 = 46, XY [AN].

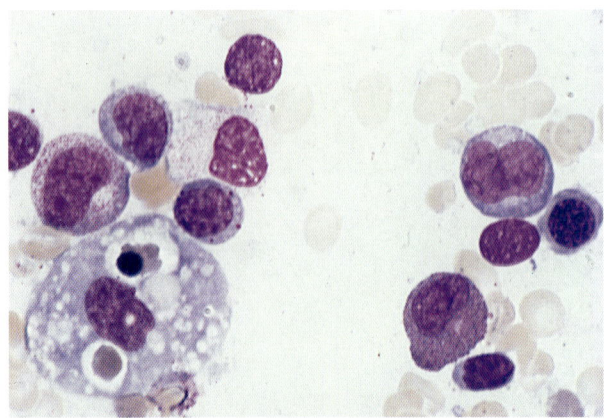

CASE 47-1. A marrow smear showed hemophagocytic histiocytes and a few atypical lymphoid cells (Wright's stain, ×1000). These atypcial lymphoid cells were negative for peroxidase.

Comments. Many patients with peripheral T-cell lymphoma present with B symptoms and an aggressive clinical course. Certain subgroups are also characterized by paraneoplastic complications that are likely due to lymphokines or other humoral factors produced by the neoplastic T cells.

This patient had clincial features of profound rhabdomyolysis, with no significant lymphomatous infiltration demonstrated on the muscle biopsy specimen. He was treated parenterally with hydrocortisone and a single parenteral dose of mechlorethamine hydrochloride. He responded over the next 14 days with normalization of peripheral blood cell counts and lactate dehydrogenase. Unfortunately, the initial clinical picture returned 1 week later, and the patient died of a massive gastrointestinal hemorrhage.

Awareness of the unusual clinical spectrum of this disease and early diagnosis may permit the use of aggressive chemotherapy before liver and kidney complications preclude effective treatment.

SUGGESTED READING

Diéz-Marín JL, Lust JA, Witzig TE, et al: Unusual presentation of extranodal peripheral T-cell lymphomas with multiple paraneoplastic features. *Cancer* 68:834–841, 1991.

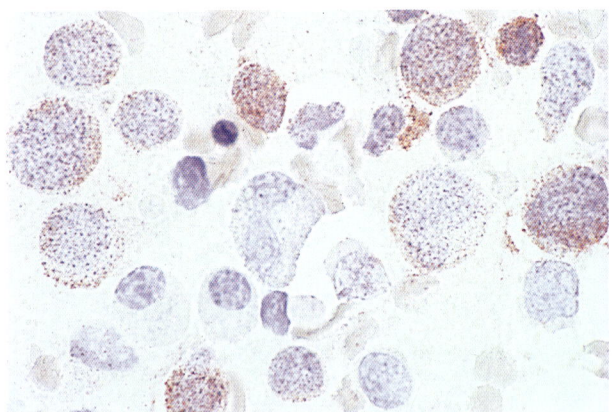

CASE 47-2. Another marrow smear showed positive immunostaining (brownish red granular staining) of CD2 on the surface of many atypical lymphoid cells, establishing the diagnosis of T-cell lymphoma (indirect immunoperoxidase stain for CD2 using monoclonal antibody Leu-5b, ×1000). These atypical lymphoid cells stained negatively for CD3, CD4, CD5, CD7, and CD20.

CASE 48 Metastatic Undifferentiated Prostatic Carcinoma

A 69-year-old man was admitted for evaluation of left lower quadrant abdominal pain of 3 months' duration. Physical examination revealed 1 to 2 cm palpable nodes in the left scalene area. An intravenous pyelogram and a CT scan of the abdomen demonstrated a large, diffuse retroperitoneal mass in the upper abdomen. This finding was suggestive of malignant lymphoma. Blood examination yielded the following data: RBC 4.84×10^{12}/L (4.84×10^{6}/μL); hemoglobin 142.0 g/L (14.2 g/dL); hematocrit 0.421 (42.1%); platelets 226.0×10^{9}/L (226.0×10^{3}/μL); and WBC 4.6×10^{9}/L (4.6×10^{3}/μL) with 66.5% neutrophils, 26.5% lymphocytes, 3.5% monocytes, 3% eosinophils, and 0.5% basophils.

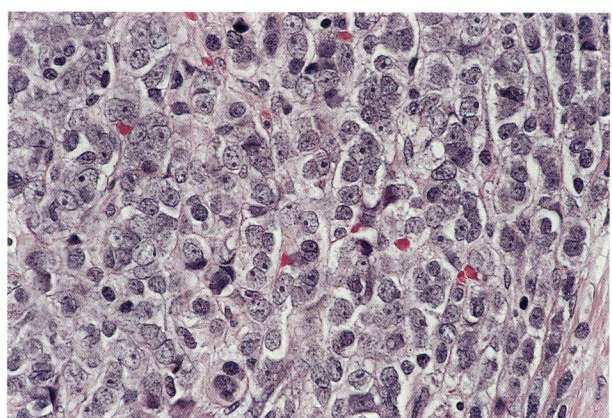

CASE 48-1. A section of a left scalene node showed total replacement of the node by large, anaplastic tumor cells (H&E stain, ×400). The major differential diagnoses included malignant lymphoma, retroperitoneal seminoma, and undifferentiated carcinoma. Immunohistochemical stains for immunoglobulin, fetoprotein, and β-human chorionic gonadotropin were negative.

Comments. Undifferentiated carcinomas may simulate malignant lymphoma in presentation. Again, the proper application of immunohistochemical stains is helpful in making the difficult differential diagnosis.

This patient was treated with diethylstilbestrol and continued to feel well in general at the 8½ year follow-up.

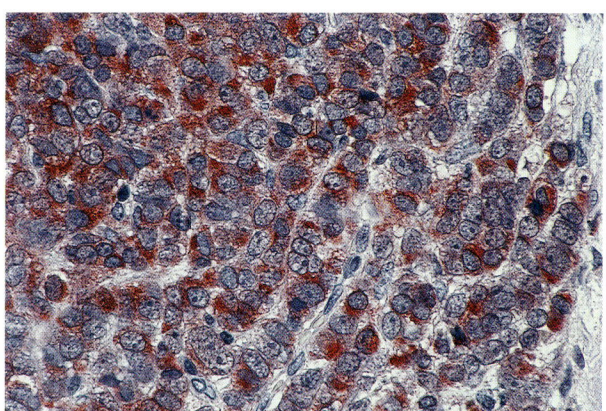

CASE 48-2. Another section of the same node showed strongly positive staining (brownish red granular staining) of prostatic acid phosphatase in the cytoplasm of the tumor cells (immunoperoxidase stain for prostatic acid phosphatase, ×400). This finding indicated the prostatic origin of the tumor cells and established the diagnosis of metastatic undifferentiated prostatic carcinoma.

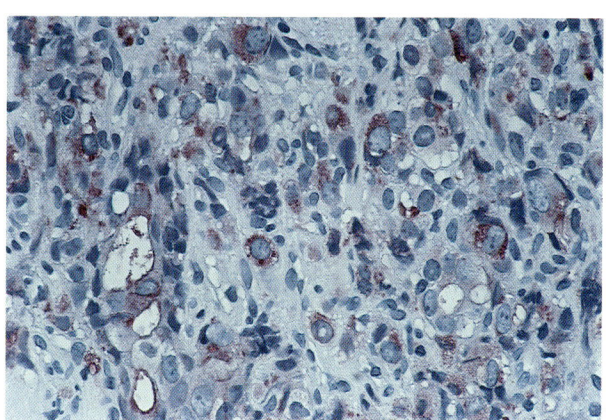

CASE 48-3. A section of the prostatic needle biopsy specimen showed poorly differentiated adenocarcinoma that was also positive (brownish red granular staining in the cytoplasm) for prostatic acid phosphatase (immunoperoxidase stain for prostatic acid phosphatase, ×400). This finding further confirmed the diagnosis of prostatic carcinoma with metastasis.

CASE 49 Granulocytic Sarcoma

A 45-year-old man was initially seen because of an 8-week history of epigastric pain and progressive dysphagia. Findings of the physical examination were normal. Blood examination yielded the following data: RBC 3.82×10^{12}/L (3.82×10^6/μL); hemoglobin 96.0 g/L (9.6 g/dL); hematocrit 0.29 (29.0%); and WBC 7.0×10^9/L (7.0×10^3/μL). An upper gastrointestinal tract series revealed high-grade obstruction of the distal portion of the esophagus at the level of the cardia. Abdominal exploration revealed a very large, malignant neoplasm in the upper half of the stomach. Partial esophagectomy, total gastrectomy, partial duodenectomy, omentectomy, splenectomy, resection of the tail of the pancreas, esophagojejunostomy, and jejunojejunostomy with closure of the duodenal stump were performed.

Comments. This case illustrates the characteristic histochemical and immunohistochemical features of granulocytic sarcoma and its morphologic similarity to the diffuse large-cell lymphomas.

This patient developed acute granulocytic leukemia 2 months after the operation.

Because of wide variations in clinical presentation, infrequent occurrence, and morphologic similarity to diffuse large-cell lymphoma, the diagnosis of granulocytic sarcoma is one of the most difficult to make. Fortunately, the chloroacetate esterase stain, useful in identifying granulocytic sarcoma, is relatively simple to perform and is easily applicable to paraffin sections. It is important to do this stain routinely in all cases with morphologic features of diffuse large-cell lymphoma to identify or rule out the possibility of granulocytic sarcoma.

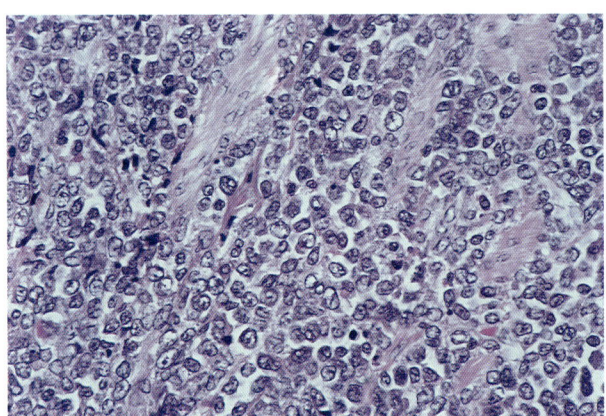

CASE 49-1. A section of the stomach showed transmural infiltration by large neoplastic cells (H&E stain, ×400). This finding simulated diffuse large-cell lymphoma.

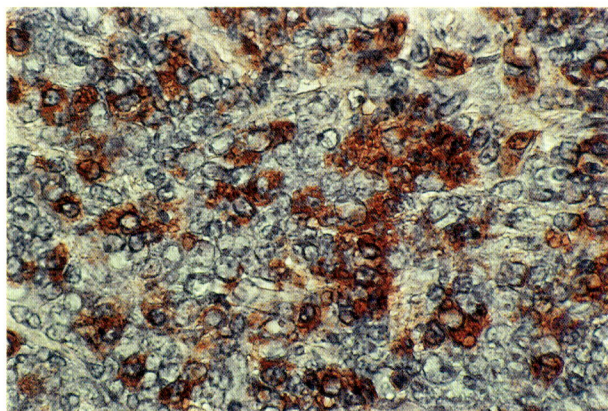

CASE 49-3. Another section of the stomach showed positive lysozyme staining (brownish red granular staining) in the cytoplasm of the neoplastic cells (immunoperoxidase stain for lysozyme, ×400). This finding further confirmed the diagnosis of granulocytic sarcoma.

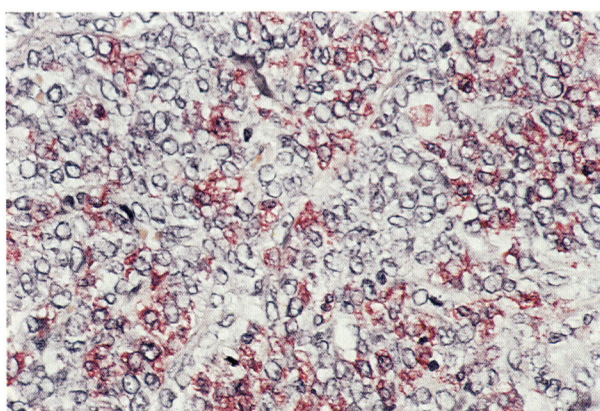

CASE 49-2. Another section of the stomach showed positive chloroacetate esterase staining (reddish granular staining) in the cytoplasm of many of the infiltrating neoplastic cells (chloroacetate esterase stain, ×400). This finding established the diagnosis of granulocytic sarcoma.

CASE 50 Gamma Heavy Chain Disease

A 78-year-old man was initially seen because of progressive weakness of 2 weeks' duration. He had a history of angina for 10 years and had had a resection for bladder carcinoma 10 years ago. Physical examination revealed lymph nodes enlarged to 2 to 4 cm throughout the cervical, axillary, and inguinal regions. The spleen tip was also palpable. Blood examination yielded the following data: RBC 3.92×10^{12}/L (3.92×10^6/μL); hemoglobin 112.0 g/L (11.2 g/dL); hematocrit 0.329 (32.9%); platelets 300.0×10^9/L (300.0×10^3/μL); and WBC 9.2×10^9/L (9.2×10^3/μL) with 76% neutrophils, 14% lymphocytes, 8% monocytes, and 2% eosinophils. Bone marrow examination revealed mild erythroid hyperplasia.

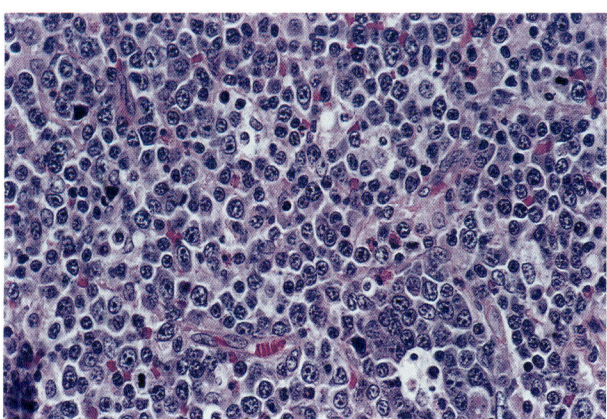

CASE 50-1. A section of a left axillary lymph node showed diffuse replacement of the node by various-sized lymphoid cells with some plasmacytoid differentiation (H&E stain, ×400). The differential diagnoses included non-Hodgkin's lymphoma and angioimmunoblastic lymphadenopathy.

Comments. This case illustrates the characteristic immunohistochemical features of γ heavy chain disease. However, this disease has no specific histopathologic pattern and is extremely diverse in regard to clinical presentation, distribution of disease, and histopathologic features.

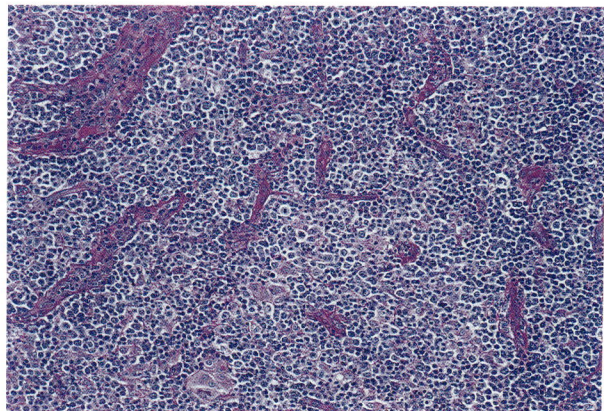

CASE 50-2. Another section of the same node showed increased vascularity among the lymphoid infiltrates (PAS stain, ×160).

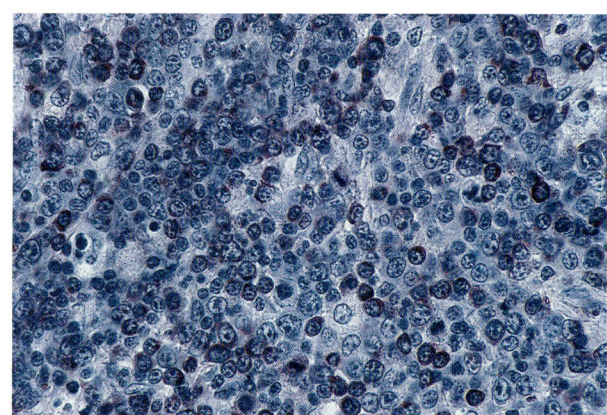

CASE 50-3. Another section of the same node showed positive staining (brownish red staining) of γ heavy chains in the cytoplasm of most of the lymphoid cells (immunoperoxidase stain for γ heavy chains, ×400). Staining for κ and λ light chains, as well as for α and μ heavy chains, was negative, establishing the diagnosis of γ heavy chain disease. Subsequent immunoelectrophoretic studies of serum and urine also demonstrated the presence of monoclonal γ heavy chains, which further confirmed the diagnosis.

CASE 51 Cutaneous T-Cell Lymphoma—Mycosis Fungoides

An 85-year-old man was initially seen because of extensive erythematous plaque and nodular skin lesions that had developed during the past 3½ years. Two months later, right inguinal lymphadenopathy developed.

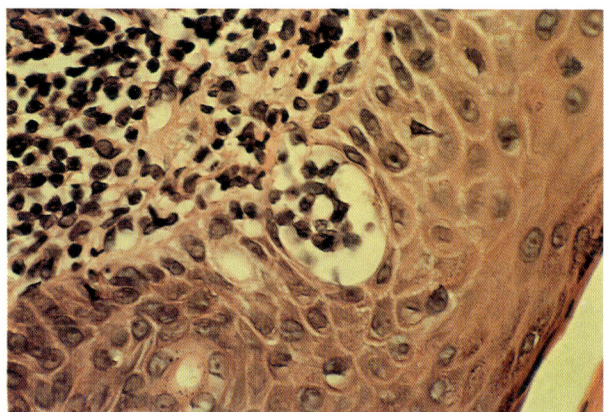

CASE 51-1. A section of the skin biopsy specimen showed a band-like lymphocytic infiltrate in the upper dermis and the presence of Pautrier's microabscesses in the epidermis (H&E stain, ×400). These findings are characteristic of cutaneous T-cell lymphoma (mycosis fungoides).

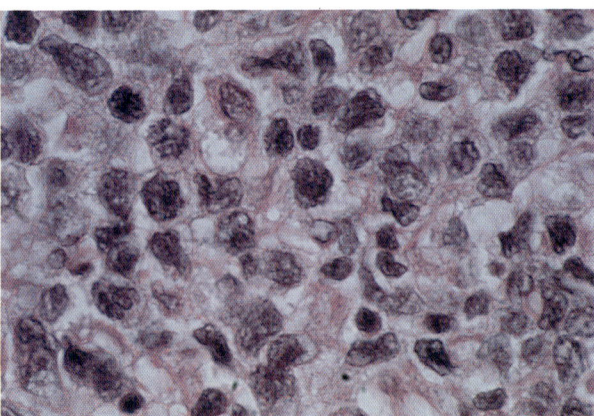

CASE 51-2. A section of a right inguinal lymph node showed diffuse replacement of the node by large lymphoid cells with irregular cerebriform nuclei (H&E stain, ×1000). These cells stained negatively for nonspecific esterase.

Comments. This case illustrates the characteristic morphologic and histochemical features of cutaneous T-cell lymphoma. The neoplastic cells of cutaneous T-cell lymphoma have been further characterized as the T-helper cell subtype.

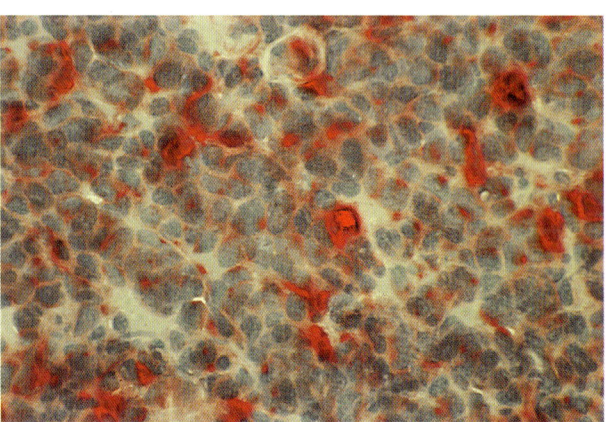

CASE 51-3. A cryostat section of the same node showed positive focal acid phosphatase staining (reddish staining) in the Golgi areas of the tumor cells (acid phosphatase stain, ×400). This finding confirmed the T-cell nature of the tumor cells. The T-cell identity of the tumor cells was further confirmed when E-rosettes were found in a cell suspension for sheep erythrocyte rosette formation.

CASE 52 Cutaneous B-Cell Lymphoma

A 22-year-old man was initially seen with lumps over his scalp and back of 6 months' duration. Physical examination revealed multiple large (1 × 1 cm to 3 × 2 cm), erythematous, firm, ill-defined plaques over his forehead, cheeks, scalp, neck, and back. No lymphadenopathy or hepatosplenomegaly was noted. Results of a bone marrow biopsy specimen, a lymphangiogram, and a CT scan were negative.

Comments. This case illustrates the immunohistochemical features of cutaneous B-cell lymphoma and its characteristic infiltration pattern.

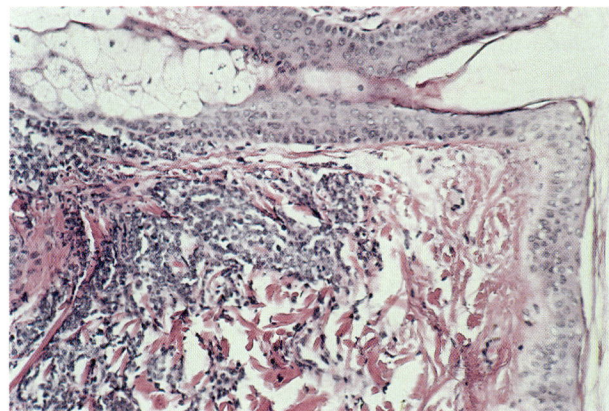

CASE 52-1. A section of the skin biopsy specimen from his forehead showed monomorphic lymphoid infiltrates around the skin appendage in the middle dermis, but the infiltrates spared the epidermis and subepidermal layer (H&E stain, ×160).

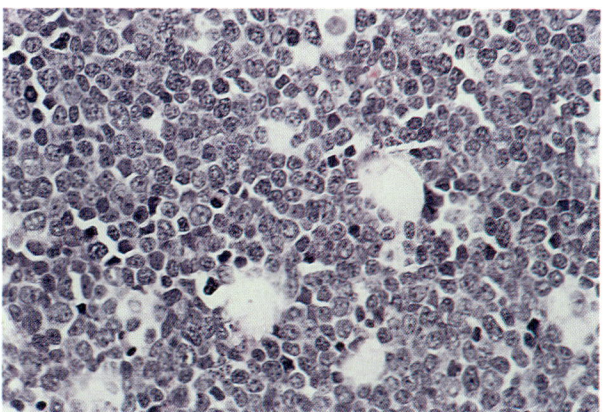

CASE 52-2. Another section of the same tissue showed dense lymphoid infiltrates in the deeper dermis extending into the subcutaneous fat (H&E stain, ×400).

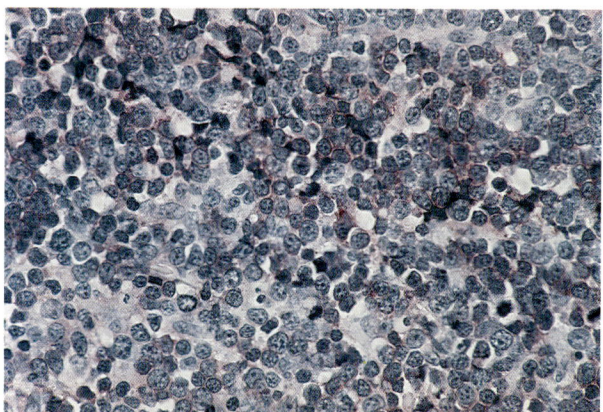

CASE 52-3. Another section of the same tissue showed positive staining for λ light chains (brownish red granular staining) in the cytoplasm of most of the large lymphoid cells (immunoperoxidase stain for λ light chains, ×400). Staining for κ light chains was negative. This finding established the diagnosis of B-cell lymphoma of the large noncleaved follicular center cell type.

CASE 53 Small Lymphocytic Lymphoma of Lung

A 40-year-old woman had been experiencing fatigue for 5 months. Findings of the physical examination were normal. Blood examination yielded the following data: RBC 4.37×10^{12}/L (4.37×10^6/µL); hemoglobin 119.0 g/L (11.9 g/dL); hematocrit 0.369 (36.9%); platelets 250.0×10^9/L (250.0×10^3/µL); and WBC 4.7×10^9/L (4.7×10^3/µL) with 55.5% neutrophils, 22.5% lymphocytes, 18% monocytes, 2% eosinophils, and 2% basophils. A chest roentgenogram and CT scans revealed a poorly defined nodule in the superior segment of the lower lobe of the right lung. Segmental resection of the right lower lobe revealed a subpleural lesion measuring 2.5 cm in diameter.

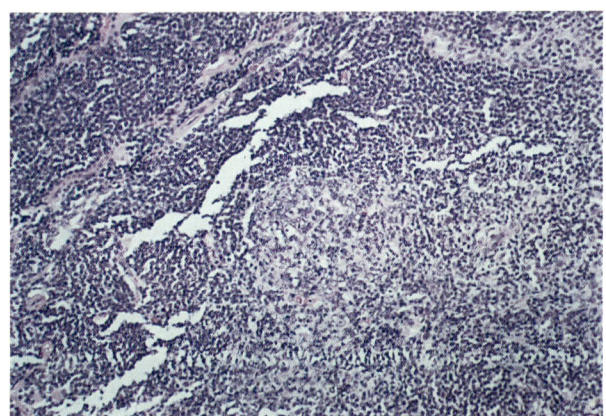

CASE 53-1. A section of the lesion showed a germinal center among the monomorphic lymphocytic infiltrates (H&E stain, ×100). The major differential diagnoses included extranodal lymphoma of the small lymphocytic type and inflammatory pseudolymphoma.

Comments. Making a differential diagnosis between inflammatory pseudolymphoma and extranodal, small lymphocytic lymphoma may be difficult. The presence of a germinal center in the lesion has been considered one of the morphologic features that indicates an inflammatory pseudolymphoma; however, it may also be present in the lymphoma lesion. Immunoperoxidase stains for κ and λ light chains are most helpful in determining the monoclonal nature of the B-cell neoplasm in contrast to the polyclonal nature of a reactive inflammatory pseudolymphoma.

This patient developed a similar lesion in the middle lobe of the right lung 2 years later and was treated with combination chemotherapy consisting of cyclophosphamide, vincristine, procarbazine, and prednisone after surgical resection of the lesion. She was doing well, with no evidence of further recurrence, 21 years after the diagnosis was made.

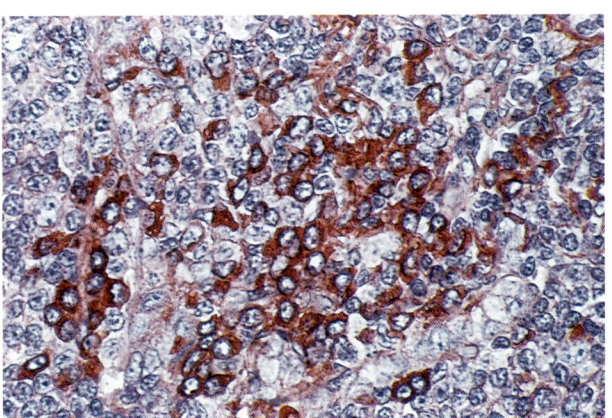

CASE 53-2. Another section of the lesion showed positive staining for λ light chains (brownish red granular staining) in the cytoplasm of many of the infiltrating lymphocytes (immunoperoxidase stain for λ light chains, ×400). Staining for κ light chains was negative. This finding indicated monoclonal proliferation and established the diagnosis of small lymphocytic lymphoma with plasmacytoid differentiation rather than inflammatory pseudolymphoma.

CASE 54 B-Cell Lymphoma with High Content of Epithelioid Histiocytes

A 50-year-old man had a 4-year history of collagen vascular disease manifested by generalized, intermittent macular rash, sicca, and intermittent joint pains. Cervical adenopathy had developed during the past 6 weeks. Physical examination revealed bilateral cervical adenopathy and a macular rash over the lower extremities. Blood examination yielded the following data: RBC 4.7×10^{12}/L (4.7×10^{6}/μL); hemoglobin 127.0 g/L (12.7 g/dL); hematocrit 0.363 (36.3%); platelets 270.0×10^{9}/L (270.0×10^{3}/μL); and WBC 3.9×10^{9}/L (3.9×10^{3}/μL) with 67.1% neutrophils, 23.9% lymphocytes, 8% monocytes, 0.5% eosinophils, and 0.2% basophils. Bone marrow examination showed granulocytic hyperplasia. A chest roentgenogram revealed multiple small nodules throughout both lungs and bilateral hilar adenopathy.

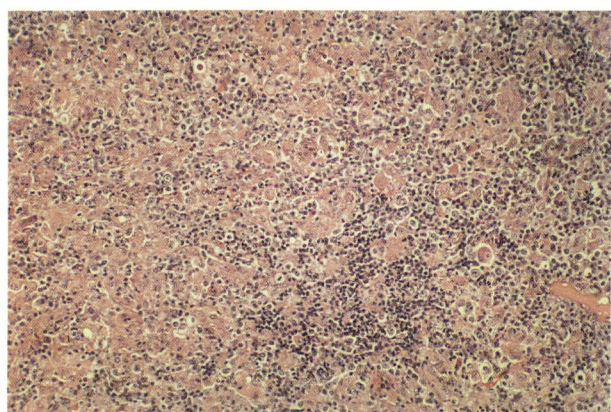

CASE 54-1. A section of the left cervical lymph node showed diffuse replacement of the node by mixed cellular infiltrates that were predominantly epithelioid histiocytes (H&E stain, ×100).

Comments. Lymphoepithelioid cell lymphoma was first described by Lennert, who regarded it as a mixed entity including some cases of Hodgkin's disease. Most of these lymphomas were subsequently characterized as neoplasms of CD4-positive T cells. Although it is rare, non-Hodgkin's lymphoma of the B-cell type with a high content of epithelioid histiocytes also exists, as illustrated in this case. The cytologic appearance of the lymphoid cells comprising these neoplasms and the B-cell phenotype differentiates them from lymphoepithelioid cell lymphoma (Lennert's lymphoma).

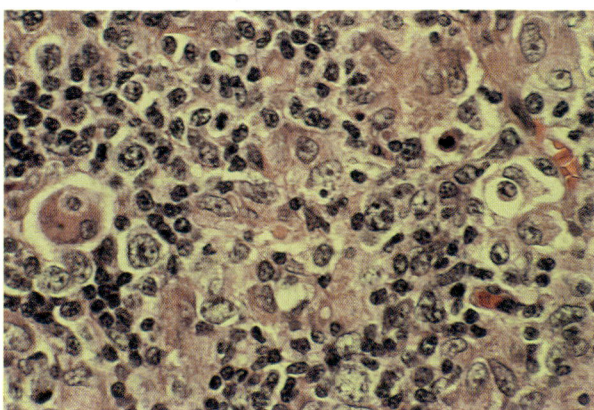

CASE 54-2. A higher-magnification view showed mixed lymphoid and histiocytic infiltrates (H&E stain, ×400). The major differential diagnoses included lymphocyte- and histiocyte-predominant Hodgkin's disease, Lennert's lymphoma, and mixed cell-type diffuse non-Hodgkin's lymphoma.

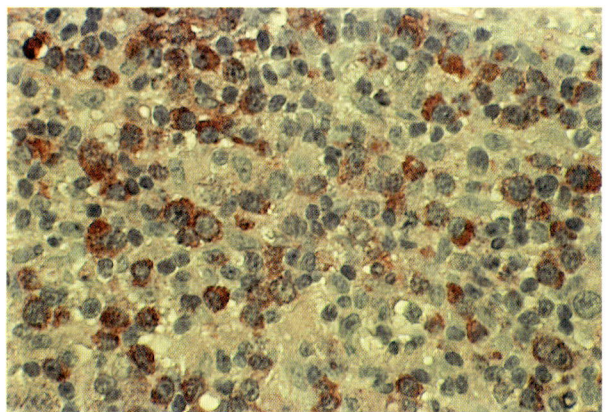

CASE 54-3. Another section of the same node showed intense staining (brownish red granular staining) of κ light chains in the cytoplasm of most of the lymphoid cells (immunoperoxidase stain for κ light chains, ×400). Staining for λ light chains was negative, indicating a monoclonal B-cell neoplasm and establishing the diagnosis of B-cell lymphoma (non-Hodgkin's lymphoma) associated with a histiocytic reaction.

CASE 55 Plasmacytoma

A 70-year-old woman was initially seen because of a 2-year history of oropharyngeal discomfort and changes in her voice. Physical examination revealed that the soft and hard palates were enlarged and appeared to be chronically inflamed. An ear, nose, and throat examination revealed a left parapharyngeal mass that was pushing the palate medially. Blood examination yielded the following data: RBC 4.43×10^{12}/L (4.43×10^{6}/μL); hemoglobin 134.0 g/L (13.4 g/dL); hematocrit 0.401 (40.1%); platelets 289.0×10^{9}/L (289.0×10^{3}/μL); and WBC 5.2×10^{9}/L (5.2×10^{3}/μL) with 67.1% neutrophils, 22.3% lymphocytes, 5.6% monocytes, 2.9% eosinophils, and 0.9% basophils. An exploration and biopsy of the left side of the neck were performed.

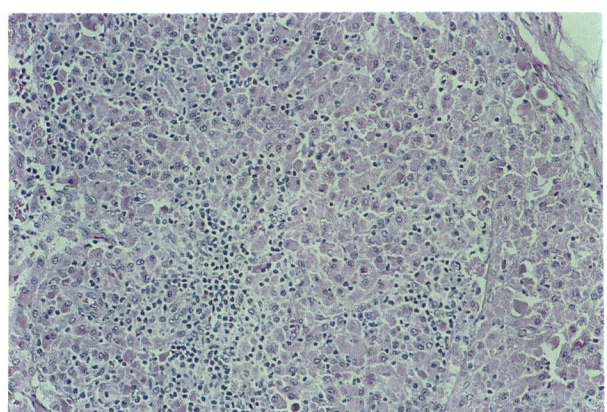

CASE 55-1. A section of a left cervical lymph node showed massive replacement of the node by what appeared to be histiocytes (H&E stain, ×160). Major differential diagnoses included sinus histiocytosis with massive lymphadenopathy, histiocytic lymphoma, and plasmacytoma with an unusal morphology.

Comments. This patient received radiation therapy to the nasopharynx. Two years later, multiple myeloma developed. The disease progressed slowly, and the patient eventually died with the complication of pleural effusion 4 years after the diagnosis of multiple myeloma.

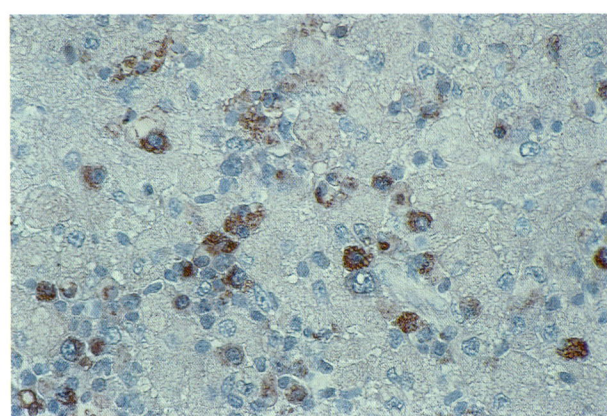

CASE 55-2. Another section of the same node showed positive staining (brownish red granular staining) of κ light chains in the cytoplasm of the plasma cells and histiocytoid cells (immunoperoxidase stain for κ light chains, ×400). Staining of λ light chains was negative. This finding indicated a monoclonal plasmaproliferative disease and established the diagnosis of extramedullary plasmacytoma.

CASE 56 Multiple Myeloma

A 60-year-old man was initially seen because of a 6-month history of back pain. Roentgenographic examination demonstrated a probable destructive lesion involving the left lateral aspect of L1. Blood examination yielded the following data: RBC 3.09×10^{12}/L ($3.09 \times 10^{6}/\mu$L); hemoglobin 89.0 g/L (8.9 g/dL); hematocrit 0.255 (25.5%); platelets 58.0×10^{9}/L ($58.0 \times 10^{3}/\mu$L); and WBC 3.2×10^{9}/L ($3.2 \times 10^{3}/\mu$L) with 66.5% neutrophils, 17.5% lymphocytes, 11% monocytes, 2% eosinophils, 1% basophils, 1.5% myelocytes, and 0.5% normoblasts.

Comments. This case illustrates the characteristic immunohistochemical features of multiple myeloma. No monoclonal protein was detected in the serum, but a monoclonal κ protein was demonstrated in the urine by immunoelectrophoresis.

The patient had an excellent response to combination chemotherapy that consisted of melphalan and prednisone. His condition remained stable for 4 years, but he eventually died of progressive disease 4½ years after the diagnosis.

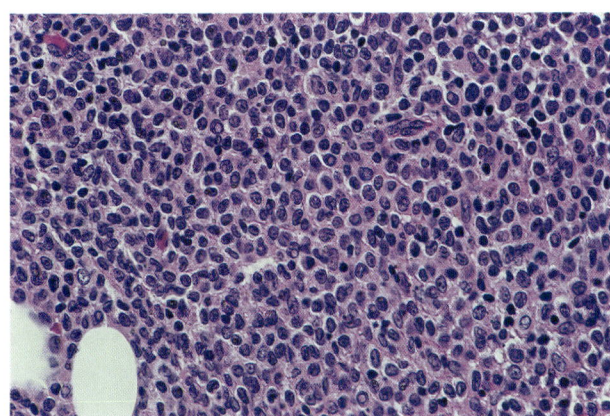

CASE 56-1. A section of a marrow biopsy specimen showed extensive replacement of the marrow by atypical plasma cells (H&E stain, ×400). This finding was consistent with multiple myeloma.

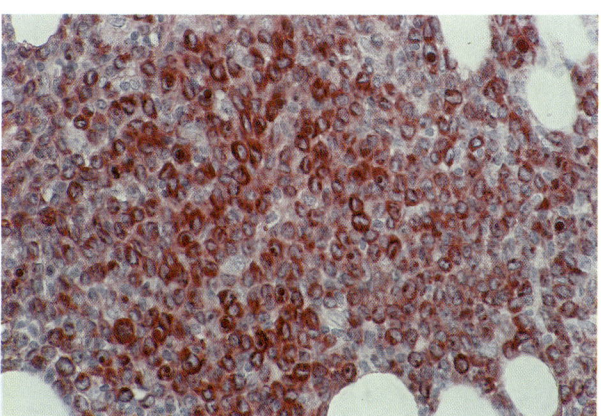

CASE 56-2. Another section of the same specimen showed intense staining (brownish red granular staining) of κ light chains in the cytoplasm of most of the atypical plasma cells (immunoperoxidase stain for κ light chains, ×400). Staining of λ light chains was negative. This finding indicated a monoclonal plasmaproliferative disease and confirmed the diagnosis of multiple myeloma.

CASE 57 Signet-Ring-Cell Myeloma

A 59-year-old man had experienced periodic episodes of back pain for the past year and persistent pain in the upper lumbar and lower thoracic areas for the past 4 weeks. The pain was aggravated by bending and certain other movements. He had lost 6.8 kg in the past 10 months. Physical examination revealed tenderness over the vertebral spinous processes in the area of T1 through L3. The prostate was moderately enlarged and firm but symmetric. Blood examination yielded the following data: RBC 3.73×10^{12}/L ($3.73 \times 10^6/\mu$L); hemoglobin 104.0 g/L (10.4 g/dL); hematocrit 0.32 (32.0%); platelets 274.0×10^9/L ($274.0 \times 10^3/\mu$L); and WBC 4.0×10^9/L ($4.0 \times 10^3/\mu$L) with 43% neutrophils, 47.5% lymphocytes, 8% monocytes, 1% eosinophils, and 0.5% basophils. A roentgenogram examination of the bone revealed demineralization of the spine and compression fractures, as well as several lytic lesions in the pelvis and right femoral neck.

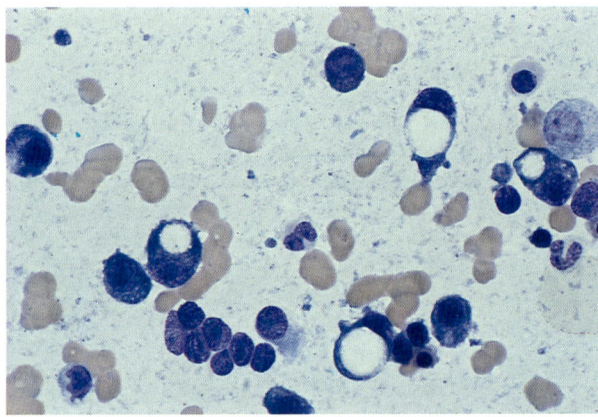

CASE 57-1. A marrow smear showed tumor cells with a signet-ring appearance (Wright's stain, ×1000).

Comments. The signet-ring cell is most commonly seen in mucin-producing adenocarcinoma. However, signet-ring cell lymphoma and myeloma (as in this case) have been recognized.

Further laboratory studies of this patient disclosed a γ spike in the serum, consisting of 43.2 g/L (4.32 g/dL) of an IgG-λ monoclonal protein, and a urine sample that contained 8.83 g/d of protein, which was almost entirely a monoclonal λ protein.

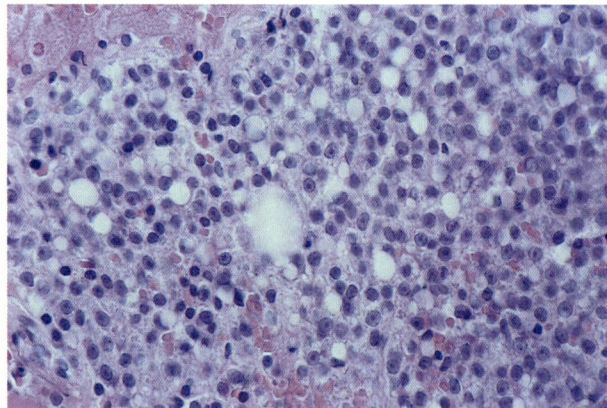

CASE 57-2. A section of the marrow biopsy specimen showed extensive replacement of the marrow by tumor cells, including some signet-ring cells (arrows) (H&E stain, ×400). The major differential diagnoses included metastatic adenocarcinoma and signet-ring-cell myeloma.

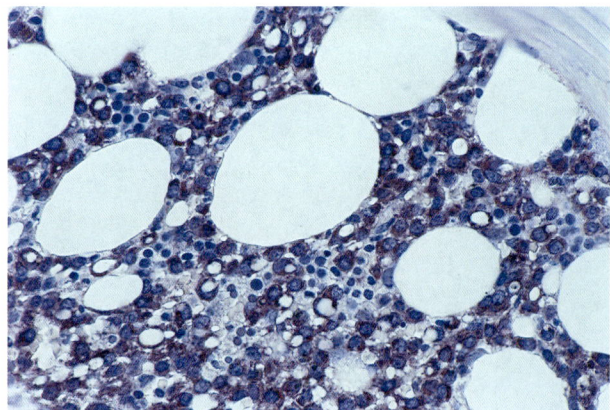

CASE 57-3. Another section of the same marrow biopsy specimen showed intense λ light chain staining (brownish red granular staining) in the cytoplasm of most of the tumor cells (immunoperoxidase stain for λ light chains, ×400). When stained for κ light chains, these plasma cells stained negatively. This finding established the diagnosis of myeloma rather than metastatic adenocarcinoma.

CASE 58 Undifferentiated Myeloma

A 76-year-old man was hospitalized because of increasing fatigue, lethargy, and anorexia of 1 week's duration. He had been followed up periodically for benign monoclonal gammopathy of the IgM -κ type for the past 11 years. He had been receiving melphalan and prednisone for the past 5 years after a bone marrow examination showed diffuse plasmacytoid lymphocytic infiltration and a renal biopsy specimen showed amyloidosis. Physical examination revealed marked hepatomegaly down to 7 cm below the right costal margin, but the spleen was not palpable. Blood examination yielded the following data: RBC $2.43 \times 10^{12}/L$ ($2.43 \times 10^6/\mu L$); hemoglobin 81.0 g/L (8.1 g/dL); hematocrit 0.227 (22.7%); platelets $113.0 \times 10^9/L$ ($113.0 \times 10^3/\mu L$); and WBC $2.4 \times 10^9/L$ ($2.4 \times 10^3/\mu L$) with 63.5% neutrophils, 18.5% lymphocytes, 15.5% monocytes, 0.5% basophils, 0.5% progranulocytes, and 1.5% blasts.

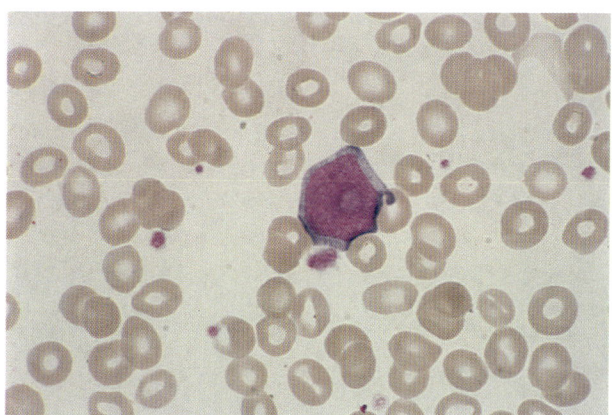

CASE 58-1. A blood smear showed blasts (Wright's stain, ×1000).

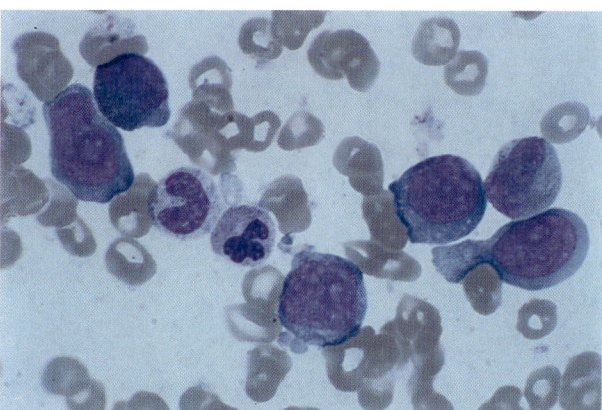

CASE 58-2. A marrow smear showed replacement of the marrow by blast-like cells (Wright's stain, ×1000). The major differential diagnoses included acute nonlymphocytic leukemia and undifferentiated myeloma. The blast-like cells stained negatively for peroxidase and lysozyme.

Comments. Common clinical problems in patients being treated for plasma cell dyscrasia include the recurrence or development of refractory plasma cell dyscrasia or the development of treatment-related myelodysplasia or acute nonlymphocytic leukemia. In this case, the presence of blast-like cells suggested the possibility of either undifferentiated myeloma or treatment-related secondary acute nonlymphocytic leukemia. Appropriate cytochemical and immunohistochemical studies were helpful in establishing the diagnosis, as illustrated in this case.

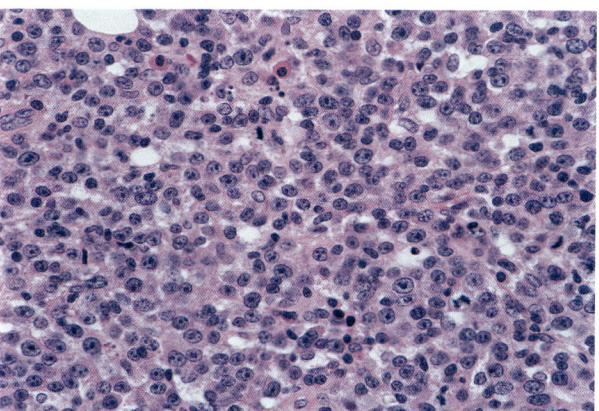

CASE 58-3. A section of a marrow biopsy specimen showed extensive replacement of the marrow by large, primitive cells with prominent central nucleoli (H&E stain, ×400).

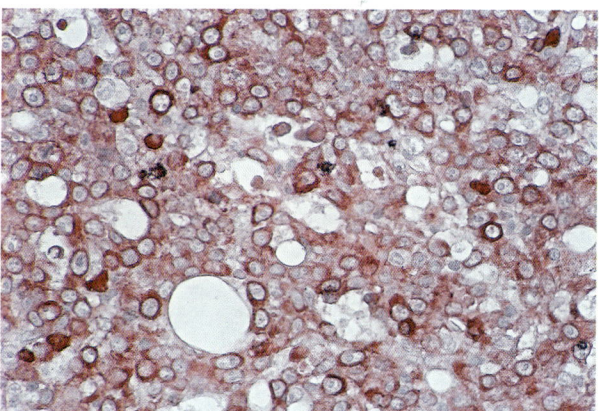

CASE 58-4. Another section of the same specimen showed strong λ light chain staining (brownish red granular staining) in the cytoplasm of most of the primitive cells (immunoperoxidase stain for λ light chains, ×400). Kappa light chain staining was negative. This finding established the diagnosis of undifferentiated myeloma rather than acute nonlymphocytic leukemia.

CASE 59 Primary Amyloidosis

A 76-year-old man was initially seen because of a 1-year history of progressive weakness, anorexia, edema, and a 13.6 kg weight loss. Physical examination revealed mild pedal edema up to the level of the knees, venous stasis in the lower extremitites, and decreased vibratory sense in the lower extremities.

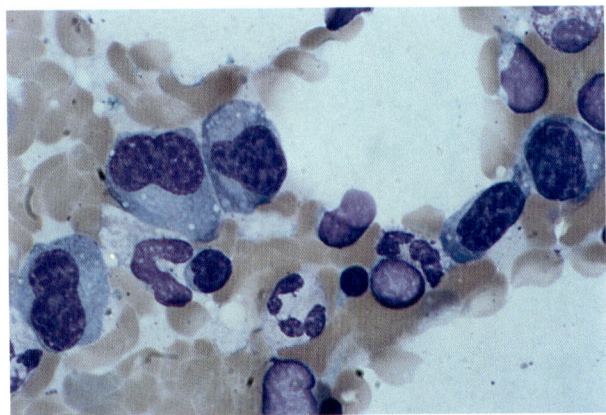

CASE 59-1. A marrow smear showed occasional atypical plasma cell (Wright's stain, ×1000). These cells were positive for λ light chains but negative for κ light chains by immunoperoxidase stain.

Comments. This case illustrates the characteristic morphologic and immunohistochemical features of primary amyloidosis.

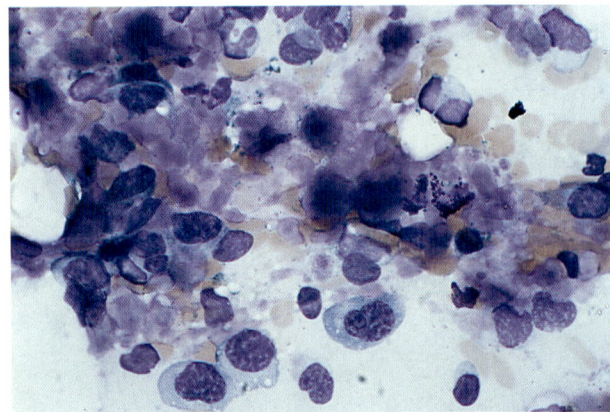

CASE 59-2. Another area of the same marrow smear showed aggregates of amorphous purple materials that were suggestive of amyloidosis (Wright's stain, ×1000).

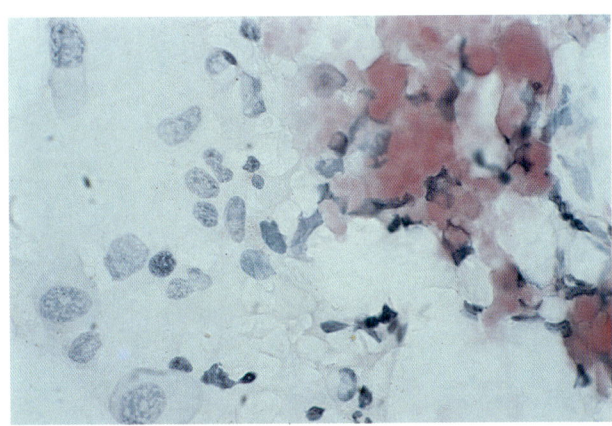

CASE 59-3. Another marrow smear showed positive (orange-red) Congo red staining (Congo red stain, ×1000). This finding confirmed the diagnosis of amyloidosis.

CASE 60 Primary Amyloidosis with Cardiomyopathy

A 54-year-old man was referred for general malaise, shortness of breath, and weight loss over the past 18 months. Physical examination revealed that the breath sounds were clear and the cardiac sounds normal. The blood pressure was 120/80 mmHg, and the pulse was regular at 78 beats per minute. A chest roentgenogram showed mild cardiac enlargement. Echocardiography showed thickened left and right ventricular walls, and a Doppler study showed tricuspid regurgitation. Electrocardiogram showed a flutter fibrillation pattern with a 4:1 block. Left axis deviation and relatively low voltage, especially in the anterior forces, were present. This was believed to be related to a cardiomyopathy in which amyloid disease is common. Results of a deep rectal biopsy, however, were negative. Results of urinalysis, complete blood cell count, chemistry group tests, protein electrophoresis, immunoelectrophoresis of serum and urine, and immunodiffusion of concentrated urine were all normal or negative. An immunofixation with antisera to κ and λ showed a faint κ band. Right ventricular endomyocardial biopsy showed extensive endocardial and interstitial myocardial amyloid.

Comments. This case illustrates the characteristic clinical presentation and immunohistochemical features of primary amyloidosis with cardiomyopathy.

This patient was given a regimen of melphalan, prednisone, and colchicine according to an amyloidosis protocol. He eventually died of amyloid heart disease 1 year later.

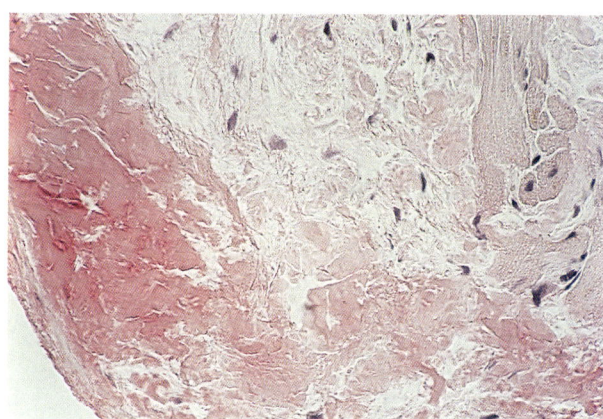

CASE 60-1. A section of the endomyocardial biopsy specimen showed positive immunostaining (pink granular staining) of κ light chains at the site of amyloid deposition (indirect immunoalkaline phosphatase stain for κ light chains, ×400). Immunostaining of λ light chains was negative. This finding confirmed the diagnosis of primary amyloidosis with cardiomyopathy.

CASE 61 Secondary Amyloidosis

A 39-year-old man with a 20-year history of multifocal eosinophilic granuloma of bone had been treated with methotrexate, vinblastine sulfate, and radiation therapy. He also had had intermittent edema during the past 2 to 3 years, and renal amyloidosis was diagnosed by renal biopsy. Physical examination revealed a hearing aid on the right and a scar from a prior right radical mastoidectomy. He had loss of mandibular teeth from eosinophilic granuloma. Radiation pigmentation was present over his sternum and thoracic spine, and a healed sinus tract was present over his sternum. His ribs flared anteriorly. He was kyphotic and had moderate edema in both lower extremities. A chest roentgenogram revealed pleural thickening in the right lower lung laterally. The sixth and seventh ribs were slightly widened bilaterally. Degenerative changes were present throughout his thoracic spine, with partial anklyosis and slight kyphosis. The bone survey showed lytic areas through the ilium bilaterally. Roentgenographic examination of both mastoids showed diffuse sclerosis due to chronic mastoiditis, with postoperative changes on the right and a surgical defect extending into the antra. Blood examination yielded the following data: RBC 2.67×10^{12}/L ($2.67 \times 10^6/\mu L$); hemoglobin 80.0 g/L (8.0 g/dL); hematocrit 0.239 (23.9%); mean corpuscular volume 89.7 fL (89.7 μm^3); reticulocytes 0.008 (0.8%); erythrocyte sedimentation rate 140.0 mm/hr; platelets 714.0×10^9/L ($714.0 \times 10^3/\mu L$); and WBC 6.4×10^9/L ($6.4 \times 10^3/\mu L$) with 80% neutrophils, 17% lymphocytes, 2% monocytes, and 1% eosinophils. Serum protein electrophoresis and serum and urine immunoelectrophoresis failed to show monoclonal protein. An echocardiogram showed no evidence of cardiac amyloidosis.

Comments. This case illustrates the characteristic clinical presentation and morphologic, histochemical, and immunohistochemical features of secondary amyloidosis. Recommendations for treatment of this patient included initiation of a diet for patients with renal disease; erythropoietin treatment for anemia; a trail of colchicine treatment for secondary amyloidosis; and dialysis for renal failure when indicated.

The patient was on a hemodialysis program for his chronic renal failure and was receiving an erythropoietin treatment for his anemia at a local hospital. He eventually died of complications with bronchopneumonia 3½ years after the diagnosis of secondary amyloidosis. Autopsy revealed extensive amyloidosis involving the kidney, heart, liver, spleen, lung, pancreas, adrenals, thyroid, diaphragm, and small arteries of the gastrointestinal tract and urinary bladder.

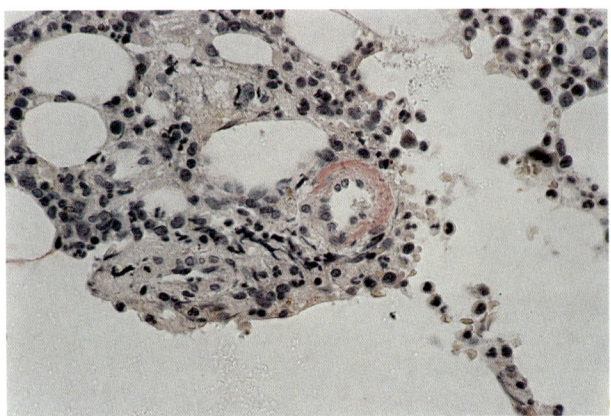

CASE 61-2. Another marrow biopsy section showed positive Congo red staining (orange-red staining) on the vascular wall of a small vessel, consistent with amyloidosis (Congo red stain, ×400).

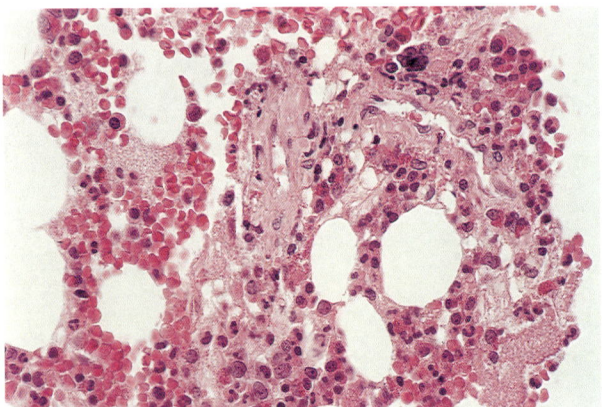

CASE 61-1. A marrow biopsy section showed thickening of the vascular wall suggestive of amyloidosis (H&E stain, ×400).

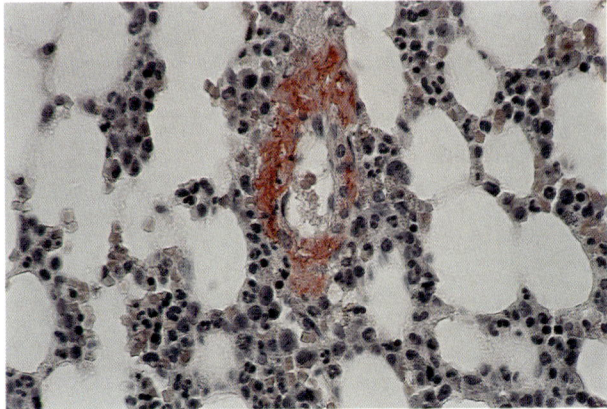

CASE 61-3. Another marrow biopsy section showed positive immunostaining (brownish red granular staining) of amyloid A protein at the site of amyloid deposition, confirming the diagnosis of secondary amyloidosis (indirect immunoperoxidase stain for amyloid A protein, ×400).

CASE 62 Large-Cell Lymphoma, B-Cell Type, with Features of "Malignant Histiocytosis"

A 60-year-old man was initially seen because of a 6-month history of increasing weakness, night sweats, chills, and fever. A thorough medical evaluation had revealed no etiology for his persistent fever. Physical examination revealed splenomegaly extending to 4 cm below the left costal margin. Blood examination yielded the following data: RBC $3.75 \times 10^{12}/L$ ($3.75 \times 10^6/\mu L$); hemoglobin 109.0 g/L (10.9 g/dL); hematocrit 0.327 (32.7%); platelets $116.0 \times 10^9/L$ ($116.0 \times 10^3/\mu L$); and WBC $8.1 \times 10^9/L$ ($8.1 \times 10^3/\mu L$) with 64% neutrophils, 32% lymphocytes, and 4% monocytes. Findings of a bone marrow examination were within normal limits. Exploratory laparotomy and splenectomy were performed.

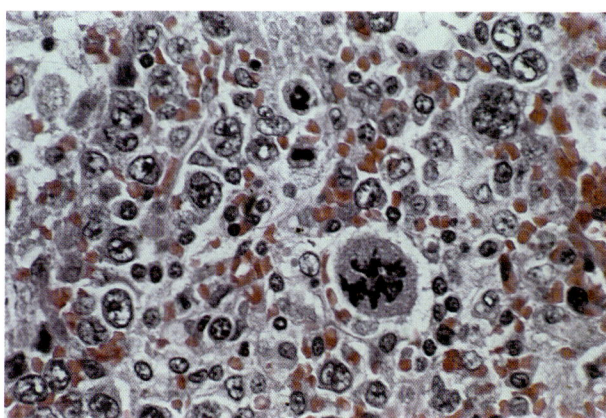

CASE 62-1. A paraffin section of the spleen showed diffuse infiltration of the red pulp by atypical, pleomorphic, large cells (H&E stain, ×400). This finding was suggestive of malignant histiocytosis. These cells stained negatively for chloroacetate esterase.

Comments. The recent availability of immunohistochemical markers useful for identification of T lymphocytes (CD45RO), B lymphocytes (CD20), and histiocytes (CD68) has made it easier to correlate the cell lineage markers and atypical neoplastic cells within a background of normal or reactive cells. Using these immunohistochemical markers to reexamine cases previously considered to be malignant histiocytosis on the basis of morphologic criteria or enzyme histochemical markers on frozen sections has led to a new understanding that some of the cases are in fact T- or B-cell neoplasms rather than true histiocytic neoplasms. It was proposed that these disorders should be more accurately described as *sinusoidal large-cell lymphoma*.

SUGGESTED READINGS

Arai E, Su WPD, Roche PC, et al: Cutaneous histiocytic malignancy. Immunohistochemical re-examination of cases previously diagnosed as cutaneous "histiocytic lymphoma" and "malignant histiocytosis." *J Cutan Pathol* 20:115–120, 1993.

Wilson MS, Weiss LM, Gatter KC, et al: Malignant histiocytosis: A reassessment of cases previously reported in 1975 based on paraffin section immunophenotyping studies. *Cancer* 66:530–536, 1990.

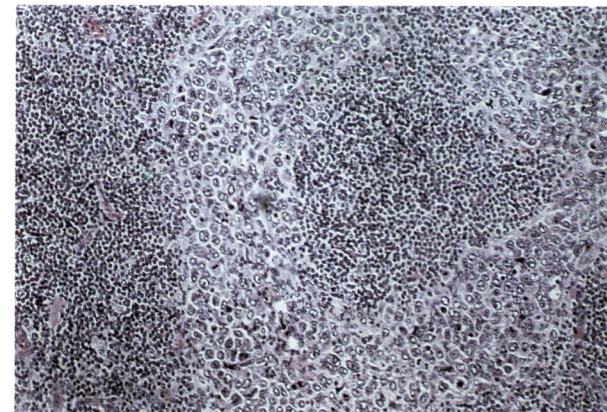

CASE 62-2. A paraffin section of an aortic lymph node showed an atypical large-cell infiltration that was predominantly located in the sinuses (H&E stain, ×100). This finding was consistent with malignant histiocytosis (histiocytic medullary reticulosis).

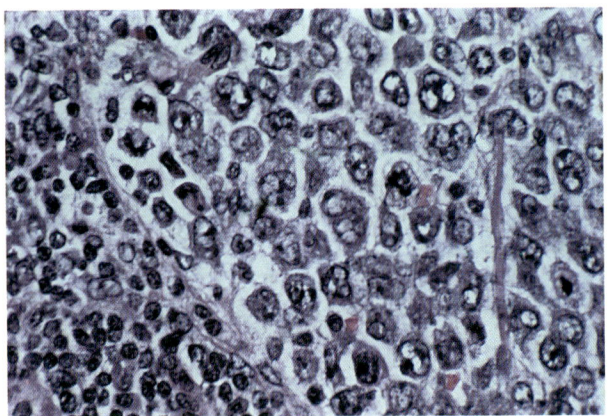

CASE 62-3. A higher-magnification view of the aortic lymph node section showed neoplastic cell morphology similar to that seen in the section of the spleen (H&E stain, ×400).

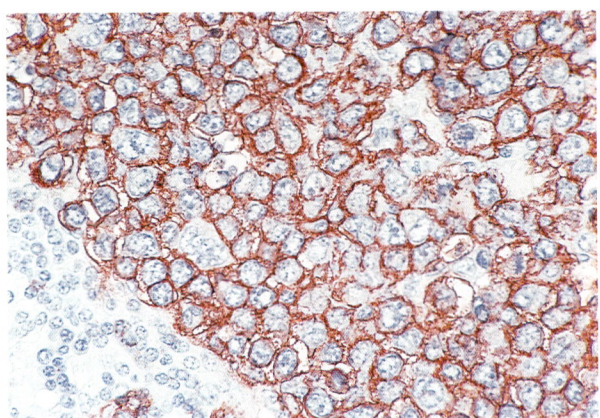

CASE 62-5. Another section of the same node showed strong positive CD20 staining (brownish red granular staining) on the surface of the neoplastic cells (immunoperoxidase stain for CD20 using monoclonal antibody L26, ×400). The neoplastic cells were also weakly positive for cytoplasmic κ light chains and negative for λ light chains. These findings indicate the monoclonal B-cell nature of the neoplastic cells rather than true histiocytic cells.

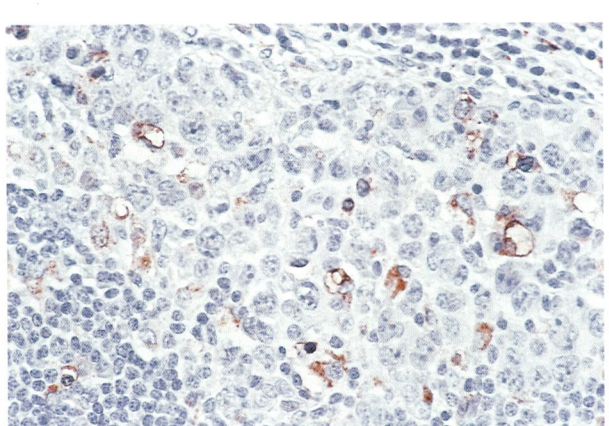

CASE 62-4. Another section of the same node showed positive CD68 staining (brownish red granular staining) in the cytoplasm of scattered, benign-appearing histiocytes but negative staining in the large, atypical neoplastic cells (immunoperoxidase stain for CD68 using monoclonal antibody KP-1, ×400).

CASE 63 Composite Lymphoma—B-Cell Type

A 35-year-old man was initially seen because of a 3-year history of progressive lymphadenopathy. Several lymph node biopsy specimens showed atypical follicular hyperplasia. He was otherwise well and had no fever or other symptoms. Physical examination revealed massive lymphadenopathy (up to 7 cm in diameter) in the cervical, axillary, and inguinal areas and severe pitting edema of the legs. Extensive retroperitoneal adenopathy was demonstrated on a CT scan, and obstruction of the left ureter was seen on an excretory urogram. Blood examination yielded the following data: RBC 4.88×10^{12}/L (4.88×10^{6}/µL); hemoglobin 156.0 g/L (15.6 g/dL); hematocrit 0.435 (43.5%); platelets 246.0×10^{9}/L (246.0×10^{3}/µL); and WBC 8.2×10^{9}/L (8.2×10^{3}/µL) with 85% neutrophils, 8% lymphocytes, 2% monocytes, and 5% eosinophils. Findings of a bone marrow examination were normal.

Comments. The results of immunohistochemical studies helped to exclude the possibility of malignant histiocytosis or metastatic carcinoma and established the diagnosis of composite lymphoma. The neoplastic cells in this tumor were monoclonal B cells (κ chain) but with two morphologic expressions, namely, follicular small cleaved cell lymphoma and diffuse large-cell lymphoma involving the sinuses.

This patient responded well to initial combination chemotherapy that included cyclophosphamide, vincristine, doxorubicin hydrochloride, and prednisone. His disease was well under control for 2 years. However, the lymphoma eventually recurred, and he died 2½ years after the diagnosis.

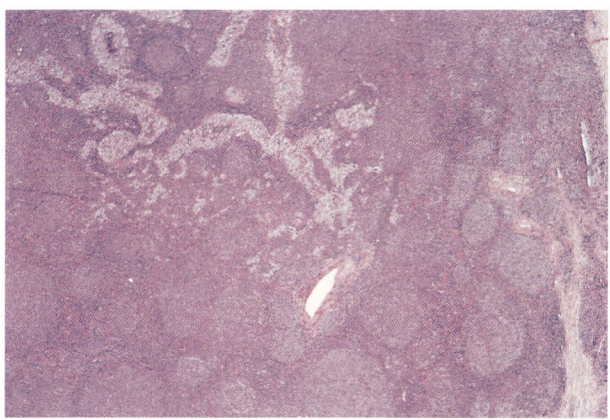

CASE 63-1. A section of a left cervical lymph node biopsy specimen showed extensive replacement of the node by nodular lymphoma and infiltration of sinuses by large, atypical cells in the left upper corner of the field (H&E stain, ×25). The major morphologic differential diagnoses included composite lymphoma, nodular lymphoma with malignant histiocytosis, and nodular lymphoma with metastatic carcinoma.

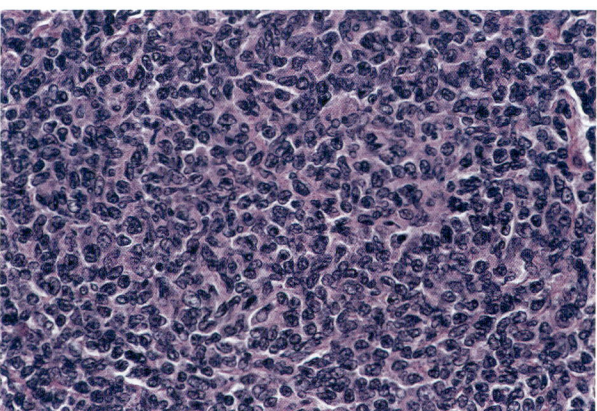

CASE 63-2. A higher-magnification view of the same lymph node section showed an area of nodular lymphoma consisting mainly of small, cleaved follicular center cells (H&E stain, ×400). This finding was characteristic of nodular, poorly differentiated lymphocytic lymphoma of Rappaport or small cleaved follicular center cell lymphoma of Lukes.

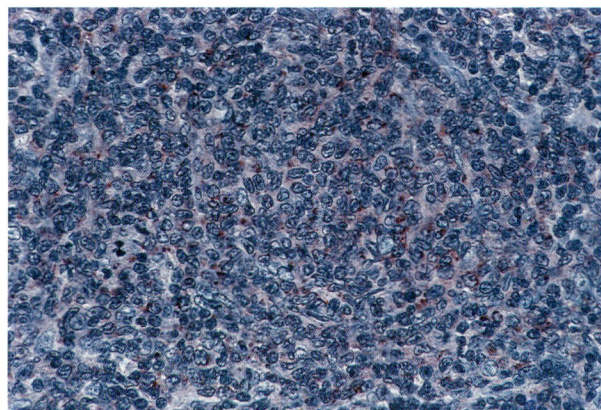

CASE 63-3. Another section of the same lymph node showed positive κ light chain staining (brownish red granular staining) in the cytoplasm of most of the neoplastic small, cleaved follicular center cells (immunoperoxidase stain for κ light chains, ×400). The same area stained negatively for λ light chains.

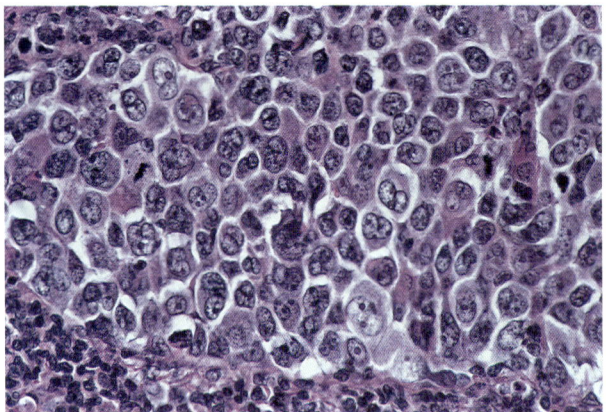

CASE 63-4. Another higher-magnification view of the same lymph node section showed another area of sinusoidal involvement by large, atypical neoplastic cells (H&E stain, ×400).

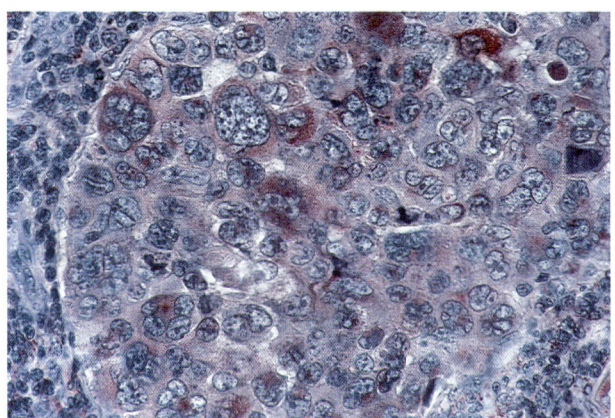

CASE 63-5. Another section of the same lymph node showed that the large, atypical cells in the sinuses were also positive for κ light chain staining (brownish red granular staining) in the cytoplasm (immunoperoxidase stain for κ light chain, ×400). The same area stained negatively for λ light chains and lysozyme.

INDEX

A

Acetate buffer, 103–104
Acetate-tartrate buffer, 104
Acid α-naphthyl acetate esterase for T lymphocytes, 119–120
Acid α-naphthyl acetate esterase reaction, 10, 22
Acid phosphatase, 121
  tartrate-resistant, 121–122
Acid phosphatase reaction, 11, 23
  tartrate-resistant, 11–12, 23
Acid phosphatase and tartrate-resistant acid phosphatase (TRAP), 137–138
Alkaline phosphatase
  anti-alkaline phosphatase (APAAP) method for cytologic materials, 153–154
  method (modified after Leary et al), 124
  reaction, 10–11, 23
Alkaline phosphatase, 138
ALL antigen (CD10), common, and null-cell markers, 42
ALLs, markers used for subclassification of, t84
aminoalkylsilane-treated (silanized) glass slides, 111
Aminocaproate esterase reaction, 10, 22–23
Aminocaproate esterase (Trypsin-like enzyme), 126, 139
Aminocaproate esterase reaction, 22–23
Amyloidosis, 92
  markers useful for subclassification of, t92
Antigen receptor genes, structure and rearrangement of, 61–63
Artifacts in immunophenotyping by FCM, potential sources of, t58
Avidin-biotin complex system, 29–30

B

Baker's formol-calcium solution, 107
B-cell acute lymphoblastic leukemia (L3), marrow similar to Burkitt's lymphoma (H&E stain), f185
B-cell acute lymphoblastic leukemia (L3), marrow replacement by lymphoid cells (Wright's stain), f185
B-cell acute lympoblastic leukemia (L3), Sudan black B staining of leukemic blasts, f185
B-cell chronic lymphocytic leukemia
  globular cytoplasmic inclusion (Wright's stain), f191
  positive staining of HLA-DR, f191
  small lymphocytes (Wright's stain), f191
B-cell differentiation, f39
B-cell lymphoma with high content of epithelioid histiocytes
  κ-light chains staining, f239
  lymphoid/histiocytic, f239
  node replacement by infiltrates, f239
B-cell tumors involving translocation of putative oncogenes and heavy chain gene, 74–75
B-5 fixative, 108
B-lineage ALL, classification of, t42
B small cleaved cell leukemia
  immunostaining, f192
  immunostaining of CD20, f193
  immunostaining of HLA-DR, f192
  lymphocytes and cleaved cells (Wright's stain), f192
Buffered 60% acetone in citrate, 106
Buffered formol-acetone, 106
Buffered gum sucrose solution, 110
Buffered 0.5% neutral red solution, 109
Buffered methanol-acetone, 106
Buffered 1% methyl green solution, 109
Buffer solutions, 103–105
Burkitt's lymphoma, 73–74
  morphologic similarity with lymphoblasts of L3-ALL, f216
  neoplasm of B lymphoblasts, f216
  positive λ-light chain staining in cytoplasm, f216

C

Cacodylate buffer, 104
CD68 antigen (KPI) detections, 31
Cell cycles, 53
Cell populations and phases of cell cycle, f53
Chlorazol fast pink, 139
Chloroacetate esterase, 135–136
  new Fuchsin method, 117–118
  reaction, 9, 22
Chromosomal
  abnormalities, prognostic significance of, 77
  translocation by DNA hybridization technique, identification of, 67
  translocation in lymphoid neoplasms, t73
  translocations and oncogenes, 73–74
Chromosomes, structural and numerical anomalies in, 72
CIg, immunofluorescence technique for, 148
Colon tissue, detection of TGFβ-1 message with riboprobe, f166
Complement receptor, 40–41
Contourgram
  showing blood specimen stained with monocyte and panleukocyte markers, f57
  showing one cell population in each of four quadrants, f56
  showing results of overcompensation, f57
  showing result of spectral overlap, f56
Counterstains, 109
Cross-lineage rearrangement, lineage infidelity or promiscuity, 67

251

Cryostat sections for enzyme
  histochemistry, preparation of, 129
Cutaneous B-cell lymphoma
  dense lymphoid infiltrates in deeper
    dermis, f237
  monomorphic lymphoid infiltrates in
    middle dermis, f237
  positive staining for λ-light chains in
    cytoplasm, f237
Cutaneous T-cell lymphoma-mycosis
  fungoides
  lymphocytic infiltrate in upperdermis,
    f236
  node replacement by large lymphoid
    cells, f236
  positive focal acid phosphatase staining,
    f236
Cytochemical, histochemical,
  immunologic and immunochemical
  markers, t81
Cytochemical and immunochemical
  markers applied to various types of
  specimens, t80
Cytochemical features of blood cells,
  summary of, t13
Cytochemical reactions, cell specificity
  and clinical applications of, t14
Cytochemistry, 7–19
  definition of, 7
  miscellaneous reactions, 14–15
Cytodiagnosis
  preparation of cerebrospinal fluid for,
    114
  preparation of effusions for, 113
Cytogenetics and oncogenes, 72–78
Cytogenetic studies
  of bone marrow (direct method),
    158–159
  of peripheral blood, 159–160
Cytogenetic techniques, 158–162
Cytology and cytochemistry, 112–127
Cytometric immunophenotyping and
  immunogenotyping, comparison of,
  t62
Cytoplasmic immunoglobulin, 40

D

Diagnostic techniques, special, technical
  considerations of, 79–82
DNA cell cycle analysis of lymph node,
  f53
DNA ploidy analysis: rapid nuclear
  isolation and staining, 161–162
DNA/RNA analysis, 53–55

E

Epstein-Barr virus
  in brain lymphoma, f165
  gene detected in Doudi cell line, f165
  receptor for, 41
Erythroleukemia, acute (M6)
  erythroid hyperplasia (Wright's stain),
    f176
  vs. myelodysplastic syndrome, 85
  PAS positivity (PAS stain), f176
  positive immunostain of erythroid
    antigen (immunoperoxidase stain),
    f176
Esterase
  nonspecific, 118
    and chloroacetate esterase, combined
      method for, 119, 136–137
    and fluoride-resistant esterase, 136
Esterase reaction, nonspecific, 9–10, 22
Ewing's sarcoma
  cells in clumps (wright's stain), f188
  marrow with PAS positivity in tumor
    cells (PAS stain), f188
  marrow replaced by blast-like
    malignant cells (Wright's stain),
    f188
Extranodal lymphocytic lymphoma vs.
  pseudolymphoma, 89–90
Extranodal peripheral T-cell lymphoma
  with paraneoplastic complications,
  f232

F

Factor VIII antigen detection, 32
FC receptor, 40
Fixatives, 106–108
Flow cytometric studies, pitfalls of, 55–58
Flow cytometry
  basic principles of, 48–52
  basic structure of, f49
  cell sorter, 52
  computer system, 50–52
    contourgram, 51–52
    isometric plot, 52
    scattergram, 50–51
    single histogram, 51
  contourgram of CLL, f51
  electronic system, 50
  fluid transport system, 48
  monoclonal antibody panel, 52–53
  monoclonal antibody panels for
    hematologic neoplasms, t52
  optical system, 48–50
  single histogram of κ-antigen-negative
    population, f51
  single histogram of lymphoma, f51
  summary of, 58
  wavelength and color of fluorochromes,
    t50
  wavelength of light source and choice
    of fluorochrome, t50
Fluorochrome combination, wavelength
  of light source and, t50
Fluorochromes, wavelength and color of,
  t50
Formol-calcium in cadodylate buffer, pH
  7.4, 107
Formol-ethanol, 106–107
Formol-methanol, 106

G

Gamma heavy chain disease
  increased vascularity among lymphoid
    infiltrates, f235
  node replacement by lymphoid cells,
    f235
  staining of γ-heavy chains, f235
Gene rearrangement
  in lymphoid neoplasms, 64–65
  as markers of clonal origin and
    recurrent tumors, 65–66
  in nonneoplastic conditions, 66–67
Germline genomic and chromosomal
  locations of human immunoglobulin
  genes, f62
Germline heavy chain genes, f63
Giemsa
  C-banding, 160–161
  trypsin banding, 160
Gomori's method for reticulum, 133
Granulocytic
  disorders, diagnosis of, 88
  sarcoma, 88
    infiltration by large neoplastic cells,
      f234
    lysozyme staining of neoplastic cells,
      f234
    positive chloroacetate esterase
      staining of neoplastic cells, f234

H

Hairy cell leukemia, 87
  blood and marrow
    reticulin network around
      mononuclear cell infiltrates, f205
    monomorphic loose mononuclear
      cell infiltration, f205
    mononuclear cells with indented
      nuclei, f205
    TRAP activity, f205
  spleen and liver
    mononuclear cells with cytoplasm
      (Wright-Giemsa stain), f206
    hairy cell infiltration and trapping of
      RBCs, f206

infiltration by monomorphic mononuclear cells, f207
infiltration of red pulp by hairy cells (H&E stain), f206
positive staining with TRAP, f207
TRAP activity in cytoplasm (TRAP stain), f206
Heavy chain diseases, 91–92
Hematologic neoplasms, diagnosis of, 79–99
Hematoxylin and eosin (H&E) stain, 129–130
Histiocytosis, malignant, diagnosis of, 92–93
Histochemical reactions, cell specificity and possible clinical applications of, t21
Histochemistry, 20–26
 definition of, 20
 miscellaneous reactions, 24
Histogram
 showing granulocyte peak and monocyte peak, f55
 showing granulocyte peak as negative due to underadjustment, f55
 showing result of overadjustment of photomultiplier tube, f56
 showing small- and large-cell lymphoma, f56
Histology and histochemistry, 128–140
HLA-DR, 41
Hodgkin's disease
 diagnosis and classification of, 90–91
 nodular sclerosing
  immunostaining of CD15, f212
  negative immunostaining of CD45, f213
  pleomorphic lymphoid infiltrates, f212
Holt's gum sucrose solution, 110
Human T-cell lymphotropic virus type I (HTLV-I) signal, f166
Human T-lymphocyte antigen, 41–42
Hybridization
 in situ, 69
 technique
  in situ, 163–166
  in situ hybridization, 164–165
  materials and equipment, 163
  preparation of probe, 163
  preparation of slide and section, 163

I

Immunoalkaline phosphatase method, 29, 151–153
Immunochemistry
 enzyme, 28–30

miscellaneous markers, 32
Immunocytochemistry and immunohistochemistry, 150–157
Immunofluorescence techniques, 27–28
Immunogenotyping
 and polymerase chain reaction, 61–71
 results, problems with interpretation of, 68
Immunoglobulin, 37–40
 detection, cytoplasmic, 30–31
 in heavy chain, light chain and TCR genes and segments, t63
 and TCR gene rearrangement in lymphoproliferative disorders, t67
Immunology and immunofluorescence, 141–149
Immunoperoxidase technique, 28–29, 150–151
Immunophenotyping of AML, t45
Intravascular lymphomatosis
 blast-like neoplastic cells (H&E stain), f180
 negative immunostaining of UEA-1, f181
 positive immunostaining of CD20 in cytoplasm, f181
 positive staining of factor VIII antigen, f181
Iron stain (Perls' reaction), 12–14, 126, 132
Isometric plot, composite, f52

L

Labeled streptavidin-biotin (LSAB) method for
 cytologic materials, 156–157
 tissue sections, 155–156
Large-cell lymphoma
 B-cell type
  basophilic cytoplasm (Wright's stain), f222
  with features of malignant histiocytosis
   large-cells, f247
   neoplastic cells, f248
   positive CD20, f248
   negative CD68 stain, f248
   red pulp infiltration, f247
  interstitial infiltration by large cells (H&E stain), f223
  lymphoma cells in capillaries of alveolar septi, f223
  positive immunostaining of κ-immunoglobulin, f223
  positive immunostaining of CD22, f222
Leukemia

acute
 classification of, 82–85
 using cytochemical stains, f82
acute megakaryocytic (M7), positive immunostaining of glycoprotein, f179
acute megakaryocytic (M7), blasts and increased platelets (Wright's stain), f179
acute monoblastic (M5)
 α-naphthyl butyrate esterase stain, f175
 cytoplasm and nucleoli (Wright's stain), f175
acute myeloblastic (M1)
 marrow replaced by myeloblasts (Wright's stain), f171
 positive for chloracetate esterase, f171
 positive peroxidase staining, f171
acute myelogenous (AML), 76–77
acute myeloid
 acute lymphoblastic leukemia (ALL) (Wright's stain), f169
 blasts with cytoplasmic vacuolization (Giemsa stain), f169
 blasts replacing marrow (Wright's stain), f177
 immunohistochemical stain for lysozyme, f170
 large-cell infiltration (H&E stain), f169
 leukemic blasts replacing marrow (Wright's stain), f178
 markers useful for subclassification of, t84
 positive for chloroacetate estrase, f169
 positive cyanide-resistant peroxidase staining, f178
 positive for lysozyme indicating myeloid, f170
 positive toluidine blue staining in cytoplasm, f177
acute myelomonocytic (M4)
 monocytoid cells (Wright's stain), f173
 positive for chloroacetate esterase, f173
acute myelomonocytic (M4 variant)
 chloroacetate esterase and α-naphthyl butyrate, f174
 monocytoid cells (Wright's stain), f174
acute promyelocytic (M3)
 hypercellular marrow (Wright's stain), f172

Leukemia, acute promyelocytic (M3) (contd.)
   peroxidase staining, f172
   positive chloroacetate esterase staining, f172
  chronic basophilic with erythroblastic transformation
   blasts (Wright's stain), f203
   erythroid antigen, f204
   metachromatic granules, f203
   Wright's stain, f203
  chronic lymphocytic, classification of, 85–87
  chronic lymphoid, markers useful for subclassification of, t86
  chronic myelocytic
   low alkaline phosphatase activity, f200
   marked neutrophilia (Wright's stain), f200
   positive control smear for alkaline phosphatase, f200
  chronic myeloid and unclassified myeloproliferative disorders, 88
  chronic myelomonocytic in transition to M4
   granulocytic hyperplasia, f201
   increased blasts indicates acute, f202
   leukocytosis (Wright's stain), f201
   positive α-naphthyl butyrate esterase, f202
   positive immunostaining of CD14, f202
   positive alkaline phosphatase staining, f201
  common acute lymphoblastic
   hypercellular marrow with blasts (Wright's stain), f184
   positive staining of common ALL surface antigens, f184
   positive staining of HLA-DR antigens, f184
  helper T-cell chronic lymphocytic
   E-rosettes (Wright's stain), f197
   focal acid phosphatase, f197
   lymphocytosis (Wright's stain), f197
  helper T-cell chronic lymphocytic focal globular α-naphthyl acetate esterase, f197
Leukemias
  acute
   lymphatic vs. nonlymphatic, 83
   nonlymphatic, subclassification of, 83–85
   peroxidase and esterase-negative, classification of, f83
Leukocyte alkaline phosphatase
  Kaplow's method, 122–123
  Rutenberg's method, 123–124
Leukocyte concentrate (buffy coat), capillary method for, 113
Light scatter and cell size/structure, relationship of, f49
Lymphoblastic leukemias, subclassification of, 85
Lymphoblastic vs. small noncleaved follicular center cell lymphoma (undifferentiated lymphoma), 88
Lymphoepithelioid cell lymphoma (Lennert's lymphoma), 90
Lymphoma
  bone marrow staging for, 91
  composite B-cell type
   node replaced by nodular lymphoma, f249
   positive for κ-light chain staining, f250
   positive κ-light chain staining in cytoplasm, f249
   sinusoidal involvement by large, atypical neoplastic cells, f249
   small, cleaved follicular cells, f249
  diffuse large-cell
   markers useful for subclassification of, t89
   subclassification of, 88–89
  diffuse large-cell B-cell immunoblastic lymphoma, f218
   staining for κ-light chains, f218
  diffuse large-cell follicular center cell type
   large, noncleaved cells, f217
   positive for λ-light chains, f217
  diffuse large-cell histiocytic type
   α-naphthyl butyrate esterase activity, f221
   cells with elongated nuclei, f221
   lysozyme in cytoplasm, f221
  diffuse large-cell T-cell immunoblastic lymphoma
   focal acid phosphatase activity, f220
   lymphoid cells, f220
  diffuse large-cell T-cell type
   focal acid phosphatase activity, f219
   node replacement by large lymphoid cells, f219
   wide variation in cell size, f219
  lymphoepithelioid cell (Lennert's lymphoma), 90
  malignant lymphoblastic
   focal acid phosphatase pattern, f215
   indistinguishable from morphology of lymphoblasts of ALL, f214
   lymphoblastic lymphoma early involvement, f215
   node replacement by lymphoid cells, f214
   positive immunostaining of CD7, f215
   positive immunostaining of TdT, f215
  small cleaved follicular center cell with bone marrow involvement
   CD20 staining, f224
   CD45RO immunostain, f224
   lymphoid lesion, f224
  small lymphocytic, germinal center among monomorphic lymphocytic infiltrates, f238
  small lymphocytic B-cell type with marrow involvement
   lymphocyte increase, f226
   negative immunostain of CD45RO, f227
   positive immunostain of LN2, f226
  small lymphocytic of lung, positive staining for λ light chains in cytoplasm, f238
  small lymphocytic with plasmacytoid differentiation
   focal aggregate of lymphocytes, f225
   positive immunostaining of κ-immunoglobulin, f225
  small noncleaved cell-leukemic phase (L3)
   blasts with L3 type of ALL, f186
   light chain staining, f186
   starry-sky appearance (H&E stain), f186
Lymphoma/leukemia
  small lymphocytic helper T-cell with marrow involvement
   lymphocytes, f228
   OPD4 staining, f228
Lymphomas, malignant, (non-Hodgkin's) classification of, 88
Lymphoproliferative disorder
  chronic classification of, using immunocytochemical methods, f86
  of granular lymphocytes
   CD57 staining on lymphocytes, f229
   left-shifted granulopoiesis, f229
   normal biopsy for comparison, f229
   positive immunostaining of CD57, f229
Lysozyme detection, 31

M

Mast cell disease, diagnosis of, 87–88
Mast cell leukemia
  degranulated cells with elongated nuclei (Wright's stain), f210

diffuse red pulp infiltration, f211
marrow replacement by mononuclear cells (H&E stain), f211
marrow replacement by mononuclear cells with basophilic granules, f210
metachromatic granules in cytoplasm, f210
positive aminocaproate esterase staining, f211
positive chloroacetate esterase staining, f210
positive chloroacetate staining in cytoplasm, f211
Mayer's hematoxylin, 109
Metastatic undifferentiated prostatic carcinoma
  node replacement by anaplastic tumor cells, f233
  prostatic acid phosphatase staining, f233
Methenamine silver stain, 134
Methyl green-pyronine
  reaction, 24
  stain (paraffin), 131
Monoamine oxidase (method of Glenner et al), 127
Monoclonal antibodies, 42–45
  cell specificity and clinical applications of, t44
  to human blood cells, reactions of, t43
Mota's fixative, 107
Mounting media, 111
Mouse erythrocyte receptor, 41
Multiple myeloma
  intense staining of κ-light chains in cytoplasm, f241
  marrow replacement by atypical plasma cells, f241
  and Waldenstom's macroglobulinemia, 91
Myeloma with unusual morphology, 91
Myeloperoxidase detection, 31–32

N
Naphthol
  AS acetate esterase, 139–140
  AS acetate esterase reaction, 23
Neoplastic vs. reactive, 91
Neuroblastoma
  focal acid phosphatase staining, f187
  marrow replaced by blast-like cells (Wright's stain), f187
  positive monoamine oxidase staining, f187
Neutral buffered formaldehyde, 107
New Fuchsin solution, 4%, 110

P
Paraffin-embedded tissue sections, preparation of, 128
Paraformaldehyde-glutaraldehyde-acrolein buffer, 107–108
Pararosaniline solution, 4%, 110
Periodic acid-Schiff (PAS) reaction, 12, 23–24, 120
  paraffin, 131–132
Peripheral blood smears, preparation of, 112
Peripheral T-cell lymphoma with multiorgan failure
  dense granules in cytoplasm, f230
  interstitial atypical cell infiltration, f230
  positive immunostaining of CD45RO, f231
Peroxidase
  and cyanide-resistant peroxidase, 134–135
  for eosinophils, cyanide-resistant, 117
  method
    Hanker's method, 116
    modified after Graham et al, 115–116
    modified after Graham & Karnovsky, 115
    for PHI bodies
      modified after Hanker et al, 116
  reaction, 8, 21–22
Persistant polyclonal B lymphocytosis
  binucleated lymphocytes, f195
  hybridization of Epstein-Barr virus genome, f196
  lymphocytes (Wright's stain), f195
  positive immunostaining of CD20, f195
  positive immunostaining of κ-immunoglobulin, f196
Philadelphia chromosome-positive chronic myelogenous leukemia, 74
Phosphate-buffered saline (PBS), 105
Phosphate buffers, 103
Plasma cell leukemia
  marrow replacement by plasmacytoid cells (H&E stain), f194
  plasmacytoid cells with basophilic cytoplasm, f194
  positive immunostaining of λ-immunoglobulin, f194
Plasmacytoma
  node replacement by histiocytes, f240
  positive staining of κ-light chains in cytoplasm, f240
Plasmaproliferative disorders, diagnosis of, 91–92

Plastic-embedded tissue sections, preparation of, 128–129
Ploidy, 53–54
Polymerase chain reaction (PCR), 68–69
  process, f69
Pre-T-cell acute lymphoblastic leukemia blasts with L1 morphology (Wright's stain), f182
  positive immunostaining of CD5, f183
  positive immunostaining of CD7, f182
  positive immunostaining of CD10, f182
  positive immunostaining of TdT, f182
Primary amyloidosis
  amorphous purple materials (Wright's stain), f244
  with cardiomyopathy, positive κ-light chain staining, f245
  positive for λ-light chains, negative for κ light chains, f244
  positive Congo red staining of marrow smear, f244
Propanediol buffer, 104
Prostatic carcinoma, metastatic undifferentiated, adenocarcinoma, f233
Prostatic specific antigen (PSA) mRNA in prostate carcinoma, f165
Pseudoperoxidase for hemoglobin, 135

Q
Quinacrine fluorescent stain, 161

R
Reagents for cytogenetic studies, preparation of, 158
Reed-Sternberg cell, f90
Reticulin stain, 24
Rhabdomyosarcoma
  cross-striation after chemotherapy-trichrome stain, f190
  immunostaining of desmin in cytoplasm, f189
  immunostaining of muscle actin-indirect immunoproxidase stain, f190
  malignant cells with erythrophagocytosis (Wright's stain), f189
  marrow replaced by round, clear cells (H&E stain), f189
Riu's stain, 114
RNA index, 54–55
Round cell tumors
  diagnosis of, 92–93
  markers useful for characterization of, t93

S

Scattergram
  of lymph node, 51
  of lysed whole blood, f50
Secondary amyloidosis
  Congo red staining of small vessel in vascular wall, f246
  positive immunostaining of amyloid A protein, f246
  thickening of vascular wall, f246
Sézary syndrome and mycosis fungoides, 90
Sheep erythrocyte rosettes, 41
Signet-ring-cell myeloma
  intense λ-light chain staining in cytoplasm of most tumor cells, f242
  marrow replacement by tumor cells-some signet ring cells, f242
  marrow smear of tumor cells signet-with ring appearance, f242
Smears of marrow aspirate, preparation of, 112
Solutions, miscellaneous, 110–111
Southern blot hybridization, 63–64
  analysis of immunoglobulin heavy chain gene, f65–f66
  procedure, f64
Specimens, preparation of, 7–8
S-phase, 54
Stains
  Giemsa, 109, 160
    paraffin, 130
    plastic, 130
  hematoxylin and eosin (H&E), 129–130
  iron (Perl's reaction), 12–14, 126, 132
  Mayer's hematoxylin, 109
  methyl green-pyronine (paraffin), 131
  quinacrine fluorescent, 161
  reticulin, 24
  Riu's, 114
  Sudan black B, 8–9, 22, 120–121
  Wright-Giemsa, 114
Sudan black B stain, 8–9, 22, 120–121
Suppressor T-cell chronic lymphocytic leukemia
  lymphocytosis-Wright's stain, f199
  positive staining of suppressor T-cell antigens, f199
Surface markers
  for human blood cells, t38
  other than monoclonal antibodies, t38
Systemic mast cell disease-marrow
  mast cells (Wright's stain), f208
  monomorphic mononuclear cells with eosinophils (H&E stain), f208
  paratrabecular mast cell lesion, f208
  perifollicular infiltration of mast cells, f209
  perivascular infiltration of mast cells, f209
  perivascular mast cell lesion, f208

T

Tartrate-resistant acid phosphatase reaction, 11–12
Terminal deoxynucleotidyl transferase (TdT)
  detection, 31–32
  indirect immunofluorescence for, 147–148
T-cell and B-cell identification and quantitation, 141–147
  0.83% ammonium chloride treatment, 143
  B-cell SIg, 144
  cell cryopreservation, 146–147
  cell suspension from body fluids, prep., 142–143
  cell viability, determination of, 143
  monoclonal antibody panel, 145
  mononuclear cell suspension, preparation of, 141
  single cell suspensions from lymphoid tissue, 142
  staining for T- and B-cell surface markers, 143
  whole blood lysis technique, 145–146
T-cell differentiation, f39
T-cell lymphoma/leukemia, 75–76
Tγ-lymphoproliferative disorder, 85–87
TGFβ-1 message in Bouin's-fixed, paraffin-embedded colon tissue, f166
Tissues
  embedded in parafin, 20
  embedded in plastics, 21
  fixed and cryostat sectioning, 20–21
  fresh frozen, 20
  imprints, preparation of, 112–113
  preparation of, 20–21, 27
Toluidine blue O stain, 14, 132–133
  for basophils, 125
Topoisomerase II mRNA in blood smear in patient with acute myelocytic leukemia, f165
Tris buffers, 103

U

Undifferentiated myeloma
  blasts in blood smear (Wright's stain), f243
  marrow replacement by blast-like cells (Wright's stain), f243
  marrow replacement by large, primitive cells, f243
  strong λ-light chain staining in cytoplasm, f243

V

Veronal buffer, 104

W

Wright-Giemsa stain, 114